Autism Spectrum Disorder in the Ontario Context

Autism Spectrum Disorder in the Ontario Context

An Introduction

Kimberly Maich and Carmen Hall

Canadian Scholars' Press Inc.
Toronto

Autism Spectrum Disorder in the Ontario Context: An Introduction
by Kimberly Maich and Carmen Hall

First published in 2016 by
Canadian Scholars' Press Inc.
425 Adelaide Street West, Suite 200
Toronto, Ontario
M5V 3C1

www.cspi.org

Library and Archives Canada Cataloguing in Publication

Maich, Kimberly, 1969-, author
        Autism spectrum disorder in the Ontario context : an introduction / Kimberly Maich and Carmen Hall.

Includes bibliographical references and index.
Issued in print and electronic formats.
ISBN 978-1-55130-912-5 (paperback).--ISBN 978-1-55130-914-9 (epub).--ISBN 978-1-55130-913-2 (pdf)

        1. Autism spectrum disorders--Treatment--Ontario. 2. Autism spectrum disorders. I. Hall, Carmen L., author II. Title.

RC553.A88M33 2016   616.85'882009713   C2016-901447-9   C2016-901448-7

Text design by Brad Horning
Cover design by Em Dash Design
Cover art by Grace Culliton

Printed and bound in Canada by Webcom.

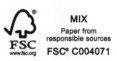

MIX
Paper from responsible sources
FSC® C004071

TABLE OF CONTENTS

PREFACE

Autism spectrum disorder (ASD) has undergone a remarkably complex history, from being misunderstood as a form of schizophrenia to its current recognition as a complex spectrum disorder, allowing for multiple levels of functioning and individuality. One current understanding of ASD describes the disorder as one that is "characterized by impairments in social communication and the presence of restricted and repetitive behaviours" (Veatch, Veenstra-VanderWheele, Potter, Pericak-Vance, & Haines, 2014, p. 276) with significant heterogeneous genetic underpinnings and wide clinical variability. Throughout this long and ever-changing history, we, the authors (Kimberly Maich and Carmen Hall), have noted not only that ASD is known for its clinical and educational implications, but also that it has become a common topic in the popular media. We often see ASD highlighted in the local newspaper or the nightly news, and when we ask someone about ASD, most people know of someone with the disorder or someone who has a son, daughter, other relative, or friend with ASD. Indeed, Kimberly Maich herself has an adult son with ASD. This increased cultural consciousness, however, while positive for raising awareness, has led to misconceptions about what causes autism, what the most effective interventions are, and what services are available. In our professional lives and our personal experiences, we see this more often than not.

Autism Spectrum Disorder in the Ontario Context was written to provide a broad perspective of ASD, including its historical roots and an explanation of the current diagnostic criteria, which we believe is critical to understanding its nature. By understanding this historical context as well as current views in the popular media, we hope that many misconceptions can be dispelled. The consistent framing we have developed within the Ontario context provides a local understanding of how the development of knowledge about the disorder influenced Ontario provincial government policies, procedures, and services (section I). We have also built this book on the foundation of evidence-based interventions (EBI), a term commonly used in the field to validate that interventions and their claims are founded on empirical, controlled research. This is essential for protecting those of us in the ASD community, whether we are intervening, teaching, parenting, or simply living in the world. We have seen that ASD is a diagnosis particularly susceptible to pseudoscience and companies advertising "a cure," leading to individuals being harmed and families spending endless amounts of money on treatments that do not show results. Hence, section II focuses on understanding how EBIs are established and the most current identified EBIs for ASD. By providing a summary of effective interventions, interventions that show some evidence of effectiveness, and interventions shown to be ineffective or harmful, we hope that clinicians, practitioners, educators, families, and individuals with ASD can become more aware of new interventions and more knowledgeable about their history of success before implementation. We provide an overview on each EBI, using a practical approach to allow for those working with individuals with ASD to understand the most common and effective treatment approaches. We have also included overviews of interventions that are somewhat supported and interventions that are not supported to inform the reader of the intervention and explain why it is not considered an EBI. We note that further research is needed to run these interventions in their entirety. We also provide information on where to research individual strategies and obtain additional training. Locating all this information in one place is essential for anyone working with individuals with ASD; therefore, we have been careful to feature Ontario examples, research, and interventions whenever possible throughout all of the following chapters.

Lastly, a look at ASD across the lifespan in Ontario is something that is rarely found comprehensively in one resource (section III). Rather, the majority of resources and information are specific to either the context or the age of the individual with ASD. In focusing this section on the lifespan from childhood to adulthood and on services from child-care centres to supports for adults with ASD, we have underscored the different needs of individuals with ASD at each age. In addition, we have highlighted services and funding models for each age group and area of interest. Although these will differ regionally throughout Ontario, we have included major services and funding sources mandated consistently by the provincial government. Where there are still gaps in services, we have presented creative ideas and unique models from regional centres, as well as models of support and services to assist families of individuals with ASD. We hope this approach will provide a sense of the continuity of services and experiences—both helpful and challenging—that individuals with ASD and their families, and those who support them, face across the lifespan.

STRUCTURE

This book is an introductory-level textbook on the topic of ASD, comprising three main sections: An Introduction to ASD, Interventions, and A Look across the Lifespan. Throughout the book, three main themes are emphasized: the emerging nature of the field of ASD; the importance of using evidence-based interventions in clinical, school, and community-based interventions; and the importance of supporting individuals with ASD across the lifespan.

Where possible, this book focuses on Ontario-based practices, resources, and research. When Ontario-specific information is not possible or preferable, a broader perspective complemented with provincial information supplements such topics. For example, chapter 3: Evidence-Based Interventions (EBIs) relies on definitions of—and a framework for—EBIs from a broader North American base of research, and is supplemented with provincial examples of practices, resources, and research related to the use of EBIs in the Ontario context.

Each chapter features a range of figures, definitions, and questions designed to deepen understanding and elicit reflection on the topics presented through supporting literature in the ASD field. In addition, most chapters include multiple feature boxes, with detailed perspectives provided by varied members of Ontario's ASD community.

ABOUT THE AUTHORS

Dr. Kimberly Maich, PhD, OCT, is an assistant professor in Brock University's Department of Teacher Education, and is affiliated with the Centre for Applied Disability Studies. Her teaching, research, and writing are typically focused around school-based special education, specifically education of students with ASD. She has worked in the field of ASD as a teacher, professor, clinician, and parent since 1998.

Carmen Hall, MC, CCC, BCBA, is the coordinator and a professor in the Autism & Behavioural Science Graduate Certificate Program at Fanshawe College. She has worked with children with ASD in a number of different environments, including the school setting and intensive behavioural intervention. She has also been involved in consulting roles at schools and in clinical environments. Her work has focused on social skills research, including peer-mediated social skills in child care, school, and camp settings. For the past four years, Carmen's passion for technology was fostered with the introduction of the iPad, both in her private practice working with children with ASD and as a college instructor teaching with the iPad in a flipped classroom. In 2013, she was named an Apple Distinguished Educator for this work, and she has completed numerous research studies on utilizing iPads in various clinical and school settings.

ACKNOWLEDGEMENTS

Kimberly thanks her husband, John, for his encouragement and support; her son, Robert, for the motivation for this book; and her daughters, Grace and Hannah, for loving their mother even though she never cooks supper. This text is also in memory of her late father, Garry Davidson (1940–2015), proud grandfather to two grandsons with ASD.

Carmen thanks her family and friends for their unconditional support during this journey. Her husband, Tony, and son, Julian, provided considerable patience and inspiration throughout the process. She also thanks her mentors throughout her career who have always inspired her and believed in the possibilities.

REFERENCE

Veatch, O. J., Veenstra-VanderWeele, J., Potter, M., Pericak-Vance, M. A., & Haines, J. L. (2014). Genetically meaningful phenotypic subgroups in Autism Spectrum Disorder. *Genes, Brain & Behavior, 13*(3), 276–285. doi:10.1111/gbb.12117

SECTION I

AN INTRODUCTION TO AUTISM SPECTRUM DISORDER

SECTION I, AN INTRODUCTION TO AUTISM SPECTRUM Disorder, focuses on the historical and current context of autism spectrum disorder (ASD). Key individuals who have contributed to the description and identification of ASD are discussed in chapter 1. Included are service provisions and a brief history of autism services in the province of Ontario. Chapter 2 focuses on the diagnostic criteria in both the *Diagnostic and Statistical Manual (DSM)—IV* and *DSM-5*, highlighting significant changes in the name and diagnosis of ASD. In addition, this chapter explains various services in Ontario and explores views of the disorder in the popular media. The chapter is designed to provide a context for the current and past events that have shaped services, interventions, and understandings of the disorder.

CHAPTER 1

A BRIEF HISTORY
OF AUTISM SPECTRUM DISORDER

IN THIS CHAPTER:

- Contributors to the Field of ASD
  - Leo Kanner and Hans Asperger
  - Bruno Bettelheim
  - Lorna Wing
  - O. Ivar Lovaas
- Elasticity of Terminology
- Highlights from the Ontario Context

This chapter provides a short historical look at autism spectrum disorder (ASD). First, some of the pioneering contributors to the field are introduced, from those constructing the diagnosis and characteristics of ASD itself, to those developing effective interventions, to those embroiled in controversy, namely, Leo Kanner, Hans Asperger, Bruno Bettelheim, Lorna Wing, and Ivar Lovaas. Those individuals and their contributions do not represent a comprehensive examination of the field of ASD and its history, but rather some figures with prominent influence. Chapter 1 also includes some key moments in the recent history of service provision for students with ASD in and beyond the school system, from ministry directives to collaborative initiatives, research, publications, and resources. The chapter traces the journey from the first described characteristics to the current *Diagnostic and Statistical Manual of Mental Disorders—5 (DSM-5)*, which defines autism spectrum disorder as presenting persistent deficits in social communication and social interaction, as well as repetitive and restricted patterns of behaviour, interests, and activities that are present in the early developmental period, cause clinically significant impairments in areas of daily functioning, and cannot be better described by an intellectual disability or global developmental delay (American Psychiatric Association [APA], 2013).

CONTRIBUTORS TO THE FIELD OF ASD

Leo Kanner and Hans Asperger

Although some controversy remains as to the identity of the primary figure who first recognized autism (Chown, 2012), infantile autism, or early infantile autism, as a distinct diagnostic name, the two figures who stand out in the history of ASD as prominent are Leo Kanner and Hans Asperger. Wing and Potter (2002) refer to Kanner and Asperger this way: "Of all the early workers in this field, Leo Kanner in the USA and Hans Asperger in Austria are the only ones whose names are now legitimately famous" (p. 152). Commonly referred to as the "two pioneers of autism" (Lyons & Fitzgerald, 2007, p. 2002), each published simultaneous and similar descriptions of small groups of children with unusual social and behavioural characteristics, differentiating these groups from children with the (then) better-known diagnosis of childhood schizophrenia (Blacher & Christensen, 2011; Neumärker, 2003). Kanner's writing was titled *Autistic Disturbances of Affective Contact* (published in 1943), and Asperger's publication was called *Autistic Psychopathology in Childhood* (published in 1944). Given its simultaneous use, it is

clear that neither Kanner nor Asperger coined the word "autism," but rather brought it into public significance. Kanner accomplished this more quickly than Asperger due to a multitude of social, cultural, and political factors occurring at the time of publication, such as the fact that Kanner published in English (Lyons & Fitzgerald, 2007; Neumärker, 2003). Perhaps this explains why the term *Kanner syndrome* came to be documented quite quickly, while *Asperger's disorder*, used synonymously, did not find its way into the diagnostic manual for decades.

Kanner described this first group of children in careful detail, following a clinical, systematic approach (Thompson, 2013), introducing them as those who "[differ] so markedly and uniquely from anything reported so far, that each case merits ... a detailed consideration of its fascinating

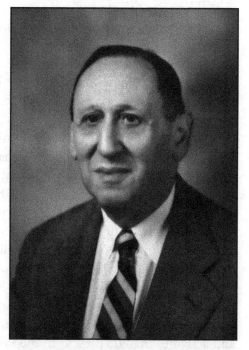

Figure 1.1: Psychiatrist Leo Kanner, Pioneer of Autism
Source: Johns Hopkins University, via Wikipedia Commons.

peculiarities" (Kanner, 1968, p. 217). Some characteristics of his *Autistic Disturbances of Affective Contact* that may be still familiar today include somewhat positive references to the cognitive capabilities of the involved children and the so-called "cold-hearted" yet "highly intelligent families" (Neumärker, 2003, p. 207; Kanner, 1968), as well as the use of terms such as *echolalia, solitude, sameness, obsession,* and *stereotypy*. Following the initial work of Kanner and Asperger, little literature was published that moved the field of ASD forward in a hopeful and positive manner until the 1960s (Thompson, 2013).

Child-Onset Schizophrenia: A rare and severe form of schizophrenia, defined by psychosis, or thoughts and beliefs that differ from reality, that appears before age 13 (Rapoport, Chavez, Greenstein, Addington, & Gogtay, 2009).

Decades later, Blacher and Christensen (2011) published a detailed overview of Kanner's originally characterized children, along with descriptions of the characteristics or symptoms Kanner had noted while claiming to develop the term himself. One of these children was referred to as Donald T. (see Table 1.1 for Kanner's description of Donald T.'s behaviour), whose father wrote extensively to Kanner and thus assisted with these first descriptive terms (Donvan & Zucker, 2010). Almost simultaneously, the *Atlantic* published a magazine article about the life of Donald Gray Triplett (also known as Donald T.) as a 77-year-old adult, more than six decades after

Echolalia: Repetition of verbal language in an echoic manner, looping words and phrases around in a recurring way (Arora, 2012). For example, an inclusive classroom teacher says "pretty flower," and the student with ASD repeats "pretty flower," perhaps multiple times. As a child, Donald Triplett endlessly repeated "chrysanthemum" (see Table 1.1) (Donvan & Zucker, 2010).

Stereotypy: Most commonly recognized stereotypies are motor stereotypies, which are "rhythmic movements that have a predictable pattern and location, seem purposeful but serve no obvious function, tend to be prolonged, and can be suppressed" (Thilinie & Tamara, 2010, p. 255). For example, a young girl with ASD sits at her desk in the classroom reading a book on dog breeds while repeatedly rocking her body from front to back. Other examples are waving one's hands, flapping one's arms, and nodding one's head (Thilinie & Tamara, 2010).

Table 1.1: Kanner's Original Symptoms Describing Donald T. as a Child

Kanner's symptoms	Other: Predictive Donald T. (age 1–5)
Does not look at the person while speaking	"Obsessive detail" from father's typewritten history
Does not use communicative gestures	Eating always a problem for Donald; sweets not a temptation
Not interested in playing with other children; ignores other children	Walked at 13 months
Prefers objects to people	Excellent rote memory for song lyrics, alphabet, and numbers
Father reports that he appears to "draw into his shell and live within himself." He does not seem to notice the coming or going of other people nor react to their coming with pleasure.	Had temper tantrums in which he was destructive
Does not come when called	Had difficulty associating his punishment with his behavior
Regards other people as an interference or plays with their hands/feet as an object	Showed learning—better contact with the environment, became more imaginative over time
Delay in use of questions and ability to answer questions	Later learned to read and play the piano
Conversation obsessive in nature—inexhaustible questioning	No initiation of activities other than the limited interests in which he was absorbed; mother had to direct him in all other activities
Ejaculating words and sentences such as "chrysanthemum"	
Inflexible use of language	
Pronoun reversal	
A "mania" for spinning round objects	
Arranging beads, blocks, etc., in a certain manner	

Verbal rituals requiring others to repeat certain phrases during particular activities (e.g., bedtime)	
Stereotyped finger movements, shaking his head and whispering or singing the same three-note tune	
Difficulty in social communication (learning to ask and respond to questions) present at age 2	

Source: Blacher & Christensen, 2011, p. 174.

Kanner's original description. This publication refers to Donald as "Autism's First Child" (Donvan & Zucker, 2010), and answers the self-posed question, "What happened to Donald?" After being briefly institutionalized as a child, he was raised on a farm, went to college, and became employed. Although he was teased mildly as a child and regarded as eccentric as an adult, he developed and sustained connections with his family and community, as well as activities, interests, and hobbies in the context of "freedom, independence & good health" (Donvan & Zucker, 2010, p. 81). Refer to Table 1.2 for a full listing of Donald Triplett's characteristics as an adult with ASD.

Table 1.2: Characteristics of Donald T. as an Adult with ASD

Repetitive behaviours	Legendary skills
Prefers being alone	Appears content
Unusual gait	Active community life
Reliance on rituals	Engages in conversation
Conversation limited to pragmatics	Develops new skills into adulthood (e.g., driving, international travel)
Thinks concretely	Has activities, interests, and hobbies (e.g., golf)
No romantic relationships	Attended college
Needs financial support	Employed

Source: Donvan & Zucker, 2010.

Read about it. Think about it. Write about it.

If Kanner had written a letter to his mother about what he imagined Donald T. might be like as an adult, what would that letter say?

What recorded similarities are there between Donald T. as a child, and Donald as an adult?

When we document the characteristics of a child who may or may not yet be diagnosed with ASD, what characteristics should be recorded? Should the focus be on strengths or deficits? Why?

Hans Asperger, a paediatrician in Vienna, also described a group of boys he labelled as having autistic psychopathy (AP). These boys had high intellectual functioning but difficulties with learning, attention, and social behaviour, and seemed to have impairments in emotions and instincts (Hippler & Klicpera, 2003). Asperger published his work about 4 children in 1943, the same year as Kanner described 11 others (Lyons & Fitzgerald, 2007). Hans Asperger's work did not become well known, as it was written in German and was not translated into English until 1991, by Uta Frith (Lyons & Fitzgerald, 2007). Lorna Wing, mentioned later in this chapter, first coined the term *Asperger's syndrome* in 1981, when she used Hans Asperger's description of the individuals with a slight extension (Hippler & Klicpera, 2003). Later, with the publication of the *Diagnostic and Statistical Manual of Mental Disorders (DSM)-IV* in 1994, the term *Asperger's disorder* first appeared officially in the manual that many clinicians turn to when making a diagnosis. In this manual, the diagnosis was slightly different than first described, and included two criteria in social impairments and one in repetitive and restricted patterns of behaviour from Kanner's description of autistic disorder (Hippler & Klicpera, 2003). In 2013, with the introduction of the *DSM-5*, Asperger's disorder no longer appeared as a separate diagnosis, but was grouped under the umbrella term *autism spectrum disorder*.

Bruno Bettelheim

With a diverse career that encompassed far more than principles and practices related to autism, Bruno Bettelheim, a doctoral graduate of psychology and philosophy and a later proponent of the then-dominant psychoanalytic approach (Fleck & Müller, 1997), affected the direction of the field of ASD from the 1950s onward. His prominence was even to the point of holding what was described as "celebrity status" (Adelson, 1997, p. 67), a large departure from his early experiences as a concentration camp prisoner (Fleck & Müller, 1997). In 1959, he described children with autism as "unable to relate themselves in the ordinary way to people and situations" (p. 455), comparing them to children raised in the wild, who had suffered total abandonment and extreme environmental deprivation. He saw children with autism as victims of emotionally isolating, disengaged, rejecting parents whose "efforts to find their lost children have been more than lax" (Bettelheim, 1959, p. 457). In the 1976 publication *The Empty Fortress: Infantile Autism and the Birth of the Self*, Bettelheim compares and contrasts children with ASD to "victims of concentration camps" (p. 7). He notes, however, that "autistic children withdraw from the world before their humanity ever really develops" (p. 7), this withdrawal being either chosen by the infants themselves, a withdrawal to what Bettelheim terms the "autistic position" (p. 46), or even the outcome of hostility repression: a protective reversal of humanity (Bettelheim, 1959).

Whittaker (1976) explained this with the family etiology hypothesis—common for the era—assuming that the parental "pain and strain" (p. 91) in families of "troubled children" (p. 91), especially the mother, influence the development of such children and are, in fact, directly or unconsciously, a pathological cause. One of the outcomes of such a view was the separation or severing of the "refrigerator mother" relationship, where the disorder was believed to be caused by cold, unaffectionate mothers (Barbera, 2010, p. 56). Bettelheim called this a parentectomy. A parentectomy demanded separation, including residential separation. In Bettelheim's treatments, this meant a relocation to his well-known orthogenic schools, where intensive treatment could be implemented without interruption (Whittaker, 1976).

Bettelheim's reputation disintegrated after his death, as his background, experiences, credentials, and methodology were found to be more myth than reality (Adelson, 1997). However, this influential man (Raines, 2002) sowed the seeds of a dubious yet undeniable influence, reflected in his biographies (e.g., *Rising to the Light: A Portrait of Bruno Bettelheim* [Raines, 2002]) and the stories those who had their own encounters with him (e.g., *Not the Thing I Was: Thirteen Years at Bruno Bettelheim's Orthogenic School* [Eliot, 2002]).

Refrigerator Mothers: Refrigerator mothers were described as typically cold, aloof, intellectual, professional maternal figures, whose rejecting demeanour was posited to cause the social withdrawal seen in children with autism. Such views are commonly attributed to Bettelheim, but are also present in Kanner's work (Whittaker, 1976).

> ### Read about it. Think about it. Write about it.
>
> Do you see any reflections of Bettelheim's work in the perception of autism today and the treatment of parents of children with ASD? If so, explain.
>
> Outline the main ways in which the understanding of ASD has changed since Kanner and Asperger's time.

Lorna Wing

Lorna Wing, a highly respected UK-based psychiatrist and parent of a daughter diagnosed with ASD at the age of three, is credited with many significant advances through her pioneering work expanding on and popularizing more modern notions of ASD. In particular, she popularized the term *Asperger's disorder* and widened the narrow definition of autism into a continuum of characteristics, describing it as including a "spectrum" of diagnoses and a "triad" of characteristics that make up the disorder (Hebert, 2014; Leekam, 2014). In her description of Asperger's disorder, she named the triad of characteristics differentiating Kanner's syndrome from Asperger's disorder (Wing, 1993). The three main characteristics that she described as notable in the disorder and across diagnoses were deficits in social interactions, difficulties with communication, and impairments in imagination, which most often were accompanied by repetitive and restricted patterns of behaviour (Wing, 1993). Later, when the triad of characteristics was published in the *DSM-IV*, impairments in imagination were removed, and repetitive and restricted patterns of behaviour became the third characteristic of the triad. Wing also advocated for a continuum of diagnoses, indicating the similarities of the disorders Kanner and Asperger described.

Her most well-known, foundational writing is entitled *Autistic Children: A Guide for Parents and Professionals* (Wing, 1972), which emphasized that parents should first remember the positives: "He is first and foremost a child, with the same need as every other child for a home and family, love, security, guidance and a chance to develop his skills and positive assets to the full" (p. 13). This differed significantly from other authors at the time, such as Bruno Bettelheim and others, who negatively characterized the parents of children with autism in their work. One of her best-known publications, written with Judith Gould (1979), was an epidemiological survey of children, helping to resolve the complexities of classifying social, language, and behavioural issues in the field. Importantly, "all the children with social impairments had repetitive stereotyped behavior and almost all had absence or abnormalities of language and symbolic activities. Thus the study showed a marked tendency for these problems to occur together" (Wing & Gould, 1979, p. 25). This tendency was also referred to as a "cluster of abnormalities" (p. 26), and led to a recommendation that the "full range of conditions" (p. 27) must be included in a future system of classification—something "more suitable than 'autism' or 'psychosis'" (p. 27). With the current usage of

Triad: The term *triad of impairments* was coined by Lorna Wing and Judith Gould (1979) and is described as an "abnormality of social interaction ... closely associated with impairment of communication and imagination, the latter resulting in a narrow, repetitive pattern of activities" (Wing, 1993, p. 70).

spectrum and *triad* as commonly understood descriptors in the field, Wing's leadership toward new terminology and understanding (Wing, 1993, p. 70) was solidified, marking a broadened understanding of autism as an "autistic continuum" (Wing, 1993, p. 70).

Read about it. Think about it. Write about it.

Where do you think the field of ASD would be today without Wing's advocacy, research, and writing?

O. Ivar Lovaas

O. Ivar Lovaas, another significant figure in the field of ASD, is considered a groundbreaking, transformative, and extraordinary pioneer of both applied behaviour analysis (ABA) applications for language development and challenging behaviour and interventions for children with ASD (Smith & Eikeseth, 2011). Born in Norway in 1927 and educated in the US, he worked in his field from the 1960s until his death in 2010, and was seen by his students as a "charismatic, passionate, breath-taking, and gifted man" (Smith & Eikeseth, 2011, p. 378). One listed achievement of many included a change in our understanding of children with autism (e.g., reducing serious self-injurious behaviours):

> The rapid reduction of even the most horrifying behavior—children's punching themselves hard in the face thousands of times every hour, chewing off their fingertips, smashing their heads against the sharpest object available, or poking their eyes—helped prove that children with

autism were sensitive to consequences, contrary to the conventional wisdom in the 1960s. (Smith & Eikeseth, p. 376)

Lovaas built the foundation for successful, early, and intensive behaviour intervention focused on skill building for young children with ASD, which he developed using principles of behaviour modification. His foundational work was titled the *UCLA Young Autism Project* (Lovaas, 1987; Smith & Eikeseth, 2011). In this publication, Lovaas reported on his unique intervention project, which "sought to maximize behavioural treatment by treating autistic children during most of their waking hours for many years" (Lovaas, 1987, p. 3) in a "special, intense, and comprehensive learning environment" (p. 4). His design included an experimental group that received 40 hours of individualized therapy per week (intensive treatment) using ABA intervention and two control groups, the first of which received 10 or fewer hours of individualized intervention, and the second of which received no treatment. Each group had between 19 and 21 children, all aged 46 or fewer months at the beginning of this two-year or longer intervention plan. Multiple interventions, including aversives, were utilized, and data were recorded in multiple ways. Some significant findings included that 47 percent of the intensive treatment experimental group were successful in a "normal first grade in a public school" (p. 6), and the average gain of 30 intelligence quotient points in the intensive treatment group. In other words, many students who received this intensive therapy "achieved normal intellectual and educational functioning" (p. 7), with widespread improvement in multiple domains (such as language). Lovaas concluded:

Given a group of children who show the kinds of behavioral deficits and excesses evident in our pretreatment measures, such children will continue to manifest similar severe psychological handicaps later in life unless subjected to intensive behavioral treatment that can indeed significantly alter that outcome. (Lovaas, 1987, p. 9)

Since this publication, the subject of much debate and criticism (Smith & Eikeseth, 2011), Lovaas and many others (e.g., Strauss, Mancini, & Fava, 2013) have modelled multiple programs upon components of Lovaas's intensive early-intervention treatments. The goal of such programs has been to change the developmental trajectory of children with ASD by intervening with ABA principles in intensive behaviour intervention programs early. Since this groundbreaking and seminal study, such programs—including Ontario's ministry-provided programs—have been similarly evaluated. The foundation of Lovaas's work continues to be strongly evident in Ontario's current Autism Intervention Program (AIP) (Ontario Ministry of Children and Youth Services, 2007).

ELASTICITY OF TERMINOLOGY

Leaping ahead 40 years from Leo Kanner's original 1943 term *early infantile autism*, which included features of echolalia, stereotypy, and differentiation from childhood schizophrenia (Neumärker, 2003), it is clear that the terminology around autism spectrum disorder can be described as elastic; in other words, it changes its shape to accommodate needs, but maintains its function. Since the second-most-recent iteration of the *Diagnostic and Statistical Manual IV-TR* (2000), the language has continued to shift, reflecting changes in our academic understanding, our professional approaches, and our everyday language emerging from published literature around ASD; this language remains differentiated by geographical region (Jacobsen, 2010). Perhaps this is unsurprising given the significant time lapse between revisions of the DSM, which guides our language around psychological disorders. In the meantime, there is a tug-of-war between formal language and everyday terminology. For example, the *DSM-IV-TR* used the term *Asperger's disorder* (Neumärker, 2003), but the terms *Asperger's syndrome*, *Asperger syndrome*, and simply *Asperger's* are also commonly utilized. When the term *autism*, for example, is heard or used in everyday conversation, it is often unclear whether the speaker is referencing a specific former diagnosis (i.e., autistic disorder), a previous umbrella term (i.e., PDD), or the current all-encompassing diagnosis (i.e., ASD).

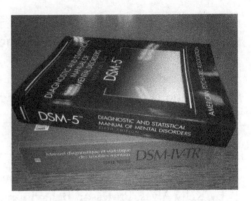

Figure 1.2: Diagnostic Statistical Manuals
Source: F.RdeC (CC BY-SA 3.0), via Wikimedia Commons.

Read about it. Think about it. Write about it.

What terminology around ASD is the most familiar to you? How did you learn these terms? What were your sources?

HIGHLIGHTS FROM THE ONTARIO CONTEXT

All the historical figures noted above who influenced the field of ASD have also made their mark on the legislation, services, education, and interventions for individuals with ASD in Ontario. One of the earliest relevant information pieces put forth by the Special Education and Provincial Schools Branch of the Ontario Ministry of Education was the *Special Education Monograph 4* (1990). This informational paper supplied educators with an introduction to autism, as well as further readings and direction to additional materials. Introductory information included the characteristics, categories, and prevalence of autistic disorders, as well as specific symptoms associated with ASD, including: social issues (e.g., trouble making friends); problems communicating (both verbally and nonverbally); receptive communication problems (e.g., difficulty understanding abstractions); challenges with expressive communication (e.g., trouble with conversational turn-taking); unique patterns of behaviour (e.g., difficulty with change); commonly associated features (e.g., sensory issues); and associated learning difficulties (e.g., problems with group-based teaching and learning). The paper also supplied narrative case descriptions to demonstrate a range of family perspectives.

Read about it. Think about it. Write about it.

Is there any language or information on ASD that has changed between the publication of *Monograph 4* and now? Explain.

Box 1.1: Intensive Behaviour Intervention: What Is It? Who Is Involved?
By Kelly Alves, Professor, Behavioural Sciences Program, Seneca College

In 2000, the Ontario Ministry of Children and Youth Services (MCYS) provided funding to lead agencies in nine geographic regions to begin planning and delivering an intervention program for young children diagnosed with moderate to severe ASD (Perry, 2002). The treatment provided through these agencies was termed *intensive behaviour intervention* (IBI). IBI is a systematic, intense behaviour analytic treatment used to improve the behavioural repertoires of young children with ASD (Ontario Ministry of Children and Youth Services, 2006). The goal of this treatment is to improve the developmental trajectory for children with ASD so it can more closely match that of their same-age, typically developing peers. The framework of this intervention is based on research carried out by Ivar Lovaas and his students at the University of California at Los Angeles for children under age six. Lovaas and his students published an article titled "Behavioral Treatment and Normal Educational and Intellectual

Functioning in Young Autistic Children" in the *Journal of Consulting and Clinical Psychology* (1987). This article presented the results of a controlled trial investigating the intensive application of behavioural intervention on young children with ASD. It was Lovaas's hypothesis that "construction of a special, intense, and comprehensive learning environment for very young autistic children would allow some of them to catch up with their normal peers by Grade One" (1987, p. 4). A variety of clinical positions are involved in the provision of IBI. The roles and responsibilities associated with these positions are described in detail in the MCYS's *ASD Intervention Program Guidelines*. The guidelines included in this public document "govern the delivery of intensive behavioural intervention and associated services to children with autism by the Regional Program Providers delivering the Autism Intervention Program" (Ontario Ministry of Children and Youth Services, 2007, p. 4).

Typically, an IBI treatment team comprises eight to nine children, each assigned one primary instructor therapist. An instructor therapist's primary responsibility is to deliver individual or small-group instruction to the clients on their caseload. Additional tasks within the instructor therapist role include creating necessary program materials, maintaining the primary client's programming binder, data collection, graphing, and program revisions. To be employed as an instructor therapist, an individual typically requires a community college diploma or university degree in a relevant field (e.g., behavioural science, psychology, early childhood education, child and youth work).

A supervising therapist directly oversees a child's IBI program. A supervising therapist's role often includes a combination of clinical and administrative responsibilities, such as implementing the clinical recommendations provided by the clinical supervisor, staffing, scheduling, and training.

A clinical supervisor is responsible for overseeing, monitoring, and evaluating the overall quality and consistency of a child's behavioural program (Ontario Ministry of Children and Youth Services, 2007). Ideally, a clinical supervisor would have a doctoral degree in psychology and be a board-certified behaviour analyst. However, due to the limited number of clinicians meeting these qualifications in the province of Ontario, clinical supervisors often possess a master's degree plus extensive relevant experience. Often, a clinical supervisor oversees between two and four treatment teams. The instructor therapist, supervising therapist, and clinical supervisor work together to deliver high-quality, intensive behavioural intervention to young children with moderate to severe ASD.

Box 1.2: ABA Differentiated from IBI

ABA ≠ IBI
By Jo-Ann Reitzel, Clinical Director, Hamilton-Niagara Regional Autism Initiative

Intensive behavioural intervention (IBI) is an evidence-based program designed to change a child's developmental trajectory. IBI also increases readiness for participation in an educational program by teaching learning and developmental skills. IBI is based on the principles of applied behaviour analysis (ABA); however, the model of service delivery for IBI is intensive. A child with ASD may be in one-on-one sessions for 20 to 40 hours a week, receiving comprehensive programming in many developmental domains. In schools, ABA uses approaches that fit with the needs and resources of the classroom. ABA is concerned with changing behaviours in a manner that is socially valid and results in lasting benefit.

Source: McMaster Children's Hospital ASD School Support Program (n.d.)

The Ontario Ministry of Education issued an information bulletin in 2007: *Policy/Program Memorandum No. 140 (PPM 140), Incorporating Methods of Applied Behaviour Analysis (ABA) into Programs for Students with Autism Spectrum Disorder (ASD)*. Its communicated purpose was to provide "a policy framework to support incorporation of ABA methods into school boards' practices" and to give "direction to school boards to support their use of applied behaviour analysis (ABA) as an effective instructional approach in the education of many students with Autism Spectrum Disorder (ASD)" (Ontario Ministry of Education, 2007b, para. 1). *PPM 140* focused on the following:

- Describing ABA practices in the school setting; and
- Explaining the foundational principles of ABA-based programming (e.g., individualization, data collection, positive reinforcement, generalization).

Two specific directives are provided within its text:

- "School boards must offer students with ASD special education programs and services, including, where appropriate, special education programs using ABA methods" (para.13)

- "School board staff must plan for the transition between various activities and settings involving students with ASD" (para. 20).

In *Autism Matters*, Laurie Pearce (2008) clarifies what this memorandum means at a practical level, stating, "The PPM makes it possible for you to insist that ABA strategies be included in your child's IEP [individual education plan]: it does not make it possible for you to insist that a board-certified behaviour analyst or other behavioural expert be involved in developing (or delivering) your child's education" (p. 6).

Instead, each school board employs staff with ABA expertise, which may or may not include an external behaviour consultant or board-certified behaviour analyst who will assist the team working with the individual to incorporate ABA programming into his or her individual education plan (IEP). Pearce (2008) also clarifies that this

Intensive Behavioural Intervention: Intensive behavioural interventions (IBIs) are defined as "programs based on the principles of ABA that have been designed specifically to help children with autism" (de Rivera, 2008, p. 4). IBI is intensive and individualized, focused on individually assessed needs, and managed by nine centres across Ontario using either the Direct Service Option (program delivery through the regional programs) or the Direct Funding Option (private program delivery). In Ontario, it is known as the Regional Intensive Early Intervention Programs for Children with Autism, under the Autism Intervention Plan umbrella (de Rivera, 2008; Ontario Ministry of Children and Youth Services, n.d.).

initiative does not apply to intensive behaviour intervention and its clinical presence, or therapists in the school environment. Weiss, White, and Spoelstra (2008) followed up the implementation of *PPM 140* with an online parent survey supported by Autism Ontario that resulted in 640 responses. Among other conclusions, quantitative results showed that only 6 percent of participants rated the use of ABA principles in school environments as happening "all of the time." Forty-five percent rated its implementation as "never," 34 percent as "some of the time," and 15 percent as "most of the time." Qualitatively, "the most frequently occurring theme to emerge from parent comments involved concerns that ABA was not being implemented effectively with their children, as it is described by PPM-140" (p. 13).

The obvious direction and intention here is the movement toward strategies involving evidence-based ABA interventions, as well as the more subtle move to embed transition plans in Individual Education Plans (IEPs) for all students with ASD, previously accessible only for students 14 years of age and older (excluding those with solely a giftedness identification) (Ontario Ministry of Education, 2002; Ontario Ministry of Education, 2004). This directive became less unique when the Ontario Ministry of Education required transition plans in IEPs as a universal component for all students who are supported by an IEP, through *Policy/Program Memorandum 156 (PPM 156)* in 2013 (Ontario Ministry of Education, 2013b).

Individual Education Plan (IEP): The brief definition of an IEP for Ontario schools is a "written plan describing the special education program and/or services required by a particular student, based on a thorough assessment of the student's strengths and needs that affect the student's ability to learn and demonstrate learning" (Ontario Ministry of Education, 2013a, para. 5).

Currently, the Ministry of Children and Youth Services provides varied types of ABA-based supports, outlined in *ABA-Based Services and Supports for Children and Youth with ASD* (2011a). One issue that can be confusing, initially, is the differentiation of ABA services—specifically, the confusion between ABA-based services (e.g., "Natural, positive reinforce[rs] are utilized which are immediate, appropriate and dependent on the child's response to assist in the acquisition of skills" [para. 4]) and intensive behavioural intervention (IBI), or the Autism Intervention Program (AIP), an intensive, individualized program. IBI is defined as an "early, intensive treatment using behaviorally based methods, sometimes known as Intensive Behavioral Intervention (IBI), [which] has a much stronger empirical basis than virtually any other intervention used with children with autism and is considered 'best practice' for young children with autism" (Perry et al., 2008, p. 622). Although definitions vary, characteristic commonalities across programs exist, including highly structured, individualized interventions with typically a minimum of 25 and a maximum of 40 hours of treatment a week, lasting from one year to three years (Perry et al., 2008).

Applied Behaviour Analysis (ABA): ABA is "a scientific approach to behaviour change that uses interventions based on behavioral principles and that relies on data to verify that behavior change interventions are indeed responsible for behaviour change" (Scheuermann & Hall, 2011, p. 465).

Overall, the vision of the MCYS-supported ABA-based services is focused on "increas[ing] functional life skills and decreas[ing] interfering behaviours" in four specific areas (communication skills, social skills,

Individual Education Plan

IEP

REASON FOR DEVELOPING THE IEP

☐ Student identified as exceptional by IPRC

☐ Student not formally identified but requires special education program/services, including modified/alternative learning expectations and/or accommodations

STUDENT PROFILE

Name: _____ Gender: _____ Date of Birth: _____

School: _____

Student OEN/MIN: _____ Principal: _____

Current Grade/Special Class: _____ School Year: _____

Most Recent IPRC Date: _____ Date Annual Review Waived by Parent/Guardian: _____

Exceptionality: _____

IPRC Placement Decision (*check one*)

☐ Regular class with indirect support
☐ Regular class with resource assistance
☐ Regular class with withdrawal assistance

☐ Special education class with partial integration
☐ Special education class full-time

ASSESSMENT DATA

List relevant educational, medical/health (hearing, vision, physical, neurological), psychological, speech/language, occupational, physiotherapy, and behavioural assessments.

Information Source	Date	Summary of Results

STUDENT'S STRENGTHS AND NEEDS

Areas of Strength	Areas of Need

Health Support Services/Personal Support Required ☐ Yes (*list below*) ☐ No

1

Figure 1.3: IEP Sample: Page 1 of an Ontario IEP Template

Source: Ontario Ministry of Education, 2004, p. 52.

skills of daily living, and emotional regulation/behaviour management) and is described this way:

> The vision of the Ministry of Children and Youth Services (MCYS) is an Ontario where all children and youth have the best opportunity to succeed and reach their full potential. To support this vision, the ministry is building on and improving the continuum of services and supports for children and youth with Autism Spectrum Disorder (ASD) in Ontario, and their families by implementing Applied Behaviour Analysis (ABA)-based services and supports. (Ontario Ministry of Children and Youth Services, 2011a)

The Ontario Ministry of Children and Youth Services' guiding principles include descriptors such as *collaborative, evidence-informed, family-centred*, and *accessible*. It sets goals at the systems level, the family level, and child-focused levels. Ontario's clinic- and community-based ABA services target children from birth to adulthood—specifically, to their 18th birthday—targeting highest-priority needs in time-limited and potentially repeating interventions (i.e., two to six months, two to four hours per week), summarized in an *ABA service plan.*

One recent innovation worth highlighting is the Connections for Students initiative (Council of Ontario Directors of Education, 2014). This is defined as "multidisciplinary, student-specific and school based transition teams that are established approximately six months before a child prepares to leave [IBI] services delivered through [MCYS's] Autism Intervention Program (AIP) and starts or continues in publicly funded school" (para. 1). This initiative is designed to support the transition from intensive, clinical service provision to school-based support services (e.g., special education). Since 2007 and the increased recognition of—and emphasis on—the critical need for effective transitions (Ministers' Autism Spectrum Disorder Reference Group, 2007), school boards and AIP service providers province-wide have developed individualized plans together to support transitioning students with their individual needs as they move from the clinic to the classroom. Though individual boards are developing regionalized, collaborative materials, practices, policies, and protocols, MCYS provides capacity-building tools and communication materials. For example, they have provided a list of typical roles in Connections for Students transition teams, composed of:

ABA Service Plan: An ABA service plan includes—at minimum—target skill(s), service delivery, duration, setting, staff, goals, as well as parental agreement, and a plan for capacity building in the latter (Ontario Ministry of Children and Youth Services, 2011a).

- The team lead (principal or designate)
- Parent(s)/guardian(s)
- Teacher(s)
- School support program ASD consultant
- School board professional with ABA expertise (as required)
- Education assistants (if necessary)
- Special education resource teachers (if necessary)
- Other professionals (if necessary), such as mental health service providers, speech-language pathologists, occupational therapists, physiotherapists, and so on (Ontario Ministry of Children and Youth Services, 2011b)

Another resource is the publication *Effective Educational Practices for Students with Autism Spectrum Disorder: A Resource Guide* (Ontario Ministry of Education, 2007a).

Effective Educational Practices combines the clinical and educational foundations of ASD with practical appendices for everyday use in the school, home, and community. (It is important to note that an earlier, significantly briefer version was released; however, that version does not include the practical appendices found in the full-length manual.) The final chapter is approximately 100 pages of tools and techniques, described as follows:

> Ontario educators use a wide range of strategies, tools, and resources to provide effective educational programs for students with ASD. Some of the materials that have been developed by school boards and regional autism service providers are reproduced, with permission, in chapter, and may be used by schools and school boards across the province. (Ontario Ministry of Education, 2007a, p. 109)

Included are profiles, pamphlets, visuals, checklists, diagrams, data sheets, inventories, narratives, routines, and more. Pages 109 to 111 offer a full listing of practical resources from across Ontario.

Read about it. Think about it. Write about it.

Which of these practical tools and techniques do you think you would choose to implement first? Why?

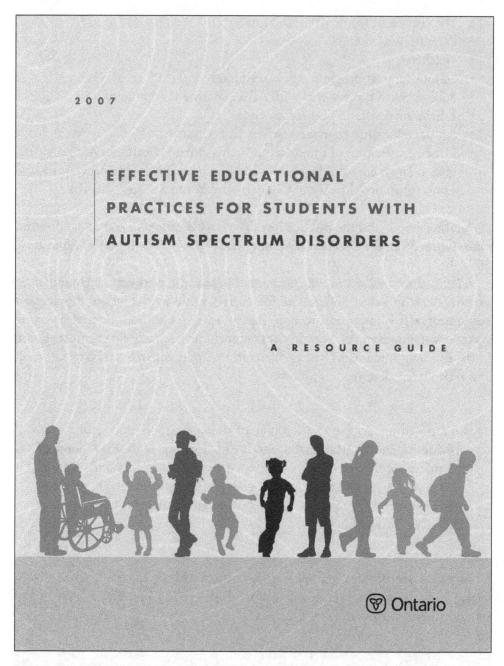

Figure 1.4: Effective Educational Practices for Students with Autism Spectrum Disorders
Source: Ontario Ministry of Education, 2007a.

Some investigation and research focuses on the implementation of Ontario's programs, typically IBI, and is published in peer-reviewed literature, through governmental venues, and through one of Ontario's strongest advocacy groups, Autism Ontario. For example, in 2004, the Office of the Provincial Auditor of Ontario released a report entitled *Report on the Review for the Standing Committee on Public Accounts: Intensive Early Intervention Program for Children with Autism*, in response to budgetary and other concerns (e.g., wait lists). This report culminated with a review of seven recommendations and seven ministry responses, with next steps related to funding, monitoring, accountability, and other issues, and noted that court cases were in progress—at the time—but no decisions had yet been made. The success of literature-based early interventions in IBI led parents of children with ASD in Ontario to a protracted—but ultimately unsuccessful—court battle with the provincial government to obtain provincially funded IBI treatments, and IBI therapy in the school environment. Until 2006, IBI was limited to children up to age six; Ontario voluntarily lifted this age ban, even though full governmental financing was denied (Top Court Halts, 2007; Pourier, 2006) in two prominent cases (*Arzem v. Ontario* [Ontario Human Rights Commission] and *Wynberg v. Ontario* [a civil case]), which found that neither age nor disability discrimination had occurred in the provision of early IBI (Hilborn, 2006). While the ministry provides funding, decisions about which children will—and do—benefit is a clinical decision, and does not apply to every child at every age and functional level who is diagnosed with an ASD. This leads some parents to fund therapy privately, which can cause significant financial distress. In fact, Ontario's IBI is targeted toward "more severe and needy children" (Perry et al., 2008, p. 625). Nevertheless, IBI is implemented in a climate that can be divisive, with "political pressure, advocacy, media attention, and litigation" (Perry et al., 2008, p. 625).

Multiple local research studies have been carried out relating to Ontario's IBI outcomes, from large, quantitatively oriented large studies examining statistical and clinical change (e.g., Perry et al., 2008) to smaller, case-study-based examinations (e.g., Blacklock & Perry, 2010). As an example of the former approach, in 2008, Perry et al. published an evaluation of the effectiveness of Ontario's IBI program, studying statistical and clinical change from program entry to discharge, focusing on "outcomes of 332 children, aged 2–7 years, enrolled in a large, community-based, publicly funded IBI Program in Ontario" (Perry et al., 2008, p. 622). This evaluation is described as the largest in the world to date, and utilized file reviews to examine outcomes. Overall, much individual progress and improvement was seen, described as an approximate doubling of developmental growth rate. As well,

Results indicated that children showed statistically significant and clinically significant reduction in autism symptom severity during the time they were involved in the IBI program. Cognitive level improved significantly for children, in some cases dramatically so. Children gained significantly in developmental skills (increased age equivalents) in all areas of adaptive behavior. (Perry et al., 2008, p. 636)

A LOOK BACK

Chapter 1, "A Brief History of Autism Spectrum Disorder," focused on:

- A history of the highlights of ASD research and understanding from its first recognition, including the work of some influential pioneers in the field (e.g., Hans Asperger and Leo Kanner);
- Discussion around the elasticity of terminology in the field of ASD over time; and
- Initiatives in the fairly recent history of service provision for those with ASD in the context of school and community, including resources, publications, research, and more.

A LOOK AHEAD

Chapter 2, "A Contemporary Understanding of Autism Spectrum Disorder," focuses on:

- Current definitions of ASD in the *DSM-TR* and the *DSM-5*, and the changes to diagnostic criteria within these;
- An overview of Ontario's clinical ASD services, supports, and issues, including the typical diagnostic pathway, and intensive behavioural intervention services;
- A discussion of perspectives on ASD found in the media, including what everyday mass media teaches about ASD; and
- The importance of self-advocacy, including a discussion of Ontario's Carly Fleischmann.

ADDITIONAL RESOURCES

- ABA Services (Ontario Ministry of Children and Youth Services, 2011a): http://www.children.gov.on.ca/htdocs/English/topics/specialneeds/autism/guidelines/guidelines-2011.aspx
- "Autism's First Child" (Donavan & Zucker, 2010): http://www.theatlantic.com/magazine/archive/2010/10/autisms-first-child/308227

- *Autistic Children: A Guide for Parents* (Wing, 1972)
- *DSM-5* (American Psychological Association, 2012):
  http://www.dsm5.org/Pages/Default.aspx
- *Effective Educational Practices for Students with ASD* (Ontario Ministry of Education, 2007):
  http://www.edu.gov.on.ca/eng/general/elemsec/speced/autismspecdis.pdf
- Leo Kanner Collection (Johns Hopkins, n.d.):
  http://www.medicalarchives.jhmi.edu/papers/kanner.html
- *Policy/Program Memorandum No. 140* (Ontario Ministry of Education, 2007):
  http://www.edu.gov.on.ca/extra/eng/ppm/140.html
- *Special Education: A Guide for Educators* (Ontario Ministry of Education, 2010):
  http://www.edu.gov.on.ca/eng/general/elemsec/speced/guide.html
- *The Individual Education Plan (IEP): A Resource Guide* (Ontario Ministry of Education, 2004):
  http://www.edu.gov.on.ca/eng/general/elemsec/speced/guide/resource/iepresguid.pdf

REFERENCES

Adelson, J. (1997). The creation of Dr. B: A biography of Bruno Bettelheim. *Commentary, 6,* 67–68.

American Psychiatric Association. (1994). *Diagnostic and statistical manual of psychiatric disorders* (4th ed.). Arlington, VA: American Psychiatric Publishing.

American Psychiatric Association. (2000). *Diagnostic and statistical manual of psychiatric disorders: Text revision* (4th ed.). Arlington, VA: American Psychiatric Publishing.

American Psychiatric Association. (2012). DSM 5 development. Retrieved from www.dsm5.org/Pages/Default.aspx

American Psychiatric Association. (2013). Highlights of changes from DSM-IV-TR to DSM-5. Retrieved from http://www.dsm5.org/Documents/changes%20from%20dsm-iv-tr%20to%20dsm-5.pdf

Arora, T. (2012). Understanding the perseveration displayed by students with an autism spectrum disorder. *Education, 132*(4), 799–808.

Asperger, H. (1944/1991). Autistic psychopathology in childhood. In Uta Frith (ed.), *Autism and Asperger syndrome* (pp. 37–92). Cambridge: Cambridge University Press.

Bahsoun, P. (2012, December 3). Changes to autism definition approved for publication in DSM V. *The Examiner*. Retrieved from http://www.examiner.com/article/changes-to-autism-definition-approved-for-publication-dsm-v

Barbera, M. L. (2010). The experiences of "autism mothers" who become behavior analysts: A qualitative study. *The Journal of Speech-Language Pathology and Applied Behavior Analysis, 4,* 56–73. Retrieved from www.baojournal.com/SLP-ABA%20WEBSITE/SLP-Best%20of%202009/Best%20Of%20SLP-ABA-2009.pdf

Bettelheim, B. (1959). Feral children and autistic children. *American Journal of Sociology, 64*(5), 455.

Bettelheim, B. (1967). *The empty fortress: Infantile autism and the birth of the self.* New York, NY: The Free Press.

Blacher, J., & Christensen, L. (2011). Sowing the seeds of the autism field: Leo Kanner (1943). *Intellectual & Developmental Disabilities, 49*(3), 172–191. doi:10.1352/1934-9556-49.3.172

Blacklock, K., & Perry, A. (2010). Testing the applications of benchmarks for children in Ontario's IBI program: Six case studies. *Journal on Developmental Disabilities, 16*(2), 33–43.

Chown, N. (2012). "History and first descriptions" of autism: A response to Michael Fitzgerald. *Journal of Autism & Developmental Disorders, 42*(10), 2263-2265. doi:10.1007/s10803-012-1529-5

Council of Ontario Directors of Education. (2014). Connections for students: Resources provided by school boards and autism intervention program providers. Retrieved from ontariodirectors. ca/ASD/asd-english.html

de Rivera, C. (2008). The use of intensive behavioural intervention for children with autism. *Journal on Developmental Disabilities,* 14(2), 1–15. Retrieved from www.oadd.org/publications/journal/issues/vol14no2/download/deRivera.pdf

Donvan, J., & Zucker, C. (2010). Autism's first child. *Atlantic Monthly (10727825), 306*(3), 78–90.

Eliot, S. (2002). *Not the thing I was: Thirteen years at Bruno Bettelheim's orthogenic school.* New York, NY: St. Martin's Press.

Fleck, C., & Müller, A. (1997). Bruno Bettelheim and the concentration camps. *Journal of the History of the Behavioural Sciences, 33*(1), 1–37.

Hebert, J. (2014, June 12). Lorna Wing; Psychiatrist whose work did much to improve the understanding of autism after her only child had the condition diagnosed. *Times,* p. 58. Retrieved from www.thetimes.co.uk/tto/opinion/obituaries/article4116049.ece

Hilborn, T. L. (2006). Age discrimination and children with autism: Two recent Ontario decisions muddy the waters. *Education Law Journal, 16*(2), 225–235. Retrieved from search.proquest.com/docview/212964455?accountid=9744

Hippler, K., & Klicpera, C. (2003). A retrospective analysis of the clinical case records of "autistic psychopaths" diagnosed by Hans Asperger and his team at the University Children's Hospital, Vienna. *Philosophical Transactions of the Royal Society B: Biological Sciences, 358*(1430), 291–301.

Jacobsen, K. (2010). Diagnostic politics: The curious case of Kanner's syndrome. *History of Psychiatry, 21*(4), 436–454. doi: 10.1177/0957154X09341438

Johns Hopkins Medical Institutions. (n.d.). Leo Kanner collection. Retrieved from www. medicalarchives.jhmi.edu/papers/kanner.html

Kanner, L. (1968). Autistic disturbances of affective contact. *Acta Paedopsychiatrica: International Journal of Child & Adolescent Psychiatry, 35*(4-8), 98–136.

Leekam, S. (2014, August). Lorna Wing (1928–2014). *Psychologist,* 564.

Lovaas, O. I. (1987). Behavioral treatment and normal educational and intellectual functioning in young autistic children. *Journal of Consulting and Clinical Psychology, 55*(1), 3–9.

Lyons, V., & Fitzgerald, M. (2007). Asperger (1906-1980) and Kanner (1894-1981), the two pioneers of autism. *Journal of Autism and Developmental Disorders, 37,* 2022–2023. doi: 10.1007/s10803-007-0383-3

McMaster Children's Hospital ASD School Support Program. (n.d.). Quick reference guide to ASD and ABA. Hamilton, ON: Author.

Ministers' Autism Spectrum Disorder Reference Group. (2007). Making a difference for students with Autism Spectrum Disorder in Ontario schools: From evidence to action. Retrieved from www.edu.gov.on.ca/eng/document/nr/07.02/autismfeb07.pdf

Neumärker, K. (2003). Leo Kanner: His years in Berlin, 1906-24. The roots of autistic disorder. *History of Psychiatry, 14*(54), 205–218.

Office of the Provincial Auditor of Ontario. (2004). *Report on the review for the standing committee on public accounts: Intensive early intervention program for children with autism.* Retrieved from www.auditor.on.ca/en/reports_en/2004_autism_en.pdf

Ontario Ministry of Children and Youth Services. (n.d.). The autism parent resource kit. Retrieved from www.children.gov.on.ca

Ontario Ministry of Children and Youth Services. (2006). McGuinty government committed to helping children and youth with autism. http://news.ontario.ca/archive/en/2006/07/07/McGuinty-Government-Committed-to-Helping-Children-and-Youth-with-Autism.html

Ontario Ministry of Children and Youth Services. (2007). Autism intervention program guideline revision. Retrieved from www.children.gov.on.ca/htdocs/English/topics/specialneeds/autism/guidelines/guidelines.aspx

Ontario Ministry of Children and Youth Services. (2011a). ABA-based services and supports for children and youth with ASD. Retrieved from www.children.gov.on.ca/htdocs/English/topics/specialneeds/autism/guidelines/guidelines-2011.aspx

Ontario Ministry of Children and Youth Services. (2011b). Educational transitions: Connections for students. Retrieved from http://www.children.gov.on.ca/htdocs/English/topics/specialneeds/autism/aprk/educational-transitions/connections-for-students.aspx

Ontario Ministry of Education. (1990). *Special education monographs, no. 4: Students with autism.* Retrieved from http://www.edu.gov.on.ca/eng/general/elemsec/speced/monog4.html

Ontario Ministry of Education. (2002). *Transition planning: A resource guide.* Toronto, ON: Queen's Printer. Retrieved from www.edu.gov.on.ca/eng/general/elemsec/speced/transiti/transition.pdf

Ontario Ministry of Education. (2004). *The individual education plan (IEP): A resource guide.* Toronto, ON: Queen's Printer. Retrieved from www.edu.gov.on.ca/eng/general/elemsec/speced/guide/resource/iepresguid.pdf

Ontario Ministry of Education. (2007a). Effective educational practices for students with Autism Spectrum Disorder: A resource guide. Retrieved from www.edu.gov.on.ca/eng/general/elemsec/speced/autismspecdis.pdf

Ontario Ministry of Education. (2007b). Policy/program memorandum no. 140: Incorporating methods of applied behaviour analysis (ABA), into programs for students with Autism Spectrum Disorder (ASD). Retrieved from www.edu.gov.on.ca/extra/eng/ppm/140.html

Ontario Ministry of Education. (2013a). An introduction to special education in Ontario. Retrieved from www.edu.gov.on.ca/eng/general/elemsec/speced/ontario.html

Ontario Ministry of Education. (2013b). *Program/policy memorandum no. 156: Supporting transitions for students with special educational needs.* Retrieved from www.edu.gov.on.ca/extra/eng/ppm/ppm156.pdf

Pearce, L. (2008, Winter). Ministry of Education ASD initiatives and what they mean for you. *Autism Matters, 5*(1), 5–7.

Perry, A. (2002). Intensive early intervention program for children with autism: Background and design of the Ontario pre-school autism initiative. *Journal on Developmental Disabilities, 9*(2), 121–128.

Perry, A., Cummings, A., Geier, J. D., Freeman, N. L., Hughes, S., LaRose, L., . . . & Williams, J. (2008). Effectiveness of intensive behavioral intervention in a large, community-based program. *Research in Autism Spectrum Disorder, 2*(4), 621–642.

Pourier, J. (2006, July 6). Ontario court of appeal decision anticipated tomorrow in Wynberg et al. v. Ontario autism cases. *Ontario Human Rights Commission.* Retrieved from www.ohrc.on.ca/en/news_centre/ontario-court-appeal-decision-anticipated-tomorrow-wynberg-et-al-v-ontario-autism-cases

Raines, T. (2002). *Rising to the light: A portrait of Bruno Bettleheim.* New York, NY: Knopf.

Rapoport, J., Chavez, A., Greenstein, D., Addington, A., & Gogtay, N. (2009). Autism spectrum disorder and childhood-onset schizophrenia: Clinical and biological contributions to a relation revisited. *Journal of the American Academy of Child & Adolescent Psychiatry, 48*(1), 10–18.

Scheuermann, B. K., & Hall, J. A. (2011). *Positive behavioral supports for the classroom.* Toronto, ON: Pearson.

Smith, T., & Eikeseth, S. (2011). O. Ivar Lovaas: Pioneer of applied behavior analysis and intervention for children with autism. *Journal of Autism and Developmental Disorders, 41*(3), 375–378. doi:10.1007/s10803-010-1162-0

Strauss, K., Mancini, F., & Fava, L. (2013). Parent inclusion in early intensive behavior interventions for young children with ASD: A synthesis of meta-analyses from 2009 to 2011. *Research in Developmental Disabilities, 34*(9), 2967–2985.

Thilinie, R., & Tamara, P. (2010). Pharmacotherapeutics of tourette syndrome and stereotypies in autism. *Seminars in Pediatric Neurology, 17*, 254–260. doi:10.1016/j.spen.2010.10.008

Thompson, T. (2013). Autism research and services for young children: History, progress and challenges. *Journal of Applied Research in Intellectual Disabilities, 26*(2), 81–107. doi:10.1111/jar.12021

Top court halts parents' autism funding appeal. (2007, April 12). *CBC News Canada.* Retrieved from www.cbc.ca/news/canada/top-court-halts-parents-autism-funding-appeal-1.647636

Weiss, J., White, S., & Spoelstra, M. (2008). *PPM-140 parent survey: An analysis on the implementation of PPM-140.* Toronto, ON: Autism Ontario.

Whittaker, J. K. (1976). Causes of childhood disorders: New findings. *Social Work, 21*(2), 91–96.

Wing, L. (1972). *Autistic children: A guide for parents and professionals.* Don Mills, ON: Musson Book Company.

Wing, L. (1993). The definition and prevalence of autism: A review. *European Child and Adolescent Psychiatry, 2*(1), 61. doi:10.1007/BF02098832

Wing, L., & Gould, J. (1979). Severe impairments of social interaction and associated abnormalities in children: Epidemiology and classification. *Journal of Autism and Developmental Disorders, 9*(1), 11–29.

Wing, L., & Potter, D. (2002). The epidemiology of autistic spectrum disorders: Is the prevalence rising? *Mental Retardation and Developmental Disabilities Research Reviews, 8*(3), 151–161.

CHAPTER 2

A CONTEMPORARY UNDERSTANDING OF AUTISM SPECTRUM DISORDER

IN THIS CHAPTER:

- Current Definitions
  - DSM IV-TR
  - DSM-5 Definition
- Diagnostic Pathway in the Province of Ontario
- Ontario's Clinical ASD Services, Supports, and Issues: An Overview
- Messages from Popular Media
  - Self-Advocacy

Chapter 2 provides a focus on recent and current definitions of ASD, as presented in the two most recent editions of the *Diagnostic and Statistical Manual (DSM)*, and the changes to diagnostic criteria that make up the disorder within these. This includes an overview of Ontario's clinical ASD services, supports, and issues, including the typical diagnostic pathway, and intensive behavioural intervention services. As well, this chapter discusses media-based perspectives on ASD, including what everyday mass media teaches its audiences about ASD, and emphasizes the importance of advocacy in today's field of ASD. Special areas of focus include Ontario's Carly Fleischmann and an Ontario-developed Diagnostic Observation Form.

CURRENT DEFINITIONS

As previously explained, definitions in the field of ASD are flexible and elastic, changing over time as knowledge and understandings of and attitudes toward ASD change. These changes are reflected in the language used in the field, the published literature on the topic of ASD, and most notably in the manuals guiding the diagnosis of ASD—most recently the fourth and fifth editions of the *DSM*.

Autism was first found in the *DSM-III*, as a distinct category called *infantile autism*; before this the characteristics of the disorder were listed under childhood schizophrenia (Watkins, n.d.). There were six characteristics listed for a diagnosis of infantile autism. Revisions to the *DSM*, for the *DSM-III-R* in 1987, renamed the term *autistic disorder*, with notable increases in the number and quality of observable and measurable characteristics to be diagnosed (Watkins, n.d.). Thompson (2013) highlights the literature of the autism diagnosis up to the mid-2000s (see Figure 2.1).

DSM IV-TR

The *DSM-IV* was published in 1994, and later the *DSM-IV-TR* in 2000, which provided additional diagnosis and the triad of characteristics earlier described by Wing (1993). The *DSM-IV-TR* included autism under the term *pervasive developmental disorders*, which encompassed five different disorders, including: autistic disorder; Asperger's disorder; pervasive developmental disorder—not otherwise specified; Rett's disorder; and childhood disintegrative disorder. Hartley and Sikora (2010) succinctly summarize two of these former subtypes, autistic disorder and pervasive developmental disorder—not otherwise specified:

> A *DSM-IV-TR* diagnosis of Autistic Disorder requires impairments in three domains, including Social Relatedness (i.e., deficits in social interest or interactions), Communication (i.e., deficits in language development or atypical speech), and Restricted/Repetitive/Stereotyped Patterns (i.e., odd or stereotyped interests or behaviors). A diagnosis of Pervasive Developmental Disorder—Not Otherwise Specified is given if some but not all criteria are met for Autistic Disorder, the onset of symptoms occurs after 3 years of age, or there is an atypical presentation of symptoms. (pp. 85–86)

Less commonly recognized were Rett's disorder—characterized by cognitive delays, atypical motor movements, social disinterest, and its presence primarily in females—and childhood disintegrative disorder, which is typically marked by a regression later in childhood (Odle, Barstow, & Cataldo, 2011). Asperger's disorder, often called Asperger's syndrome, is commonly recognized now, although this diagnosis is no longer in the *DSM-5*. A diagnosis of Asperger's disorder in the *DSM-IV* required that the individual have two deficits in social interaction and one impairment in repetitive and restricted patterns of behaviour, as for a diagnosis of autistic disorder, with no characteristics of communication impairments or no delay of language onset (American Psychological Association, 2000). Asperger's disorder is perhaps best distinguished from the other subtypes by what it lacks,

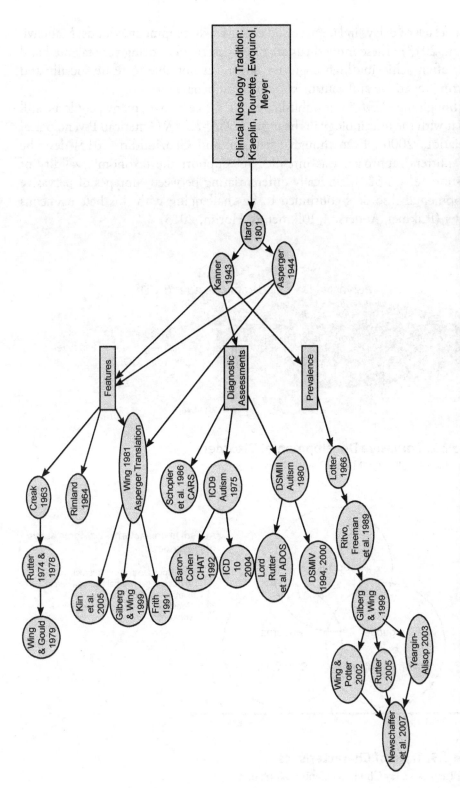

Figure 2.1: Theoretical Origins and Empirical Influences on Autism Diagnostic Classification and Prevalence

Source: Thompson, 2013, p. 87.

such as a lack of delays in language and cognitive development (Woods, Mahdavi, & Ryan, 2013). These individuals are often described as being very talented and gifted, often achieving high cognitive tasks, but not able to relate socially and preferring repetitive and routine structure and behaviour.

Although the *DSM-5* was published in 2013 (see below), many people are still familiar with the terminology in the former *DSM-IV-TR* (American Psychological Association, 2000). Even though what Tsai and Ghaziuddin (2013) describe as a "splitters" approach was intended to "support the taxonomic validity of each subtype" (p. 324), clinically differentiating between subtypes of pervasive developmental disorders continued to be challenging with this heterogeneous disorder (Falkmer, Anderson, Falkmer, & Horlin, 2013).

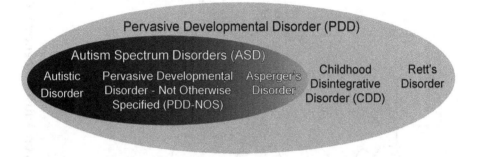

Figure 2.2: Pervasive Developmental Disorders
Source: Thames Valley Children's Centre, 2008, p. 2.

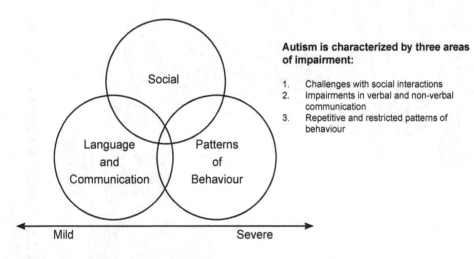

Figure 2.3: Triad of Characteristics
Source: Thames Valley Children's Centre, 2008, p. 3.

Read about it. Think about it. Write about it.

Which of these subtypes of PDD are most familiar to you? In what context did you learn about these subtypes?

What—if any—new facts about the definition of PDD subtypes in the *DSM-IV-TR* did you learn from this section?

DSM-5 Definition

In a significant shift to diagnostic categorization in the field of ASD, the *DSM-5* entered the picture in May 2013 as a newly updated diagnostic tool, after 6,000 hours of consideration through the American Psychiatric Association's Work Group on Neurodevelopmental Disorders, as well as field testing (Grzadzinski, Huerta, & Lord, 2013; Tsai & Ghaziuddin, 2013). The changes included replacing terminology (e.g., PDD), subsuming some subtypes (e.g., PDD—NOS), removing other subtypes (e.g., Rett's), and absorbing the entire category into a singular yet adaptable term: ASD (Tsai & Ghaziuddin, 2013).

The full text of ASD-related criteria is available on the Autism Speaks website (www.autismspeaks.org). A new, related addition in the *DSM-5*—though not labelled as an ASD—is social (pragmatic) communication disorder, which, as its name implies, relates to "persistent difficulties in the social use of verbal and nonverbal communication" (para. 2) (i.e., social relationships, listener-based flexibility, rule-following, and non-explicit information, or the "hidden curriculum"). Three other main diagnostic criteria are: functional limitations in a range of areas, such as academic achievement; its onset at an earlier stage of development; and the exclusion of other diagnostic possibilities (e.g., ASD).

The former five pervasive developmental disorders described in the *DSM-IV-TR* (American Psychological Association, 2000) have been collapsed and subsumed in the *DSM-5* into the single category called *autism spectrum disorder*. This reflects the common usage adopted in the field, in everyday conversation, and in recent literature (e.g., Hall, 2013), reflecting the

Hidden Curriculum: The set of implicit rules about what to do and what not to do in every context, communication, and situation (e.g., what to wear) that most children will successfully pick up through everyday interactions, without explicit instruction (Myles & Simpson, 2001).

"adapt[ation of] common practice of diagnosing to the changes in society with respect to cultural and sociologic factors" (Lauritsen, 2013, p. S37), even though the "official" terminology of pervasive developmental disorders had remained static for 14 years after its inception (Lauritsen, 2013). Perhaps, though, some of these now-common usages that reflect, for example, the community, culture, and services of Asperger's may continue, "just like the term 'high-functioning autism' (HFA) being commonly used despite the fact that it was never in the DSM" (Fung & Hardan, 2014, p. 95).

The 2013 ASD diagnosis in the *DSM-5* is also outlined by multiple diagnostic criteria, specifications, and severity levels (see Figure 2.3) (Autism Speaks, 2015). These severity levels are graded on a scale of one to three, with level one requiring support, level two requiring substantial support, and level three requiring very substantial support. Examples of how characteristics are displayed at each level for the social communication and restricted, repetitive behaviour domains are presented in Table 2.1.

Five diagnostic criteria are required for a diagnosis of ASD: (1) "persistent deficits in social communication and social interaction across multiple contexts" (Autism Speaks, 2015, para. 3), such as social-emotional reciprocity, nonverbal communication, and interpersonal relationships; (2) two indications of "restricted, repetitive patterns of behavior, interests, or activities" (ibid., para. 3), including motor movements, inflexibility, and sensory-based issues; (3) an onset early during the developmental period; (4) clinical impairment (e.g., occupational) resulting from the deficits; and (5) exclusionary considerations. Lastly, the *DSM* emphasizes that any cognitive, language, medical, genetic, or environmental factors must be indicated (Autism Speaks, 2015). It is clear that subsumed in these changes is a move to a dual-deficit model of social communication and repetitive/restricted behaviour deficits, rather than the familiar triad of characteristics (Grzadzinski, Huerta, & Lord, 2013). Another noticeable change is the lack of reference to a delay in language development (Fung & Hardan, 2014). Grzadzinski, Huerta, and Lord (2013) reference this new framework as a "dimensional approach" (p. 2), and describe it as having positive possibilities for research typologies. Interestingly, they also note the philosophical shift indicated by the change from Roman numerals (e.g., IV) to digits (e.g., 5), describing the *DSM* as now a "living document." Instead of using the Roman numeral *V* to label the fifth edition of DSM, the Arabic number *5* is used to signify that there will be updates to the *DSM-5*. Incremental updates will be identified with decimals, i.e., *DSM-5.1*, *DSM-5.2*, etc., instead of waiting for the sixth edition of the DSM to be released.

Box 2.1: ASD Diagnostic Criteria

Autism Spectrum Disorder

Diagnostic Criteria **299.00** (F84.0)

A. Persistent deficits in social communication and social interaction across multiple contexts, as manifested by the following, currently, or by history (examples are illustrative, not exhaustive):

1. Deficits in social-emotional reciprocity, ranging, for example, from abnormal social approaches to a failure of normal back-and-forth conversation; to reduced sharing of interests, emotions, or affect; to failure to initiate or respond to social interactions.
2. Deficits in nonverbal communicative behaviours used for social interaction, ranging for example from poorly integrated verbal and nonverbal communication; to abnormalities in eye contact and body language or deficits in understanding and use of gestures; to a total lack of facial expressions and nonverbal communication.
3. Deficits in developing, maintaining, and understanding relationships, ranging, for example, from difficulties adjusting behaviour to suit various social contexts; to difficulties in sharing imaginative play or in making friends; to absence of interest in peers.

Specify current severity:
Severity is based on social communication impairments and restricted, repetitive patterns of behavior.

B. Restricted, repetitive patterns of behaviour, interests, or activities, as manifested by at least two of the following, currently or by history (examples are illustrative, not exhaustive):

1. Stereotyped or repetitive motor movements, use of objects, or speech (e.g., simple motor stereotypies, lining up toys or flipping objects, echolalia, idiosyncratic phrases).
2. Insistence on sameness, inflexible adherence to routines, or ritualized patterns for verbal or nonverbal behaviour (e.g., extreme distress at small changes, difficulties with transitions, rigid thinking patterns, greeting rituals, need to take same route or eat same food every day).

3. Highly restricted, fixated interests that are abnormal in intensity or focus (e.g., strong attachment to or preoccupation with unusual objects, excessively circumscribed or perseverative interests).
4. Hyper- or hyporeactivity to sensory input or unusual interest in sensory aspects of the environment (e.g., apparent indifference to pain/temperature, adverse response to specific sounds or textures, excessive smelling or touching of objects, visual fascination with lights or movement)

Specify current severity:
Severity is based on social communication impairments and restricted, repetitive patterns of behaviour.

C. Symptoms must be present in the early developmental period (but may not become fully manifest until social demands exceed limited capacities, or may be masked by learned strategies in later life).

D. Symptoms cause clinically significant impairment in social, occupational, or other important areas of current functioning.

E. These disturbances are not better explained by intellectual disability (intellectual developmental disorder) or global developmental delay. Intellectual disability and autism spectrum disorder frequently co-occur; to make comorbid diagnosis of autism spectrum disorder and intellectual disability, social communication should be below that expected for general developmental level.

Note: Individuals with a well-established DSM-IV diagnosis of autistic disorder, Asperger's disorder, or pervasive developmental disorder not otherwise specified should be given the diagnosis of autism spectrum disorder. Individuals who have marked deficits in social communication, but whose symptoms do not otherwise meet criteria for autism spectrum disorder, should be evaluated for social (pragmatic) communication disorder.

Specify if:
With or without accompanying intellectual impairment
With or without accompanying language impairment
Associated with a known medical or genetic condition or environmental factor (Coding note: use additional code to identify the associated medical or genetic condition)

With catatonia (refer to the criteria for catatonia associated with another mental disorder, pp. 119-120, for definition) (Coding note: Use additional code, 293.89 [F06.1] catatonia associated with autism spectrum disorder to indicate the presence of the comorbid catatonia).

Source: American Psychiatric Association, 2013, pp. 50–51.

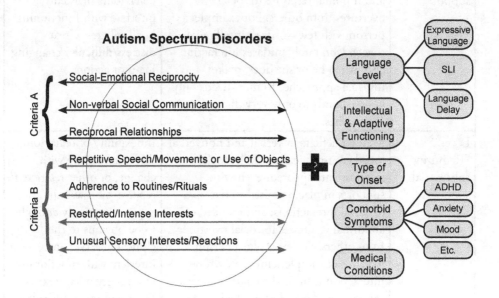

Figure 2.4: Characterization of ASD
Source: Grzadzinski, Huerta, & Lord, 2013, p. 3.

Read about it. Think about it. Write about it.

How do you think the *DSM-5*'s definition of ASD will change the field or services for those with ASD?

According to Lauritsen (2013), these changes had been "widely anticipated" (p. S37), in part due to the frustrating lack of clarity that plagues classification systems in psychiatry, as well as the diagnostic processes families endured (Fung & Hardan, 2014; Grzadzinski, Huerta, & Lord, 2013; Lord et al., 2012; Tsai & Ghaziuddin, 2013). However, it remains to be seen what the final outcomes

Table 2.1: Severity Levels for ASD in the *DSM-5*

Severity level	Social communication	Restricted, repetitive behaviours
Level 3 "Requiring very substantial support"	Severe deficits in verbal and nonverbal social communication skills cause severe impairments in functioning, very limited initiation of social interactions, and minimal response to social overtures from others. For example, a person with few words of intelligible speech who rarely initiates interaction and, when he or she does, makes unusual approaches to meet needs only and responds to only very direct social approaches.	Inflexibility of behaviour, extreme difficulty coping with change, or other restricted/repetitive behaviours markedly interfere with functioning in all spheres. Great distress/difficulty changing focus or action.
Level 2 "Requiring substantial support"	Marked deficits in verbal and nonverbal social communication skills; social impairments apparent even with supports in place; limited initiation of social interactions; and reduced or abnormal responses to social overtures from others. For example, a person who speaks simple sentences, whose interaction is limited to narrow special interests, and who has markedly odd nonverbal communication.	Inflexibility of behaviour, difficulty coping with change, or other restricted/repetitive behaviours appear frequently enough to be obvious to the clinical observer and interfere with functioning in a variety of contexts. Distress and/or difficulty changing focus or action.
Level 1 "Requiring support"	Without supports in place, deficits in social communication cause noticeable impairments. Difficulty initializing social interactions, and clear examples of atypical or unsuccessful responses to social overtures of others. May appear to have decreased interest in social interactions. For example, a person who is able to speak in full sentences and engages in communication but whose to-and-fro conversation with others fails, and whose attempts to make friends are odd and typically unsuccessful.	Inflexibility of behaviour causes significant interference with functioning in one or more contexts. Difficulty switching between activities. Problems of organization and planning hamper independence.

Source: American Psychiatric Association, 2013, p. 52.

of this dramatic—yet fully rationalized—change might be. For example, "there is a real risk that eliminating the subtypes of PDDs and creating a single ASD will have an impact on services and may actually result in some patients being denied services" (Tsai & Ghaziuddin, 2013, p. 327). Such investigations are already underway, although the new diagnostic criteria for ASD does include a comment that those with some previous diagnoses (e.g., Asperger's disorder, PDD—NOS, autistic disorder) should be rediagnosed with ASD, with the exception of those who do not meet criteria (Autism Speaks, 2015). In these cases, an examination of either the heightened restrictiveness (Fung & Hardan, 2014) or the inclusivity of "the new" ASD is needed. Taheri, Perry, and Factor (2014), for example, completed an Ontario-based file review and found that many of the 22 previously diagnosed participants would not meet *DSM-5* criteria, with a bias toward excluding those with PDD—NOS diagnoses and/ or higher cognitive scores. They conclude with some important considerations for the future:

> *People with disabilities:* The rules are changing about how professionals make a diagnosis of an autism spectrum disorder. This might mean people's diagnosis could change or maybe they won't have a diagnosis at all. This might be bad if it makes people lose the help they get because of having a certain diagnosis, but we're not sure exactly what will happen. *Professionals:* Diagnosis requires information from a variety of sources, and a comprehensive assessment process. Clinical judgment will be required with respect to using the *DSM-5* ASD criteria as part of a comprehensive assessment, especially for individuals who are higher functioning. *Policymakers:* Caution is needed with respect to using the *DSM-5* ASD criteria in isolation to determine funding or eligibility for services rather than individual need. (Taheri, Perry, & Factor, 2014, p. 120)

DIAGNOSTIC PATHWAY IN THE PROVINCE OF ONTARIO

Typical diagnostic pathways vary by diagnostician, by region, and over time; however, both typical practice and best practice do exist. In Ontario, the Ministry of Children and Youth Services (2011) has set out ASD diagnosis and treatment in an accessible, online format. It includes the following descriptions and expectations in this complex process:

- Observation-based
- Reliance on *DSM*
- Use of assessment tools

In Ontario, a range of professionals in varied roles can diagnose: psychologists or psychological associates, psychiatrists, pediatricians, or family physicians. Although diagnosis can and does happen in any geographic area—either rural or urban—some diagnostic and research centres are provincially, nationally, and internationally recognized, such as McMaster Children's Hospital and the Offord Centre for Child Studies in Hamilton, the Child and Parent Resource Institute and its ASD Clinic in London, and Toronto's Hospital for Sick Children (also known as Sick Kids). Additionally, many universities in the province are carrying out strong research programs related to ASD, such as ASD Studies at Queen's University in Kingston and the Kilee Patchell-Evans Autism Research Group and the Autism Centre of Excellence, both at Western University in London. ASD assessment, in general and according to the Ontario Ministry of Children and Youth Services, is focused on "observation of a child's communication, behavioural, and developmental levels. ASD is not diagnosed based on a single factor or symptom. Rather it is diagnosed after a confirmation of: specific behaviours, communication delays, [and] developmental disabilities" (Ontario Ministry of Children and Youth Services, 2011, para. 1). However, the assessment pathway and process vary according to the practices of local jurisdictions (see Boxes 2.2 and 2.3). At the Child and Parent Resource Institute's ASD Clinic, for example, intake is done through a screening clinic that asks parents a series of questions and passes this information on to the ASD team, which considers the appropriateness of the referral for assessment. The assessment then involves multiple observations and onsite clinical assessments, and may also include school visits (C. Hebert, personal communication, January 8, 2015). Observations focused on the items noted on the Diagnostic Observation template (see Figure 2.5).

Incontinence Supplies Grant Program: Easter Seals Ontario runs an Incontinence Supplies Grant Program for children three and older who have long-term developmental or physical disabilities and need financial support to purchase diapers.

Disability Tax Credit: The disability tax credit is described by the Canada Revenue Agency (2015) as "a non-refundable tax credit used to reduce income tax payable on the income tax and benefit return [for a] person with a severe and prolonged impairment in physical or mental functions" (para. 1).

Diagnostic Observation

Name: _____ **Date:** _____

Location: _____
Use these questions as a guide for observing the child/adolescent and your description of the child/adolescent. The description should be in narrative form rather than "yes" and "no" responses. Wherever possible, use examples.

Section	Observation Notes
(A) Free Play: *Does the child…* Spontaneously seek engagement with others (children or adults)? How does he/she do this? Does it involve joint reference to objects, such as giving and showing objects, or is limited to seeking affection or help? Play by themselves or with others (children or adults)? How does he/she play? -engage in pretend situations? -use imagination, either alone or with others? Remain with the activity for an age-appropriate/developmentally appropriate amount of time, or jump from activity to activity more quickly than expected? Become fixated on any one activity (engage in one activity when change would be expected)? Change activities willingly when asked? Engage in any repetitive motor movements?	

Figure 2.5: Diagnostic Observation Form
Source: Child and Parent Resource Institute.

Section	Observation Notes
(B) Response to Name *Call the child's name when he/she is not looking at you. Each time the child does not respond, call out his/her name slightly louder. Note if and how he/she responds. If there is no response, ask an adult who is familiar with the child to do the same. Repeat several times throughout the observation.* Does the child respond to you? Does the child respond to a familiar adult? Did you have to call his/her name several times before receiving a response? How did he/she respond (turn his/her head, make eye contact, etc.)?	
(C1) Communication General: How does the child communicate with adults? How does the child communicate with other children? Does the child use facial expression to communicate, or does facial expression remain the same regardless of the situation?	
(C2) Communication Speech: Does the child speak or use speech sounds to communicate? How much of the child's speech is directed toward others, as opposed to saying words to him/herself but not for the purpose of communicating with someone else?	

Figure 2.5: Diagnostic Observation Form (continued)

Section	Observation Notes
How long are his/her utterances (words or phrases)? In what situations does the child speak with others? Is it to get help, or for social reasons? Does his/her voice sound flat or monotonic? Is there anything unusual about his/her intonation?	
*If the child is nonverbal, bypass section C3.	
(C3) Communication Unusual or Idiosyncratic Speech: *Does the child…* Use "you" or "he/she" or his/her own name instead of "I"? Have immediate echolalia? Use rehearsed/learned speech, even if it is used in the appropriate situation? Use more repetitive speech than what would be expected for his/her developmental level?	
Pointing *During your observation, make sure there is opportunity for child to point. Ask where something is and see if he/she responds by pointing.* Does the child point to objects or people… Out of reach, or only within arm's length?	

Figure 2.5: Diagnostic Observation Form (continued)

Section	Observation Notes
With his/her index finger, or with open hand? To request something of interest or to tell someone else about something?	
Other Gestures *Gestures must have a communicative purpose and must not involve the use of other people's body parts.* Does the child use any other gestures to communicate? If he/she does, are these gestures used to describe something, such as the size of an object? Does the child use these gestures (besides pointing) to display his/her emotions? Would the child wave goodbye in response to someone waving goodbye, or does he/she need to be prompted?	
Use of Another Person's Body to Communicate Does the child take someone else's hand and lead him/her to another place? Does the child... Use his/her hand to place someone else's hand (or other part of his/her body) on an object? Move someone else's hand while the other person is holding an object to get him/her to do something with the object? Move someone else's hand to get him/her to point to something?	

Figure 2.5: Diagnostic Observation Form (continued)

Section	Observation Notes
Eye Contact *Observe the child for appropriate, socially modulated, and flexible eye contact. If the child seems shy or anxious initially but his/ her eye contact changes significantly as he/ she warms up or becomes more comfortable, use this more comfortable eye contact as the basis for description. If his/her eye contact is abnormal, note this regardless of whether it seems to be due to shyness or inattention. If it seems to be reduced due to either of these factors, make note of that as well.* Is there anything unusual about the child's eye contact? For example, is it much less than what would be expected, or look more like "staring"? In what situations does the child use eye contact? Do they use eye contact when... Someone is speaking to him/her? He/she is speaking to someone? He/she is giving something to someone or requesting help from another person?	

Figure 2.5: Diagnostic Observation Form (continued)

Special Services at Home: Special Services at Home "helps families who are caring for a child with a developmental or physical disability. It is funded and managed by the Ministry of Community and Social Services" (Ontario Ministry of Children and Youth Services, 2013, para. 1). SSAH provides families with extra funding for respite or skills building, with the amount of funding dependent on each family's situation and individual application.

Box 2.2: Lenore and Quinn

"I call it 'the day he disappeared,'" recalls Lenore, with strong emotion as she recalls this still-recent event in the life of her almost-four-year-old son, Quinn. "I could see from photos that he was a totally different kid. He went from 10 to 20 words, and those disappeared. His demeanour, his eye contact, his giggling: it all disappeared."

When Lenore and her husband took Quinn to the pediatrician for a consult around 20 months, "our pediatrician said we were just used to a more advanced child—his older sister. Or, he was being just lazy. Or, we were talking for him, and he was regressing. But we knew he was truly different. He lost his back-and-forth play. He zoned out; he wouldn't listen to commands; he wouldn't answer to his name. Before, he would do this, even when he was small. Yet, we were told repeatedly that he was fine, he would 'come along' and to 'let him be.'" After their naturopath saw some red flags, they returned for a two-year appointment, still concerned about Quinn's speech development. "Quinn was checked over again and we were told he seemed healthy." The pediatrician assumed that his speech issues were behavioural in nature and did not refer him to a specialist.

At this point, Lenore took matters into her own hands, and arranged an assessment through occupational therapy, but Quinn was not deemed eligible. She was put on a waiting list for a development assessment by local behavioural services. She successfully sought out the local children's centre for individual sessions with the speech-language pathologist, where some of her concerns were validated when she was told there were "signs of autism." "But our pediatrician still scolded us, and told us that of course the children's centre would look for 'signs of autism,' and again tried to assure us that all was well, and that no referrals were necessary, even though the children's centre wanted Quinn assessed for autism." Again Lenore went her own way. Highly anxious over this lagging potential diagnosis, she went to her family doctor, who immediately agreed to a referral. During the six-month wait for this next step in solving the mystery of Quinn, their child care centre's resource teacher also joined the voices expressing worry over his development, using the same language that Lenore did: saying that Quinn was a "different child." With Quinn's growing team accepting that a diagnosis was simply a formality, Quinn was admitted into a specialized, multidisciplinary program, and an assessment and diagnosis did indeed come from the children's centre only a short while later (at three and a half years of age), along with wait lists for IBI (four years), ABA (two years), and respite (one and a half years). Applications for Special Services and the incontinence grant quickly followed, while other processes were just beginning, such as an application for the Child Disability Credit.

Post-diagnosis, Lenore found, "the people, the therapists that we met, once they were able to open the doors to get help, the help was huge. It was so nice knowing that there were people who understood, who were willing to help, and who didn't tell you that you were crazy. Although I was teary about the diagnosis of autism, it was also a relief. Once we had the confirmation, we knew, and we could move forward. Our hands didn't feel tied anymore.

"The waiting, though," she reflected, "was horrific. That's why I started as soon I could. The waiting makes it worse—an extra stress. The assessment process itself was daunting and seemed, often, to reiterate what I shared. Even though it's clinical, it felt foreign—these people didn't even know how he is every day, *who* he is."

What haunts her still is that question: *What if I had listened to that first doctor?* It is essential, she emphasizes, to simply "know your kid. The more information you have, the more equipped you are. Know where to find it, how you can access it, and how you become aware of it. It's overwhelming, but trust your gut. Fight for what you need. Surround yourself with those who can support you, who will be realistic but supportive. Find other families who have gone through it: everyone's needs are different, but it draws you together. It's *huge*. He is a kid, first and foremost—like everyone else."

Box 2.3: Anika and Nolan

When Anika O'Connor, a mother in southern Ontario, went to her regular 18-month checkup with her husband Patrick and their 18-month-old son, Nolan, their physician didn't hold back: almost immediately, he asked if there was "something wrong" with their young son, or if she and her husband had noticed "anything odd." The doctor continued: he called Nolan's name but received no response; he asked if Nolan was talking. This was the first of many of Anika's "Aha!" moments in the next four months. Though Anika and Patrick had indeed noticed some issues, they were able to ignore most of them and convince themselves that he was fine and "just slow," encouraged by well-meaning friends with comforting platitudes such as, "Don't compare your children." When prompted to think in-depth about his development, they recalled that he had been talking—a bit—at his 12-month appointment, but had stopped. He was not blowing kisses. He was, however, affectionate and cuddly, and didn't mind eye contact. They wrote themselves a "laundry list" of reasons that he was fine, such as the development of some word approximations in the coming weeks. But it turns out that he was, indeed, quite different in development than his gifted older sister, who was close in age. These differences were underscored by this visit to the doctor, who recorded a query of "PDD?" in his notes, they later discovered.

What happened next? Anika was told to take Nolan to get his hearing tested—and it was normal. He was put on a waiting list for services with speech-language pathology. He also went on a waiting list for further assessment at the local children's centre—and Anika found out how difficult it was to obtain access to the fragmented local services. When the speech-language pathologist met with Nolan, Anika was told the assessment would take 20 minutes—but it was over an hour and a half. Though the pathologist could not diagnose, she did express her concerns, and was the first to use the word *autism*. Anika left the children's centre and vomited outside, shaken by both physical and emotional reactions to "that word." To her, it meant "worst-case scenario behaviours" and self-injurious children.

The next step was yet another referral, for that ominous "*a*-word" diagnosis, which came readily—even surprisingly—within four months. The process had its odd moments, such as the pediatrician elbowing Nolan to see his reaction. They were asked to complete standardized assessments as well. Then came their second "Aha!" moment. No further denial was possible. Anika and her husband realized this as-yet-unconfirmed diagnosis was probably correct, and likely quite severe. It only took two appointments to confirm autism. "The best part," Anika reflected, "was the pediatrician allowing *us* to go through the assessment and come to conclusions. We had already processed this conclusion by the time he confirmed it." The worst part was the questions about IQ. Anika recalls, "I did not like these; I would not answer them. Who would know this? How do you tell? This memory still hurts."

Unlike the experiences of other families, the diagnostic process was fast, and no fighting was necessary. "It fell on our laps," said Anika. "We were fortunate that our family doctor was astute, even with almost no experience in the field." However, getting services was another story: "He was on the IBI wait list for 17 months." She continued with her poignant memories of these now long-past days: "A diagnosis is like a precipice—a very scary thing. I looked for everything online. I made a list for the doctor, who went through everything with me. And it came down to IBI (we couldn't afford private), and the gluten-free, casein-free diet.

"My biggest piece of advice is that we did everything so quickly. Crying and cookies were both key. I was a stay-at-home mom, and I made it my mission to be sure that Nolan was not forgotten. I would call the centre daily, and pop in with cookies for the staff. I went to every parent-training course to avoid that awful feeling of impotence where you feel you can't help your child." Her advice for other parents? "Any financial sacrifices you make are paid back ten-fold. It helps the siblings of your child: everything is planned around that one child, it's the whole family, everyone benefits, and it changes the quality of life for everyone. As daunting and as overwhelming as it is, really look at it as your full-time job." Though Anika says she once mourned for the child she thought she would have, she never blamed herself for one second, and she continued to love, honour, value, and treasure her now 10-year-old son, who came to be a poster child and video model for other families and many students in the ASD field. As her copy of *More Than Words* (Sussman, 1999) became a dog-eared bible for helping her son, all these years later, her "head is still sore from the advocate hat," Anika laughingly explained. However, she won't have time to rest that hat or that head. She is continuing her education with a post-graduate diploma, and plans to continue to take an active role in the field as a full-time front-line worker, supporting children with ASD, as her son was—and still is—supported by the professionals around him.

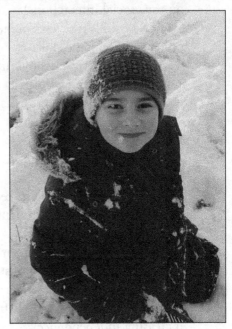

Figure 2.6: Anika's Son, Diagnosed with ASD Before Age Two

Box 2.4: Applied Behaviour Analysis (ABA)

Definition: ABA is a broad field of intervention using scientific principles of learning and behaviour to effect change by increasing desirable skills and decreasing undesirable behaviours. ABA has been proven effective with people of all ages. It is based on analysis of individual behaviours, the use of specific reinforcers, regular assessment of progress, and program modification as required, supported by collected data.

ABA includes:
- **Identifying and selecting** target behaviours you would like to see change.

- **Identifying** possible causes of the behaviour.
- **Guiding** the selection of an appropriate behavioural approach.
- **Evaluating** the outcome after implementation (Martin and Pear, 2007).

ABA in Ontario schools is used to:
- **Develop** positive behaviours (e.g., improve the ability to stay on task, improve social interactions).
- **Teach** new skills (i.e., comprehensive skills, including language, social, motor and academic skills).
- **Transfer** a positive behaviour or response from one situation to another (e.g., from completing assignments in a self-contained class to maintaining the same performance in an inclusive class).

ABA programs are:
- **Individualized**: The programs include a specific profile of strengths and needs.
- **Use positive reinforcement techniques**: These have a demonstrated motivating effect for the student and can be incorporated into academic and social routines.
- **Based on collected data**: The programs are analyzed on an ongoing basis to measure the acquisition of skills and identify new ones to be taught.
- **Emphasize generalization** or transfer of skills: Students should be taught how to transfer skills from one context or setting to another, increasing independence.

Source: McMaster Children's Hospital ASD School Support Program, n.d.

Read about it. Think about it. Write about it.

How will knowing the diagnostic pathway help you to better support the family of a child with ASD? Explain, using the above parent stories—or one of your own.

ONTARIO'S CLINICAL ASD SERVICES, SUPPORTS, AND ISSUES: AN OVERVIEW

In 2013, the annual Auditor General's report (Office of the Auditor General, 2013), one source of provincial information, included an updated audit of

"Autism Services and Supports for Children" in order to "assess whether the Ministry has adequate procedures in place to manage a system of cost-effective autism services" (p. 53). This lengthy and detailed explanation of provincial ASD-related supports and services reported the provincial prevalence of ASD as on an "upward trend" (p. 52), with a regional prevalence of 1 in 77, and underscored the multi-sectorial organizations supporting this population (e.g., the Ministry of Education). However, it focused on those services provided through the Ministry of Children and Youth Services (e.g., intensive behaviour intervention [IBI] and applied behaviour analysis [ABA]). As previously noted, this ministry funds and provides services for children and youth with ASD (and their families) through hospitals and community agencies, even though these provisions are neither legislated nor supported by the provincial health care plan (the Ontario Health Insurance Plan). Fiscally, the funding is significant: a reported $182 million in 2012/13, which represents a quadrupling over 10 years. Even so, "there are more children with autism waiting for government-funded services than there are children receiving them" (Office of the Auditor General, 2013, p. 57). A range of important observations calls attention to issues with:

- Earlier diagnosis and intervention
- Provision of IBI to children with "milder forms" of ASD (Office of the Auditor General, 2013, p. 57)
- Inconsistent fulfillment of all approved intervention hours
- Unbalanced wait lists and uneven duration of service provision
- Incorporation of ABA strategies in school-based services
- Lack of comprehensive provincial and national ASD action plans

The Autism Parent Kit describes nine types of provincial services for children and youth diagnosed with ASD and their families (see chapter 10).

Box 2.4: Ontario Autism Programs

The Ministry of Children and Youth Services (MCYS) provides a range of services and supports for children and youth with ASD. These services provide various supports for young people to meet their needs at every stage of development, from the time of diagnosis through their school years. The programs and services the Ministry funds, provides, or does both include:

Autism Intervention Program
Applied behaviour analysis (ABA)–based services and supports
Connections for Students
School Support Program

ASD Summer Camp
March Break Camp
ASD Respite Services
Potential Programme
Transitions Supports

Source: Ontario Ministry of Children and Youth Services, n.d.

MESSAGES FROM POPULAR MEDIA

Even with the regular dissemination of evidence-based interventions, many people receive, process, and accept information about disabilities, including ASD, from popular media: television, movies, and fictional books. Currently, characters with ASD or features of ASD appear to be a popular trend in entertainment-based mass media. It is difficult not to notice what appear to be traits designed to attain and maintain interest in characters portrayed as quirky, eccentric, or offbeat. Modern pop culture is exposing our society to a whole new typology of ASD, creating a new characteristic stereotype. For example, the recent release of *The Imitation Game* (Grossman et al., 2014) no doubt leaves some audience members—especially those with a background in ASD—wondering if the brilliant, troubled, and socially awkward mathematician depicted in the film, Alan Turing, should or could be retroactively diagnosed with ASD. It only takes a few moments online to see that many others have indeed wondered, investigated, and published articles in the popular media on this very topic. On the television show *The Big Bang Theory* (Lorre & Prady, 2007), the popular character Sheldon Cooper, is similarly portrayed as a socially awkward man, but a brilliant physicist. Indeed, Sheldon's character may have finally outpaced Raymond Babbit, better known as *Rain Man* (Guber et al., 1988), as the average person's go-to reference for ASD. Only one of the two, however, is directly referenced as a person with ASD (Babbit, as an "autistic savant" [Guber et al., 1988]), despite the readily available

Neurodiversity: Neurodiversity can be described as "a concept akin to biodiversity or cultural diversity that recognizes neurological disorders as a natural human variation [advocating] to promote social support systems and spotlight the value of neurological differences, in the same vein as variations in learning styles or social tendencies like introversion and extroversion" (Public Broadcasting System, 2013).

assumptions that audiences may make or that producers may intentionally or unintentionally imply. As forward-thinking as it may first appear that moviemakers are educating mass audiences about ASD, this only-somewhat-diverse depiction of neurodiversity is developing into a pattern of extremely high-functioning adult males with features of ASD-like behaviour (e.g., social difficulties) that do not impinge on everyday functioning, such as professional success. Belcher and Maich (2014, p. 98) described this recent public perception in detail.

Journalist Maggie Furlong (2013) recently noticed the rising prevalence of characters with Asperger's disorder—a former subtype of ASD—on television shows and wondered whether this is a "new, popular character quirk, or ... a sign of society's efforts to embrace and personify a disorder that has become more and more prevalent" (para. 1). Draaisma (2009) describes many media-based portrayals of ASD as misrepresentative, even potentially harmful; however, the public appears to prefer these stereotypical, fictional examples. Similarly, Kanner and Asperger, pioneers in the field of ASD (Lyons & Fitzgerald, 2007), communicated an "essence of autism" (p. 1475). Through case examples to further clinical understanding, they explained the "'Zusammenklang' or Gestalt of the child—his voice, face, body, language, intonation, gestures, gaze, expression and diction" (p. 1475). Perhaps popular media is doing the same for the everyday viewer in a stereotypical manner. Draaisma (2009) reflects,

> There is a strange discrepancy between the research that their directors, script writers and actors put in when they make a film featuring autistic persons and the actual characters they come up with ... they all want an absolutely sincere and truthful rendition of autism; what they come up with is an autistic character with freak-like savant skills, unlike anything resembling a normal autistic person. (p. 1478)

Box 2.5: Media Perspectives and ASD
By Dr. Christina Belcher, Redeemer University College, Hamilton, ON

As technological intervention in learning and the use of media becomes more evident, it is important to think about their messages. Has media technology gone too far in presenting its own perspectives (often inaccurate) regarding personhood, available every day on television and in the movies, to young minds? For example, I can remember that after seeing *Rain Man*, a movie about an autistic man starring Dustin Hoffman (Guber et al., 1988), I thought all persons with the disorder must be brilliant, savant, and would need to be managed somewhat. We learn as much from what we see as from what informed people teach us, it seems. Since my youth, I have learned not to believe everything I see.

Clinical traits of ASD are of current interest to movie and sitcom producers. This is because media, predominantly television and the big screen, educates through stereotyping. Stereotyping provides a more interesting viewer perception than reality (Draaisma, 2009). Any social screen experience is a more appealing venue to explore the ASD personality than dry clinical diagnosis. This new mediated, albeit somewhat imaginary, Asperger's person is being very welcomed within media. Thus, media has assisted greatly in providing a different portrayal of ASD than what was previously understood. A recently released paper, *Autism Spectrum Disorder in Popular Media: Storied Reflections of Societal Views* (Belcher & Maich, 2014), further explores this topic.

In sitcoms and movies, the depiction of persons on the spectrum may be viewed as suspect—not because of what is stereotypical, but rather because of what is omitted from the *real life* of a person not represented on the big screen. While physiological and psychological profiling depicts people with ASD as having specific clinical and observable traits, the traits portrayed in popular media are largely on the savant end of the scale. And savants are rare. Media depicts ASD character types who often have multiple PhDs and brilliant decision-making skills in a crisis (e.g., TV characters such as Dr. Temperance Brennan, a socially literate yet comically inept personality in her social life, on *Bones,* and Dr. Spencer Reid, an acclaimed profiler often unable to recognize social cues, on *Criminal Minds*). Such stereotyped characters are seen as brilliant and socially awkward in a lovable way (e.g., characters depicted with Asperger-"type" traits, such as Sheldon on *The Big Bang Theory*), and shine as stars in their workplaces and heroic leaders in their field. No home life traumas are included; no problematic social situations are referred to; no medication is noted; no normal daily life is seen. In the pursuit of a truthful representation, it is essential to present a balanced view—a view that realistically presents and prepares persons with ASD for life and also notes that life is a struggle at times. As the voice of reality, media is frequently mute, neglecting to include the real-life pressures and accommodations necessary for persons on the spectrum struggling with social interactions and life skills.

In the case of ASD in popular media, the truth lies not in what is included, but in what is omitted. Is media, in its portrayal, creating not only a new venue for perception, but also new kind of person entirely? Is our humanity being reformed in media's image?

While the mass media helping to educate the public on ASD can be viewed positively, perhaps it is time to go beyond a mere mass media perspective, avoiding unrealistic depictions such as "highly skilled 'superheroes'" (Belcher & Maich,

2014, p. 103), superior savants who are "worthy of awe" (p. 104), those with "comically portrayed difficulties" (p. 104), or, on the other end of the perception spectrum, excessive "fuzziness or normalization" (p. 105) of ASD-driven difficulties as something "everyone has" to some extent. The next step is a move to an individualized, authentic, insider reality.

Read about it. Think about it. Write about it.

What has a movie, television, or book character taught you about ASD?

Self-Advocacy

Likely the most well-known advocate in the field of ASD is animal behavioural scientist, and adult with ASD, Dr. Temple Grandin. Dr. Grandin is multitalented; she is a strong visual learner and a highly prolific author in her field of animal science, as well as in the field of ASD. Not only was she named to the Colorado Women's Hall of Fame (Colorado State University, 2012) and one of *Time*'s top 100 inspirational persons (TIME Magazine, 2010), but she was also the subject of an award-winning biographical movie, in which she was played by Claire Danes (Bellows et al., 2010). However, Ontario has one of its own advocates: Carly Fleischmann. Carly Fleischmann, who was born and raised in Toronto, is a young adult and a well-known figure with a strong following locally, nationally, and internationally. In her own words, Carly exemplifies self-advocacy in her online introduction:

> My name is Carly Fleischmann and as long as I can remember I've been diagnosed with autism. I am not able to talk out of my mouth, however I have found another way to communicate by spelling on my computer. (and yes that is me typing on the computer by myself) I used to think I was the only kid with autism who communicates by spelling but last year I met a group of kids that communicate the same way. In fact some are even faster at typing then I am. Last year a story about my life was shown on ABC news, CNN and CTV here in Canada. After my story was played I kept on getting lots of emails from moms, dads, kids and people from different countries asking me all sorts of questions about autism. I think people get a lot of their information from so-called experts but I think what happens is that experts can't give an explanation to certain questions. How can you explain something you have not lived or if you don't know what

it's like to have it? If a horse is sick, you don't ask a fish what's wrong with the horse. You go right to the horse's mouth. (CarlysVoice, 2013, para. 1)

Carly—and her family members—are certainly that horse's mouth. Hailed as a hero of self-advocacy in the field of ASD and beyond, Carly demonstrates, invites, and inspires independence through advocacy, struggle, and community. She represents a growing group of adults, adolescents, and even children who are turning to online social media in a movement to not only learn about others and share their stories as persons with ASD, but also to teach and preach about ASD directly, with enthusiasm and deep self-understanding.

Carly herself utilizes social media sites such as Twitter and Facebook and blogs about her journeys in ASD, from a diagnosis of severe intellectual disability to a recognition of giftedness. Some of the essential topics Carly has delved into include her struggles in advocating for using her communication device on airplane flights, promoting the successful use of assistive technology, and demonstrating what sensory overload is like to those who have not experienced it first-hand in the interactive Carly's Café. Additionally, she and Arthur Fleishmann (her father) have penned a semi-autobiographical account of Carly's life

Self-Advocacy: In the field of ASD, self-advocacy can be referred to as a group process of struggling for needs and rights: "the emergence of autistic self-advocacy movements in several Western countries in the late 1990s ... challenged the dominating views of autism and argued for their right to speak for themselves" (Bertilsdotter Rosqvist, 2014, p. 353).

and family—which includes a twin sister, Taryn—from childhood to adolescence in *Carly's Voice: Breaking through Autism* (Fleishmann & Fleishmann, 2012). Its introductory chapter includes a reminiscence of when seven-year-old Carly went, unaccompanied and naked, from her home to the park, and her father's well-practiced response for well-meaning onlookers:

One lapse in scrutiny and here we were—Carly, in the park, naked, at dusk, alone. I felt happy to have found her, but I also felt the crush of frustration and desperation, knowing that this would not be a onetime near-catastrophe. It was just a moment in our lives. And we would have many more.... "Carly has autism." Three words must suffice to explain a tome of weird behaviours and limitations. It's shorthand for Carly-is-different-she-acts-in-odd-ways-she-loves-taking-off-her-clothes-especially-if-what-she-is-wearing-has-a-spot-of-water-on-it-she-likes-repetitive-motion-like-that-of-the-swing-she-doesn't-speak. We didn't know what Carly knew and what she was incapable of knowing. She made odd movements and sounds and covered her ears when it was noisy. She cried often. And she never, ever stopped moving. Never. (p. 4-5)

Moving from a concept of ASD based on a medical model of deficits within a disorder to a neurological *difference*—even a *culture* of neurodiversity—has certainly been initiated, encouraged, and underscored by "autistic people" (Owren, 2013, p. 32), who, they say, utilize this terminology simply as a descriptor. In other words, "many autistic self-advocates reject that their autism in itself is a disorder. They claim that, apart from differences such as race, gender and sexual orientation, people are also born with different minds" (ibid.). The movement focuses not on fixing ASD, but on accessing equal rights and freedoms afforded to all human beings with diverse characteristics, and the positive attitudes and treatment that should accompany these.

In Ontario, the most recent piece of provincial legislation addressing ASD is the Accessibility for Ontarians with Disabilities Act (AODA), a provincial act designed to remove barriers to public accessibility.

According to About the AODA (Ministry of Economic Development, Employment, & Infrastructure, 2014), the AODA has five prominent accessibility elements, from physical accessibility to service accessibility and more. These five elements are: design of public spaces; transportation; information and communication; employment; and customer service. References to a 10-year history and a timeframe to ensure full compliance by 2025 are also included.

> **Accessibility for Ontarians with Disabilities Act (AODA):** AODA is provincial legislation with two main purposes: to create regulations related to accessibility and its standards (e.g., accommodation, services), and to develop these standards with multi-sectorial involvement, including those with disabilities themselves (ServiceOntario e-laws, 2009).

Read about it. Think about it. Write about it.

How will the AODA help to shape future public service supports for those with ASD?

A LOOK BACK

Chapter 2, "A Contemporary Understanding of Autism Spectrum Disorder," focused on:

- Current definitions of ASD, in the *DSM-TR* and the *DSM-5*, and the changes to diagnostic criteria within these;
- An overview of Ontario's clinical ASD services, supports, and issues, including the typical diagnostic pathway, and intensive behavioural intervention services;
- A discussion of media-based perspectives on ASD, including what everyday mass media teaches about ASD; and
- The importance of self-advocacy, including Ontario's Carly Fleischmann.

A LOOK AHEAD

Chapter 3, "Evidence-Based Interventions," focuses on:

- An overview of evidence-based interventions (EBIs), including how to find evidence, the strength of the evidence, and comparing EBI to pseudoscience;
- The most recent project evaluating EBIs for ASD;
- An overview of the established treatments, promising/emerging treatments, and unsupported/unestablished treatments for ASD; and
- Brief overviews of each intervention with some support (promising/emerging treatments), based on the most recent review of EBIs for ASD.

ADDITIONAL RESOURCES

- About the Ontarians with Disabilities Act (Ministry of Economic Development, Employment, & Infrastructure, 2014): www.mcss.gov.on.ca/en/mcss/programs/accessibility/understanding_accessibility/aoda.aspx
- ASD in the *DSM-5* (Autism Speaks, 2015): www.autismspeaks.org/what-autism/diagnosis/dsm-5-diagnostic-criteria
- ASD Studies @ Queen's University: www.queensu.ca/psychology/ASDLab/ASDHome.html
- Autism Centre of Excellence (Western University): www.autism.uwo.ca/resources.html
- Autism Spectrum Disorder Canadian-American Research Consortium: www.autismresearch.ca/
- Autism Spectrum Disorder Clinic (Child & Parent Resource Institute): www.cpri.ca/content/page.aspx?section=25

- Carly Fleischmann (ABC News, 2008):
  abcnews.go.com/Health/story?id=4311223
- Carly's Café:
  www.carlyscafe.com
- Disability Tax Credit (Canada Revenue Agency, 2015):
  www.cra-arc.gc.ca/tx/ndvdls/sgmnts/dsblts/dtc/menu-eng.html
- Incontinence Supplies Grant Program (Easter Seals Ontario):
  www.easterseals.org/services/incontinence-supplies-grant/
- Offord Centre for Child Studies:
  offordcentre.com
- Ontarians with Disabilities Act (ServiceOntario e-laws, 2009):
  www.e-laws.gov.on.ca/html/statutes/english/elaws_statutes_05a11_e.htm
- Special Services at Home (Ministry of Social and Community Services):
  www.children.gov.on.ca/htdocs/English/topics/specialneeds/specialservices/
  index.aspx
- Temple Grandin (Colorado State University):
  www.colostate.edu/templegrandin
- The Kilee Patchell-Evans Autism Research Group (Western University):
  www.queensu.ca/psychology/ASDLab/ASDHome.html

REFERENCES

American Psychiatric Association. (2013). *Diagnostic and statistical manual: DSM-5* (5th ed.). Washington, DC: Author.

American Psychological Association. (2000). *Diagnostic and statistical manual of psychiatric disorders: Text revision* (4th ed.). Arlington, VA: American Psychiatric Publishing.

Autism Speaks. (2015). DSM-5 diagnostic criteria. Retrieved from www.autismspeaks.org/what-autism/diagnosis/dsm-5-diagnostic-criteria

Belcher, C., & Maich, K. (2014). Autism Spectrum Disorder in popular media: Storied reflections of societal views. *Brock Education: A Journal of Educational Research and Practice, 23*(2), 1–19. Retrieved from brock.scholarsportal.info/journals/brocked/home/article/view/311. doi:10.1177/1088357609356094

Bellows, G., Di Loreto, D., Edwards, A., Ferguson, S., Lister, P., Owen, A., Saines, E. G., Spence, G. (Producers), & Jackson, M. (Director). (2010). *Temple Grandin* (Motion picture). United States: HBO.

Bertilsdotter Rosqvist, H. (2014). Becoming an "autistic couple": Narratives of sexuality and couplehood within the Swedish autistic self-advocacy movement. *Sexuality and Disability, 32*(3), 351–363. doi:10.1007/s11195-013-9336-2

CarlysVoice. (2013). Carly's voice: Changing the world of autism. Retrieved from carlysvoice.com/home/aboutcarly

Coello-Bannon, G., & Messer, E. (Producers). (2005). Criminal minds (Television series). Los Angeles: CBS.

Colorado State University. (2012). Grandin, Temple. Retrieved from http://ansci.agsci.colostate.edu/grandin-temple/

Draaisma, D. (2009). Stereotypes of autism. *Philosophical Transactions of the Royal Society of Biological Sciences, 364*, 1475–1480. doi:10.1098/rstb.2008.0324

Falkmer, T., Anderson, K., Falkmer, M., & Horlin, C. (2013). Diagnostic procedures in Autism Spectrum Disorder: A systematic literature review. *European Child and Adolescent Psychiatry, 22*(6), 329–340. doi:10.1007/s00787-013-0375-0

Fleischmann, A., & Fleischmann, C. (2012). *Carly's voice: Breaking through autism.* Toronto, ON: Simon & Schuster.

Fung, L. K., & Hardan, A. Y. (2014). Autism in DSM-5 under the microscope: Implications to patients, families, clinicians, and researchers. *Asian Journal of Psychiatry, 11,* 93–97. doi:10.1016/j.ajp.2014.08.010

Furlong, M. (2013, July 10). The latest trend on TV: Characters with Asperger's. *Huffington Post.* Retrieved from www.huffingtonpost.com/maggie-furlong/aspergers-on-tv_b_3574336.html?ncid=edlinkusaolp00000003

Grossman, N., Heslop, P., Moore, G., Ostrowsky, I., Schwarzman, T. (Producers), & Tyldum, M. (Director). (2014). *The imitation game* (Motion picture). United Kingdom/United States: StudioCanal/The Weinstein Company.

Grzadzinski, R., Huerta, M., & Lord, C. (2013). DSM-5 and Autism Spectrum Disorder (ASDs): An opportunity for identifying ASD subtypes. *Molecular Autism, 4*(1), 1-6. doi:10.1186/2040-2392-4-12

Guber, P., Johnson, M., McGiffert, D., Molen, G. R., Mutrux, G., Peters, J. (Producers) & Levinson, B. *Rain man.* United States: United Artists.

Hall, L. J. (2013). *Autism Spectrum Disorder: From theory to practice* (2nd ed.). Upper Saddle River, NJ: Pearson.

Hartley, S. L., & Sikora, D. M. (2010). Detecting autism spectrum disorder in children with intellectual disability: Which DSM-IV-TR criteria are most useful? *Focus on Autism and Other Developmental Disabilities, 25*(2), 85–97.

Josephson, B., & Reich, K. (2005). *Bones* (Television series). Los Angeles: Fox.

Lauritsen, M. (2013). Autism Spectrum Disorder. *European Child and Adolescent Psychiatry, 22*(Supplementary 1), S37–S42. doi:10.1007/s00787-012-0359-5

Lord, C., Petkova, E., Hus, V., Gan, W., Lu, F., Martin, D. M., … & Risi, S. (2012). A multisite study of the clinical diagnosis of different Autism Spectrum Disorder. *Archives of General Psychiatry, 3,* 306.

Lorre, C., & Prady, B. (Producers). (2007). *The big bang theory* (Television series). Los Angeles, CA: CBS.

Lyons, V., & Fitzgerald, M. (2007). Asperger (1906–1980) and Kanner (1894–1981), the two pioneers of autism. *Journal of Autism and Developmental Disorders, 37*(10), 2022–2023. doi: 10.1007/s10803-007-0383-3

Martin, G., & Pear, J. (2007). *Behavior modification: What it is and how to do it.* Prentice Hall: Upper Saddle River, NJ.

McMaster Children's Hospital ASD School Support Program. (n.d.). Quick reference guide to ASD and ABA. Hamilton, ON: Author.

Ministry of Economic Development, Employment, and Infrastructure. (2014). About the accessibility for Ontarians with disabilities act. Retrieved from www.mcss.gov.on.ca

Myles, B. S., & Simpson, R. L. (2001). Understanding the hidden curriculum: An essential social skill for children and youth with Asperger syndrome. *Intervention In School and Clinic, 36*(5), 279.

Odle, T. G., Barstow, D. G., & Cataldo, L. J. (2011). *Pervasive developmental disorders.* Independence, KY: Gale, Cengage Learning.

Office of the Auditor General of Ontario. (2013). 2013 annual report, chapter 3, section 3.1: Autism services and supports for children. Retrieved from www.auditor.on.ca/en/reports_en/en13/2013ar_en_web.pdf

Ontarians with Disabilities Act. (2009, c. 32). Retrieved from www.e-laws.gov.on.ca

Ontario Ministry of Children and Youth Services. (n.d.). The autism parent resource kit. Retrieved from www.children.gov.on.ca

Ontario Ministry of Children and Youth Services. (2011). ASD diagnosis and treatment. Retrieved from www.children.gov.on.ca

Ontario Ministry of Children and Youth Services. (2013). Special services at home. Retrieved from http://www.children.gov.on.ca/htdocs/English/topics/specialneeds/specialservices/index.aspx

Owren, T. (2013). Neurodiversity: Accepting autistic difference. *Learning Disability Practice*, *16*(4), 32–37.

Public Broadcasting System. (2013). "Neurotypical" in context: Neurodiversity. Retrieved from www.pbs.org

Sussman, F. (1999). *More than words*. Austin, TX: Pro-Ed.

Taheri, A., Perry, A., & Factor, D. C. (2014). Brief report: A further examination of the DSM-5 autism spectrum disorder criteria in practice. *Journal on Developmental Disabilities*, *20*(1), 116–121.

Thames Valley Children's Centre. (2008). *Paving the way for success: A supplementary guide for educators of students with autism spectrum disorder*. London, ON: Author.

Thompson, T. (2013). Autism research and services for young children: History, progress and challenges. *Journal of Applied Research in Intellectual Disabilities*, *26*, 81–107.

TIME Magazine. (2010). The 2010 TIME 100. Retrieved from www.time.com/time/specials/packages/completelist/0,29569,1984685,00.htm

Tsai, L., & Ghaziuddin, M. (2013). DSM-5 ASD moves forward into the past. *Journal of Autism and Developmental Disorders*, *44*(2), 321–330.

Watkins, S. (n.d.). Autism in the DSM. Retrieved from www.bdkmsw.umwblogs.org

Wing, L. (1993). The definition and prevalence of autism: A review. *European Child and Adolescent Psychiatry*, *2*(1), 61. doi:10.1007/BF02098832

Woods, A. G., Mahdavi, E., & Ryan, J. P. (2013). Treating clients with Asperger's syndrome and autism. *Child and Adolescent Psychiatry & Mental Health*, *7*(1), 1–8. doi:10.1186/1753-2000-7-32.

SECTION II

INTERVENTIONS

SECTION II, INTERVENTIONS, FOCUSES ON HOW EVIDENCE-based interventions (EBIs) are chosen in the field of autism spectrum disorder (ASD), with information on how to implement EBIs with this population. Throughout the history of ASD treatment, many unsupported and sometimes harmful treatments have been implemented in an attempt to find a cure for the disorder. As a result, the field has become very reliant on the use of EBI to guide the interventions practiced with individuals with ASD. Chapter 3 begins with a review of EBIs and information on how to differentiate and find EBIs. It also reviews pseudosciences, interventions with some support, and interventions that are unestablished or harmful. The remainder of this section is broken up so that established EBIs are reviewed in a manner that provides an introductory "how-to" for practitioners. Brief reviews of the literature are provided to explain why and how each practice became evidence-based. The EBIs are broken into three categories: 1) communication-based interventions, 2) social skills interventions, and 3) behaviour-based interventions. These categories mirror the main characteristics of the disorder according to the *Diagnostic and Statistical Manual, 5th Edition (DSM-5)*. When an EBI can fit into more than one category, this is noted, and the EBI is placed in the area where the majority of research or practitioners have used it.

CHAPTER 3

EVIDENCE-BASED INTERVENTIONS

IN THIS CHAPTER:

- Definition
  - Pseudoscience
- Finding Evidence
  - Strength of Evidence
- Different Methods to Determine Whether an Intervention is Evidence-Based
  - Current Evidence-Based Interventions in ASD
  - Established Treatments (Evidence-Based)
  - Promising/Emerging Interventions with Some Support
  - Unsupported or Unestablished Interventions
- Controversy with Evidence-Based Interventions

In chapter 3, the history and context behind the development of evidence-based interventions (EBIs) in the field of autism spectrum disorder (ASD) are examined. Pseudoscience and some of the unfortunate circumstances individuals with ASD have been placed in as a result of unsubstantiated treatments in the search for a cure are highlighted. Reports that have examined the peer-reviewed literature are evaluated, with the most recent reports highlighted, listing the interventions that are considered evidence-based. Each of these evidence-based interventions is reviewed in detail in chapters 4, 5, and 6. This chapter briefly reviews the practices with some support and practices that are unestablished or harmful, but not in depth.

DEFINITION

Evidence-based intervention is a prevalent term in the field of ASD, growing in common usage over time. This is driven, in part, by the necessity for educators to develop programs for individuals with ASD using strategies supported by scientific evidence (Odom, Collet-Klingenberg, Rogers, & Hatton, 2010). In Ontario, this initiative began with the release of *Policy/Program Memorandum No. 140* (*PPM 140*) in 2007 (Ontario Ministry of Education, 2007), which states that all school boards in Ontario must provide applied behaviour analysis (ABA) programming for students with ASD, and plan for transitions for these students. *PPM 140* was issued to provide "effective, evidence-based educational practices to meet the wide range of needs of students with ASD" (Ontario Ministry of Education, 2007, para. 2). In addition, in clinical practice, Ontario's Autism Intervention Program (AIP) mandates the use of practices supported by evidence, primarily in the use of ABA and intensive behaviour intervention (IBI) (Ontario Ministry of Children and Youth Services, 2011).

Governments and other governing bodies in psychology, nursing, and social work have collectively emphasized the importance of EBIs, defined as the use of rigorous, peer-reviewed scientific research that is replicated in order to provide safe and effective interventions. The studies that have reviewed the literature on effective practices for ASD have focused on EBIs, which inform clinicians' and educators' evidence-based practices (National Autism Center, 2015). It is important to utilize EBIs so that individuals with ASD have the best chance of making positive gains in growth and development (Simpson, 2005; Odom et al., 2010). This is perhaps even more critical when families, governments, agencies, and taxpayers are funding service provision. The notion of EBI has become even more important in the field of ASD due to the increased prevalence of ASD and the history of accepting, condoning, and implementing practices that are harmful or ineffective (Simpson, 2005).

Pseudoscience

When an individual is diagnosed with ASD, his or her parents may be devastated and search for any intervention that could potentially help their son or daughter, leaving them vulnerable to ineffective or over-promising cures (Herbert, Sharp, & Gaudiano, 2002). Families can be lured into these practices with claims of a cure, with some interventions costing

Evidence-Based Interventions (EBIs): Evidence-based interventions use peer-reviewed methodologies (where journal submissions are carefully analyzed by peers in the field) that have been replicated to determine if a practice for a certain population has enough research evidence to prove it effective. It also provides practitioners with a guide to strategies shown to be effective with particular populations, to protect consumers of various treatment approaches (McNeece & Thyer, 2004; Simpson, 2005).

large sums of money, sometimes leading to ineffective or even harmful treatment. When confronted with products or treatments claiming great results in assisting individuals with ASD, Green (1996) encourages consumers to question the source, asking how such information (e.g., research results) came to be known, and understanding the basis for any given claims that arise.

In the ASD field, a significant number of treatments have arisen that would be considered pseudoscientific. Pseudoscientific treatments are interventions that claim to be backed by scientific research, but in fact lack consistent, replicated, empirical research to support them (Green, 1996; Herbert et al., 2002). Pseudoscientific treatments often: 1) make exaggerated claims that may be outside what is possible; 2) are based on anecdotal evidence rather than empirical studies; 3) use research selectively to confirm their hypotheses; 4) are based on theories that cannot be disproven; 5) are advocated by individuals who have a financial stake in such claims; and 6) tend to be promoted on popular social media (e.g., blogs) rather than in scientific journals (Herbert et al., 2002).

Other considerations that must be made when understanding the evidence for a treatment include evaluation of the subjectivity/objectivity continuum, indirect/ direct measures used, noncomparative/comparative information, and descriptive versus experimental research. Subjective information includes information that can be biased. The goal here is to be as objective as possible, using operational definitions to remove subjectivity, using pre-existing, established measures, and hiring "blinded" observers who are unaware and/or uncommitted to particular hypothesized results to take data. In addition, the evidence needs to be evaluated by multiple, direct measures. Direct measures involve measuring the changes caused by the treatment to the person involved. These differ from indirect measures, where the person or people around the treated person are asked about perceived effects; these perceptions can be influenced by biases. Comparative information about the treatment is also critical. For example, it is insufficient to state that a child with ASD improved because of a treatment, when the child may have improved over time regardless of treatment, or the change may be due to other factors. Therefore, comparative information must be obtained to understand whether the same effect will occur in different environments, for other children, and with other variables. Lastly, just because research has evaluated a given treatment does not mean that the intervention is evidence-based. There are many different types of research that have varied levels

Operational Definition: Operational definitions involve "the process of breaking down a broad concept, such as 'aggressiveness,' into its *observable* and reliably *measurable* component behaviours" (frequency of hitting or biting others, duration of scream, and so on) (Mayer, Sulzer-Azaroff, & Wallace, 2014, p. 709).

and strengths of conclusions that can be drawn. Descriptive research, for example, is also called "uncontrolled" research and often comprises detailed information that describes the behaviour, conditions, and variables in the environment (Green, 1996). Although gathering such data is a useful and foundational step in a research project, there are many confounding variables. In order to control for these, experimental or controlled research is more rigorous and removes the chances that other variables may contribute to an area of interest. See Figure 3.1 to understand how evidence is ranked in terms of ambiguity when evaluating treatments. The EBI movement represents an effort to protect those with ASD—and their families—by ensuring that any treatments implemented are evidence-based. See Box 3.1 for an example of how a pseudoscience-based treatment has negatively affected children with ASD.

Confounding Variables: Confounding variables (e.g., a child beginning a new medication) include aspects in a research study that may contribute to the effects seen in the results, other than the intervention itself. A reduction in the number and effect of any such variables to ensure that the intervention caused, for example, a change in behaviour, is an important research goal.

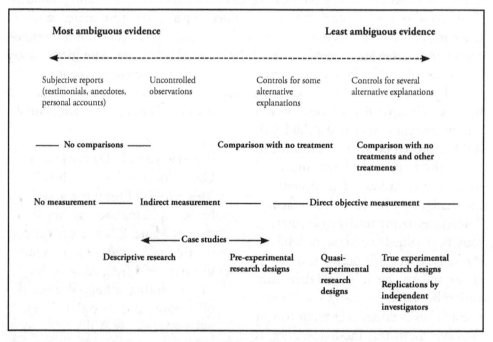

Figure 3.1: Types of Evidence about Treatment Effects
Source: Green, 1996.

Box 3.1: Chelation Therapy

A five-year-old boy, Abubakar Tariq Nadama, died August 23, 2005, after receiving intravenous chelation therapy in his doctor's office (Kane & Linn, 2005). Abubakar's family had moved from Britain to Pennsylvania to receive the treatment, touted as a cure for ASD. He had already received two treatments, but on his third, he went into cardiac arrest. He was receiving ethylenediaminetetraacetic acid (EDTA), approved by the United States Food and Drug Administration for the treatment of lead poisoning when blood tests have confirmed heavy metal poisoning (Baxter & Krenzelok, 2008; Kane & Linn, 2005). In Abubakar's case, his physician confirmed his lead levels with only a urine test, and on this basis, some have criticized the doctor for lack of care. Dr. Roy Eugene Kerry, who was an ear, nose, and throat specialist, was known in the ASD community for administering chelation therapy to children with ASD (Kane & Linn, 2005). The drug was given to the child intravenously rather than through the more common methods of pills or creams; some believe that the intravenous method decreases lead in the system more quickly (Kane & Linn, 2005). Resuscitation efforts were not successful (Baxter & Krenzelok, 2008). It was later found that Abubakar died because too much calcium was removed from his body, resulting in a heart attack (Kane, 2007).

The EDTA treatment Abubakar received included a drug called edetate disodium, which is also typically prescribed for patients diagnosed with lead poisoning (Baxter & Krenzelok, 2008). This treatment was intended to remove metals and lead from his body—thought by some in the ASD community to be the cause of ASD. Some believe that the mercury preservative used in childhood vaccines is also a cause of ASD (Baxter & Krenzelok, 2008). Therefore, the theory is that removing these heavy metals from the body will result in a decrease in symptoms and behaviours of ASD (Baxter & Krenzelok, 2008). However, there is no evidence to support this treatment in individuals with ASD, and research published to support the claim that mercury in vaccines caused autism was retracted by the journals due to falsified data (Baxter & Krenzelok, 2008).

It was later found that the wrong chemical was being used in Abubakar's treatment. The recommended form of EDTA uses edetate calcium disodium, but instead, the physician used only edetate disodium EDTA (Baxter & Krenzelok, 2008). In addition, the intravenous was administered quickly, over a number of minutes rather than via a drip over multiple hours (Kane, 2007). Dr. Kerry said that this was because he didn't think the child could remain calm for such an extended period of time (Kane, 2007). Dr. Kerry's license to practice medicine was suspended for three years in 2009 after the medical review board found that he used the wrong chelation drug, at the wrong speed for administration, for a treatment that had no supporting evidence related to ASD (Barrett, 2010). His license was reinstated in 2013, although he is barred from treating minors with chelation therapy.

> **Read about it. Think about it. Write about it.**
>
> Brainstorm or research other instances of pseudoscience that you have heard about in the popular media.

FINDING EVIDENCE

Because EBI has become a popular buzzword in the field of ASD, caution must be taken to understand what is an appropriate EBI. Too often practitioners, educators, sales representatives, and students overgeneralize the term and presume that one scientific article in a peer-reviewed journal constitutes an EBI. However, this is incorrect. Establishing an intervention as evidence-based involves reviewing outcomes from scientific, peer-reviewed journals that have been replicated numerous times by different authors. In some instances, poorly designed studies are published in order to inspire researchers to design better-controlled research studies (National Autism Center [NAC], 2009). If a study that has a poor design is published, this may mean that there are other variables causing the positive effect demonstrated in the study. Therefore, it is difficult to conclude if it was the treatment or the other confounding variables that caused the change in the intervention.

Often an intervention or a comprehensive treatment model (CTM) will not be considered evidence-based because the founders of the approach are the only researchers who have conducted research on it (Wong et al., 2014). It is necessary for multiple research groups to conduct similar studies and receive positive results. Comprehensive treatment models differ from focused intervention packages (FIPs) in that CTMs are composed of a number of practices used to address a broad range of skills and deficits typical of ASD, whereas FIPs are single practices that aim to address one skill area of an individual with ASD (Wong et al., 2014). FIPs are usually shorter in duration than CTMs and are often "considered the building blocks of educational programs for children and youth with ASD" (Wong et al., 2014, p. 3). CTMs are often excluded from some reviews of what constitutes an EBI; therefore, it is important to examine critically whether

Comprehensive Treatment Model: Comprehensive treatment models include "a set of practices designed to achieve a broad learning or developmental impact on the core deficits of ASD" (Wong et al., 2014, p. 3).

a CTM is made up of multiple FIPs that are evidence-based. Researchers also examine whether treatment approaches in combination are effective, such as early intensive behaviour intervention (EIBI), which uses various ABA skills in an intensive format for a minimum of 20 hours per week (Reichow & Wolery, 2009).

> **Focused Intervention Packages:** Focused intervention packages are treatments that focus on a single skill or a targeted goal of an individual with ASD. "These practices are operationally defined, address specific learner outcomes, and tend to occur over a shorter time period than CTM" (Wong et al., 2014, p. 3).

Read about it. Think about it. Write about it.

How would you explain the need for evidence-based interventions to a parent who comes to you with a new intervention to try with his or her son or daughter, downloaded from a website, with no research to support it?

Strength of Evidence

When professionals are determining whether a practice is evidence-based, they often examine the strength of evidence using a classification system to determine if the type of evidence available is of high quality and quantity. In a review of EBIs for autism spectrum disorder, the *National Standards Project* (NAC, 2009, 2015) used three components when determining the strength of evidence: quality of the study, quantity of evidence, and consistency or reliability over time. First, the quality of the study ensures that the study's design is strong, which includes such considerations as including multiple comparison subjects, ensuring that little data is lost in the study, the type of measurement used, and ensuring that there is substantial explanation of the different conditions in order to be credible. Second, the quantity of evidence ensures that the intervention has been replicated by multiple studies from multiple authors. The more often a particular successful

> **Strength of Evidence:** Strength of evidence is found through "the quality, quantity, and consistency of research findings" to ensure that the published studies combined support the intervention in question" (NAC, 2009, p. 31).

study is replicated, the more evidence there is to support the intervention's effectiveness. Third, reviewers evaluate consistency to ensure that the treatment shows consistent findings over time, also called reliability (see the National Standards Report [NAC, 2009, 2015] for further discussion and information on this topic).

> **Reliability:** Reliability describes the consistency of a research result. It refers to achieving the same outcome after repeated measures of a construct or intervention.

DIFFERENT METHODS TO DETERMINE WHETHER AN INTERVENTION IS EVIDENCE-BASED

▷ completo/ exhaustivo.

Determining whether an intervention is evidence-based involves using individual expertise and examining literature to see if there are substantial findings to give enough merit to an intervention (Gibbs & Gambrill, 2002). However, examining the literature each time and doing a thorough and accurate review is often not feasible or realistic for many educators, clinicians, families, and other professionals. Instead, groups of researchers have collaborated and created critical reviews of the evidence, breaking down the interventions into practices that have high, some, and little evidence to support them (Gibbs & Gambrill, 2002). It is suggested that for problems seen regularly or interventions practiced frequently, practitioners should examine the literature themselves to understand the strengths and weaknesses of available interventions, including updated information that may not be included in reviews (Gibbs & Gambrill, 2002). For less commonly encountered interventions, practitioners can often rely on the pre-existing reviews of the literature (Gibbs & Gambrill, 2002).

Several large projects undertaken in recent years that have examined the literature and provided categories of evidence-supported interventions for individuals with ASD are listed in Table 3.1. Although many of the findings are similar, differences in findings can come from the varied criteria that each review committee uses to select the articles reviewed, and the standards set to classify an intervention as an EBI. For example, comprehensive treatment models were not included in the second-latest review of the literature, but may be in other reviews (Wong et al., 2014). In addition, studies may be excluded if they are medically based, do not have an educational component, don't fit within a certain age range, or include multiple diagnoses (NAC, 2009, 2015; Wong et al., 2014). Therefore, when using these pre-existing reviews, the methods that were used to conduct the review must always be considered. If an intervention was not included, it may be because this intervention was not in the scope of the project, and additional research may be required. In addition, it is important

Table 3.1: Comparison of Large-Scale Evidence-Based Intervention Literature Reviews for Treatments for Individuals with ASD

Project	Date	Age group	Focus of interventions	Articles reviewed	Purpose	Differences from other reviews	Results
National Standards Project—Phase II (NAC, 2015)	2015	0–22 years & 22+ years	2007–2012 (ages 0–22) 1987–2012 (ages 22+)	Included behavioural and educational interventions Total of 389 articles	Update the NSP—Phase I project and include adults over 22 years	Includes adults (over age 22)	0–22 years: 14 established interventions 18 emerging interventions 13 unestablished interventions 22 years +: 1 established intervention 1 emerging intervention 4 unestablished interventions
Evidence-Based Practices for Children, Youth, and Young Adults with Autism Spectrum Disorder (Wong et al., 2014)	2014	0–22 years	1990–2011	Included behavioural, developmental, and educational interventions Total of 456 articles	Broaden the research reviewed over 20 years and use a more rigorous method to evaluate the research	5 new EBIs identified: 1. Cognitive behaviour interventions 2. Exercise 3. Modelling 4. Scripting 5. Structured play groups	27 evidence-based practices 24 practices with some support

National Professional Development Centre on ASD (Odom et al., 2010)	2010	0–22 years	1997–2007	Total of 175 articles	Understand EBIs and make strategies available to consumers	Made interventions available online in modules and fact sheets	24 evidence-based practice methods
National Standards Project (NAC, 2009)	2009	0–22 years	1957–2007	Included behavioural and educational interventions Total of 775 articles	Wide scope of research examined Created a parent manual to assist parents in understanding and navigating literature for interventions	Wide scope of research examined Created a parent manual to assist parents in understanding and navigating literature for interventions	11 established treatments 22 emerging treatments 5 ineffective/harmful treatments

to examine the methodology section to understand the dates of the literature reviewed. Newer literature may not be included in the review, due to the delay created by publishing and collating results.

Current Evidence-Based Interventions in ASD

The authors of the *National Standards Project* (NAC, 2009, 2015) created a strength of evidence classification system to evaluate studies that researched interventions for individuals with ASD. Based on the strength of the interventions, they were classified into the following categories: established treatments; emerging treatments; and unestablished treatments (ineffective or harmful treatments were included in phase 1) (see Table 3.2). In general, in the field of ASD, this language has been used to classify interventions to date. However, newer projects have used different language and classification systems to present the different evidence to support each intervention.

Established Treatments (Evidence-Based)

The *National Standards Project* (NAC, 2009) defines established interventions as having "sufficient evidence ... to confidently determine that a treatment produces beneficial treatment effects for individuals on the autism spectrum" (p. 32). In a review of the literature in 2014, 27 practices were deemed established or evidence-based, whereas a review in 2015 found that 14 practices were considered established treatments (Wong et al., 2014). This is partly due to the inclusion criteria for articles set by the authors and partly because interventions are often combined into categories whereby one title encompasses a category of similar interventions. For example, ABA strategies are the most prevalent in the literature for this population, and thus are often combined in various ways between studies (NAC, 2015). The complete chart of EBIs from the 2009, 2014, and 2015 reviews (NAC, 2015; Wong et al., 2014) is provided in Table 3.3. The majority of the practices are based on the work of ABA and include primary principles such as reinforcement, extinction, and modelling, ABA assessment tools to guide interventions, such as functional behaviour assessments, and combinations of different ABA principles such as functional communication training (FCT) and picture exchange communication system (PECS) (although FCT and PECS were found to be emerging interventions in the NAC [2015] review) (Wong et al., 2014). Therefore, ABA continues to be one of the most established treatments for individuals with ASD and continues to support such directions as *PPM 140*, which directs the use of ABA strategies for individuals with ASD in Ontario schools.

Table 3.2: Strength of Evidence Classification System

Established	Emerging	Unestablished
Several[1] published, peer-reviewed articles • SMRS[2] scores of 3, 4, or 5 • Beneficial intervention effects for a specific target These may be supplemented by studies with lower scores on the Scientific Merit Rating Scale.	Few[3] published, peer-reviewed articles • SMRS scores of 2 • Beneficial intervention effects reported for one dependent variable for a specific target These may be supplemented by studies with lower scores on the Scientific Merit Rating Scale.	May or may not be based on research • Beneficial intervention effects reported based on very poorly controlled studies (scores of 0 or 1 on the Scientific Merit Rating Scale) • Claims based on testimonials, unverified clinical observations, opinions, or speculation • Ineffective, unknown, or adverse intervention effects reported based on poorly controlled studies

[1] Several is defined as 2 group design or 4 single-subject design (SSD) studies with a minimum of 12 participants for which there are no conflicting results or at least 3 group design or 6 SSD studies with a minimum of 18 participants with no more than 10% of studies reporting conflicting results. Group and SSD methodologies may be combined.

[2] SMRS (Scientific Merit Rating Scale): Author-created scale to evaluate effectiveness of published studies for people with ASD. Experimental rigour examined on research design, measurement of dependent and independent variables, participant ascertainment, and generalization and maintenance.

[3] Few is defined as a minimum of 2 group design studies or 2 SSD studies with a minimum of 6 participants for which no more than 10% of studies reporting conflicting results are reported.
*Group and SSD methodologies may be combined.
*Conflicting results are reported when a better or equally controlled study that is assigned a score of at least 3 reports either {a} ineffective intervention effects or {b} adverse intervention effects.

Source: National Autism Center, 2015, p. 35.

Table 3.3: Summary of Evidence-Based Intervention Reviews

NAC (2009) Evidence-Based Practices from 1997 to 2007	Wong et al. (2014) Evidence-Based Practices from 1990 to 2011	NAC (2015) Evidence-Based Practices from 2007 to 2012
Antecedent-based interventions	Antecedent-based interventions	Comprehensive behavioural interventions ^
Differential reinforcement of other behaviours	Differential reinforcement of other behaviours	
Discrete trial training	Discrete trial training	
Extinction	Extinction	
Functional behaviour assessment	Functional behaviour assessment	
Prompting	Prompting	
Reinforcement	Reinforcement	
Response interruption/ redirection	Response interruption/ redirection	
Time delay	Time delay	
Functional communication training	Functional communication training	
—	Modelling	Modelling
—	Cognitive behaviour intervention	Cognitive behaviour intervention
Computer-aided instruction	—	—
—	Exercise	—
—	—	Language training (production)
Naturalistic interventions	Naturalistic interventions	Naturalistic interventions
Parent-implemented intervention	Parent-implemented intervention	Parent-implemented intervention
PECS	PECS	

Peer-mediated instruction and intervention	Peer-mediated instruction and intervention	Peer-mediated instruction and intervention
Pivotal response training	Pivotal response training	Pivotal response training
—	—	Schedules
—	Scripting	Scripting
Self-management	Self-management	Self-management
Social narrative	Social narrative	—
Speech-generating devices/ VOCA	—	—
Social skills training	Social skills training	Social skills training
—	—	Story-based intervention
—	Structured play group	—
Structured work systems	—	—
Task analysis	Task analysis	—
—	Technology-aided instruction and intervention	—
Video modelling	Video modelling	—
Visual support	Visual support	—
Adult interventions (age 22+)	—	—
Not investigated	Not investigated	Behavioural interventions

^ The NAC (2015) report grouped together behavioural interventions that had been separated in previous reports.

Sources: NAC, 2015; Wong et al., 2014.

The focus and structure for the remainder of this section will follow the recent review *Evidence-Based Practices for Children, Youth, and Young Adults with Autism Spectrum Disorder Report* (hereafter referred to as the *EBI Report*), where six new evidence-based interventions were added and two were removed from the previous edition (Wong et al., 2014). Twenty years of research was reviewed, compared to the 10 years' worth in the 2009 review, which accounts for some of the changes, including extending the scope from 2007 to include articles to 2011. The six new treatments that are now considered EBIs are cognitive behavioural interventions, exercise, modelling, scripting, structured play groups, and technology-aided instruction and intervention. All were added to the EBI list because of additional evidence (Wong et al., 2014). The two interventions that were removed were the use of speech-generating devices, which was expanded and combined within technology-aided instruction, and structured work systems, which no longer meet the EBI criteria because of the more stringent criteria used by Wong and colleagues (2014).

The remaining evidence-based strategies are covered in chapters 4, 5, and 6. Where other reports conflict with the findings used to outline these chapters, it will be noted. Fact sheets for each of the EBIs and online modules are available from the National Professional Development Center on Autism Spectrum Disorder's website. The remainder of this chapter will cover the interventions evaluated as having some support (also known as promising or emerging strategies) presented in the *EBI Report* (Wong et al., 2014).

Promising/Emerging Interventions with Some Support

There are a number of interventions that are beginning to gather some empirical support, but are not yet considered EBIs. They may not be considered EBIs because the same author group has published all of the studies, for example, or there are insufficient quantities of studies or participants (Wong et al., 2014). In the *EBI Report* (Wong et al., 2014), 24 studies demonstrated some empirical support. In the 2015 *National Standards Report—Phase II* (NAC, 2015), 18 studies explored interventions that were classified as emerging, some of which are now on the EBI list. As Wong et al. (2014) indicate, a great deal of caution is needed when discussing promising or emerging treatments, as there is no indication of levels of support: some studies almost meet the criteria for an EBI, but others may have only minimal support. In addition, there is not enough evidence to confirm that such treatments are, in fact, ineffective (NAC, 2009). Some interventions may have been found to be effective for other populations, but they are still considered emerging for the ASD population. The emerging treatments are listed in Table 3.4, and descriptions of each treatment and the reason for its exclusion from consideration as an EBI is described.

Read about it. Think about it. Write about it.

Would it be ethical to implement a strategy that is classified as having some support with a child with ASD? Why or why not?

Table 3.4: Other Focused Intervention Practices with Some Support

Practice	Description	Evidence	Exclusion
Aided language modelling	Use of several augmentative and alternative communication strategies (e.g., pointing with finger, sequential pointing, use of communication symbol and vocalization together)	Drager et al. (2006)	Insufficient evidence
Auditory integration training	Systematic exposure to modulated tones resulting in changes in parent-reported problem behaviour	Edelson et al. (1999)	Insufficient evidence
Behavioural momentum intervention	Organization of behaviour expectations in a sequence in which low probability/preference behaviours are embedded in a series of high probability/preference behaviours to increase the occurrence of the low probability/preference behaviours	Banda & Kubina (2006) Davis, Brady, Hamilton, McEvoy & Williams (1994) Davis, Brady, Williams, & Hamilton (1992) Ducharme, Lucas, & Pontes (1994) Houlihan, Jacobson, & Brandon (1994) Jung, Sainato, & Davis (2008) Patel et al. (2007) Riviere, Becquet, Peltret, Facon, & Darcheville (2011) Romano & Roll (2000)	Insufficient number of total participants

Collaborative coaching	Systematic consultation across years to promote achievement of IEP goals	Ruble, Dalrymple, & McGrew (2010)	Insufficient evidence
Cooperative learning groups	Academic learning tasks organized around joint activities and goals	Dugan et al. (1995)	Insufficient evidence
Direct instruction	Instructional package involving student choral responses, explicit signal to cue student responses, correction procedures for incorrect or non-responses, modelling correct responses, independent student responses	Flores & Ganz (2007) Ganz & Flores (2009)	Only one research group
Exposure	Increasing (for accelerating behaviours) or decreasing (for decelerating behaviours) the stimulus intensity or conditions to promote the occurrence of the desired response	Ellis, Ala'i-Rosales, Glenn, Rosales-Ruiz, & Greenspoon (2006) Shabani & Fisher (2006) Wood, Wolery, & Kaiser (2009)	Insufficient evidence
Handwriting without Tears	Multisensory activities promoting fine motor and writing skills	Carlson, McLaughlin, Derby, & Blecher (2009)	Insufficient evidence
Independent work systems	Instructional process that includes visually and spatial organized location, previously mastered work, clear specification of task(s), signal when work is finished, instructions for next activity	Bennett, Reichow, & Wolery (2011) Hume & Odom (2007) Mavropoulou, Papadopoulou, & Kakana (2011)	Insufficient evidence

Joint attention-symbolic play instruction	A combination of DTT and NI were employed to promote joint attention and symbolic play	Gulsrud, Kasari, Freeman, & Paparella (2007) Kasari, Freeman, & Paparella (2006) Kasari, Paparella, Freeman, & Jahromi (2008)	Only one research group
Music intensity	Different levels of music volume used to affect vocal stereotypy	Lanovaz, Sladeczek, & Rapp (2011)	Insufficient evidence
Music therapy	Songs and music used as a medium through which student's goals may be addressed	Kern & Aldridge (2006) Kern, Wakeford, & Aldridge (2007) Kern, Wolery, & Aldridge (2007)	Only one research group
Reciprocal imitation training	Therapist or teacher repeats the actions, vocalizations, or other behaviours of the student to promote student's imitation and other goals	Ingersoll (2010) Ingersoll (2012) Ingersoll & Lalonde (2010) Ingersoll, Lewis, & Kroman (2007)	Only one research group
Removal of restraints	Gradual removal of restraints involving application of pressure to arm, shadowing	Jennett, Hagopian, & Beaulieu (2011)	Insufficient evidence
Schema-based strategy instruction	Cognitive strategy for establishing mental representations to promote addition and subtraction	Rockwell, Griffin, & Jones (2011)	Insufficient evidence
Self-regulated strategy development writing intervention	Instructional package involving explanation of strategy and self-management to teach writing skills	Delano (2007)	Insufficient evidence
Sensory diet	Sensory-based activities integrated into child routines to meet sensory needs	Fazlioğlu & Baran (2008)	Insufficient evidence

Sensory integration and fine motor intervention	Therapeutic activities characterized by enhanced sensation, especially tactile, vestibular, and proprioceptive, active participation and adaptive interaction paired with individual fine motor instruction from OT	Pfeiffer, Koenig, Kinnealey, Sheppard, & Henderson (2011)	Insufficient evidence
Sentence-combining technique	Instructional package including teacher modelling, student practice, and worksheet to increase adjective use in writing	Rousseau, Krantz, Poulson, Kitson, & McClannahan (1994)	Insufficient evidence
Test-taking strategy instruction	Instructional package involving modelling, mnemonic devices, verbal practice sessions, controlled practice sessions, advanced practice sessions	Songlee, Miller, Tincani, Sileo, & Perkins (2008)	Insufficient evidence
Theory of Mind training	Structured training and practice of using theory of mind skills that includes a parent component	Begeer, et al. (2011)	Insufficient evidence
Toilet training	Modification of toilet training program developed by Azrin and Foxx (1971)	LeBlanc, Carr, Crossett, Bennett, & Detweiler (2005)	Insufficient evidence
Touch-point instruction	Tactile and number line materials used to introduce math and numeracy concepts	Cihak & Foust (2008) Fletcher, Boon, & Cihak (2010)	Insufficient evidence
Touch therapy	Systematic touching or massage	Field, et al. (1997)	Insufficient evidence

Source: Wong et al., 2014, pp. 25–26.

Aided Language Modelling

Aided language modelling is a method of teaching language to children in a naturalistic play setting. Children are taught to understand (receptive language/listener responding skills) and to label (expressive language skills) with a symbol board. In this strategy, the adult points to the item in the environment, and then points to the symbol on his or her board (within two seconds) while simultaneously verbally labelling the referenced item (Drager et al., 2006). At this time, there is insufficient evidence to support the intervention as an EBI due to its lack of comparative data and replicated studies across different authors and subjects.

Auditory Integration Training

Auditory integration training involves participants listening to 20 hours of music that is processed with a device to change the volume and frequency of the music in two different ways (Edelson et al., 1999). Children with ASD listen to selected music in half-hour periods over 10 to 20 days. It was initially thought that changes in behaviours that lasted after the treatment were due to reducing the individual's sensitivity to sound, but some reports have found that changes in behaviour occur in individuals not sensitive to sound (Edelson et al., 1999). There is currently insufficient evidence to support the treatment as an EBI, and some evidence has found that auditory integration training has no effect for individuals with ASD.

Behavioural Momentum Intervention

The behavioural momentum intervention approach is based on the ABA concept of behaviour momentum, where the behaviour continues after levels of reinforcement change (Romano & Roll, 2000). This is often used to increase compliance. In this approach, a high-probability request (a request that the individual is likely to respond to, e.g., "Clap your hands") is given first. This produces behaviour momentum, which then makes that person more likely to respond to a low-probability request (e.g., "Take this medicine") (Riviere, Becquet, Peltret, Facon, & Darcheville, 2011). Completing a behaviour that gained a high level of reinforcement encourages the individual to complete a behaviour that had previously met with low rates of reinforcement (Romano & Roll, 2000). Although a number of studies have demonstrated this effect across animals and humans, including those with ASD, the evidence has not demonstrated the effect across a sufficient total number of individuals with ASD (20 was the criterion) (Wong et al., 2014).

Collaborative Coaching

This approach involves specific and focused consultation with teachers serving students with ASD. In this approach, consultants with experience in ASD meet with teachers to develop skills to target and create teaching plans for each skill (Ruble, Dalrymple, & McGrew, 2010). Consulting and coaching is then provided every six weeks to help problem solve and implement skills. Although research in this area has demonstrated strong effects in teacher follow-through with consultation and coaching and student development of the identified skills, limited research is available for children with ASD. The model was taken from children's mental health approaches, and additional studies are needed to show its effectiveness for children with ASD.

Cooperative Learning Groups

Cooperative learning groups are a type of peer-mediated strategy that focuses on a group of peers working together in an educational setting for an academic outcome (i.e., to improve math skills or increase literacy) (Dugan et al., 1995). These groups have been done in numerous formats where peers work together in a team approach, such as in a game or to solve a problem, in order to attain an academic goal. The research outcomes in increasing the targeted academic skills for individuals with disabilities is somewhat mixed, with favourable outcomes not always found. There is limited research with individuals with ASD, and although positive results have been obtained in some studies, additional research is needed in this area, some of which has been completed since the publication of the *EBI Report* (Wong et al., 2014).

Direct Instruction

Direct instruction is a teaching method that uses "well-developed and carefully planned lessons designed around small learning increments and clearly defined and prescribed teaching tasks. It is based on the theory that clear instruction, eliminating misinterpretations, can greatly improve and accelerate learning" (National Institute for Direct Instruction [NIDI], 2014, para. 1). The approach is implemented in many different schools for various subjects and targets academic achievement. The learner is placed at her or his appropriate skill level, ensuring that each skill is mastered before new content is introduced, while the speed of learning is adjusted for each individual learner (NIDI, 2014). Research has demonstrated the effectiveness of this approach (e.g., Flores & Ganz, 2007; Ganz & Flores, 2009) for reading and expressive language in individuals with ASD, with positive outcomes. However, this is the only subject area targeted and it has been implemented by only one research group to date.

Exposure

Exposure, also called stimulus fading, involves gradually increasing an individual's exposure to a stimulus (Shabani & Fisher, 2006). The procedure is often completed with stimuli that the individual is averse to (e.g., needles, haircuts) to decrease a phobia (e.g., of bugs, dogs, or snakes), or to increase a skill repertoire (e.g., types of foods eaten). The procedure is often used to decrease fears and anxiety, and is often called systematic desensitization in the context of mental health literature. A number of studies have been carried out with individuals with ASD to assist with eating, reduction in needle anxiety, and increasing tolerance of creams. However, there has not been enough evidence to date for individuals with ASD to establish it as an EBI (Wong et al., 2014).

Handwriting without Tears

This commercially available program teaches handwriting in a developmentally appropriate manner by organizing letters to teach in order of least to most difficulty, making it easier to achieve (Cosby, McLaughlin, Derby, & Huewe, 2009; Carlson, McLaughlin, Derby, & Blecher, 2009). Overall, little research has been conducted on the Handwriting without Tears program, although some studies have demonstrated its effectiveness with students with ASD (Carlson et al., 2009; Wong et al., 2014).

Capital Teaching Order

Developmentally, capitals are easier so we teach them first. The capital teaching order helps teach correct formation and orientation while eliminating reversals. Learning capitals first makes it easy to transition to lowercase letters.

Frog Jump Capitals   Starting Corner Capitals   Center Starting Capitals
FEDPBRNM   HKLUVWXYZ   COQGSAITJ

Lowercase Teaching Order

We teach lowercase c, o, s, v, and w first because they are exactly the same as their capital partners, only smaller. By teaching capitals first, we have prepared children for nearly half of the lowercase letters that are similar in formation.

c o s v w   t a d g   u i e l k y j   p r n m h b   f q x z

Lowercase Cursive Teaching Order

In cursive, we teach lowercase letters first to help children learn cursive skills in the easiest, most efficient way. It's also developmentally planned to start with letters that are familiar from printing, making an easier transition from print to cursive. Children learn their lowercase letters first, and then transition to capitals.

c a d g   h t p   e l f   u y i j   k n s   o w b v   m m   x z q

Capital Cursive Teaching Order

Capitals are taught after lowercase letters because of their infrequent use and complex formations. Children usually learn capitals very quickly. The simple letter style and teaching order makes cursive capitals easy to learn.

a c o u   v w x y z   p b r n m   h k   j j   l g   d l   d g e z

Figure 3.2: Handwriting without Tears Teaching Order
Source: Handwriting without Tears, 2015, para. 2.

Independent Work Systems

Independent work systems, also called structured work systems, were created as part of the larger Treatment and Education of Autistic and Related Communication Handicapped Children (TEACCH) program. They contain multiple components, including work systems, work tasks, and visual schedules (Bennett, Reichow, & Wolery, 2011). In a work system, individuals are required to work left to right with a visual schedule where they manipulate the schedule, complete the scheduled activity, and then place it in a defined area for completed tasks, going on to the next activity independently. Research was completed in the TEACCH program as a whole and it would be considered a comprehensive treatment model, rather than an evidence-based intervention, as much of the research in this area has only been led by the authors of the TEACCH approach. As mentioned earlier, this was classified as an EBI in the past, when different criteria was used. There is some evidence to support this approach, but additional evidence is needed.

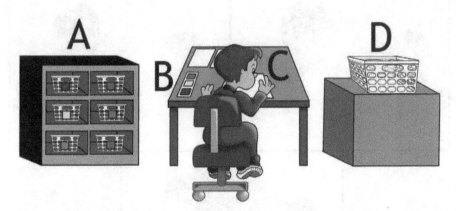

Figure 3.3: Example of a Structured Work System

Legend: **Section A** is the storage area where the work tasks are stored; **Section B** is the task schedule; **Section C** is the work task in progress; and **Section D** is the finished basket, where the tasks are put after they are completed.

Source: Thames Valley Children's Center & Greater Essex County District School Board, 2008, p. 10.

Joint Attention-Symbolic Play Instruction

Joint attention involves sharing attention with others via play and toys and showing others objects and events, and is taught to children with ASD. This approach is shown to predict language ability (Kasari, Paparella, Freeman, & Jahromi, 2008). Kasari and colleagues (2008) conclude that "[joint attention] skills may affect language outcomes because sharing a focus of attention with others allows the child to acquire the types of skills that are socially learned, such as language" (p. 125). In addition, symbolic play is taught to children both at the table in a systematic teaching format and in the natural environment during play. Although research has shown that this intervention is effective for language development in children with ASD, such results have not been expanded beyond one research group (Wong et al., 2014).

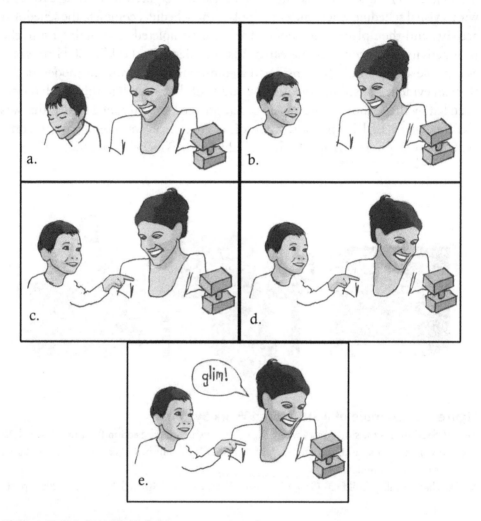

Figure 3.4: Joint Attention

Legend: In this depiction of initiation to joint attention, the child is not attending to the model (a), exhibits dyadic orienting (b), points to the object (c), directs the model's attention (d), and thus gains access to a link between a word and its referent (e).

Source: Image by David Shane Smith in Gillespie-Lynch, 2013, Figure 5.

Music Intensity

This procedure involves adjusting the volume or intensity of music, which often includes repeating words and sounds, in order to reduce vocal stereotypy (Lanovaz, Sladeczek, & Rapp, 2011). The music is thought to produce an immediate stop to the individual's production of the stereotypy and have some effect on the long-term production of the sounds. Research has shown inconsistencies, and additional research on the procedure is needed.

Music Therapy

introducir / empotrar

Music therapy involves embedding music into the teaching of a new skill, which can include transitioning, social skills, and routines (Kern & Aldridge, 2006). Research has shown that embedding music can help children with ASD improve various skills, although this has only been carried out with one research group.

Reciprocal Imitation Training

The goal of reciprocal imitation training is to teach children to imitate others through a naturalistic approach, where it is taught within a social context (Ingersoll, 2010). While playing with a child, the therapist imitates both the verbal and nonverbal actions of the child and explains the behaviours of the child with simple language (Ingersoll, 2010). In addition, the therapist provides a model of behaviour to implement with play materials about once a minute, and after three repetitions, if the child does not imitate, he or she is prompted to imitate. Research has shown positive results in children gaining imitation skills, with additional research needed with different research groups.

Removal of Restraints

For individuals who engage in self-injurious behaviours, there are situations where using a restraint can act as a negative reinforcer; restraining the body part involved in the self-injurious behaviour avoids the aversive consequence or pain that occurred when engaging behaviour (Jennett,

> **Self-Injurious Behaviours:** Self-injurious behaviours (e.g., aggressively pulling out one's own hair) involve inducing physical harm to oneself (Carr, 1977).

Hagopian, & Beaulieu, 2011). In one study, restraints acted to decrease heart rates, while removal of restraints increased heart rates, potentially signalling an increase in anxiety (Jennett et al., 2011). Increased rigorous studies to indicate a causal effect between the removal of restraints and increased anxiety is needed.

Schema-Based Strategy Instruction

This intervention is used to teach individuals to solve word problems in mathematics. Schema-based strategy instruction teaches students steps to complete when solving word problems, uses visual representations to assist in understanding and solving the problems, and includes direct instruction where the teacher provides "teacher modeling, guided practice, independent practice, and continuous teacher feedback" (Rockwell, Griffin, & Jones, 2011, p. 90). Although the procedure is used with students in academic settings, limited research has been completed with those with disabilities including ASD.

> **Negative Reinforcer:** Negative reinforcers include events, items, and stimuli that increase the likelihood that the behaviour will occur again (strengthening behaviour) when they are removed (e.g., an individual is likely to scream in the future when curfew is removed).

Self-Regulated Strategy Development

Self-regulated strategy development is used to teach writing to children with learning disabilities, although limited research has demonstrated its effect for students with ASD (Delano, 2007). The intervention involves teaching a very explicit series of steps for writing, including scaffolding and interactive back-and-forth learning with the teacher (Delano, 2007). This strategy teaches students to use self-talk to assist with planning and error correction, while using self-reinforcement strategies to avoid self-defeating statements while writing (Delano, 2007).

> **Causal Effect:** A causal effect is the likelihood that the results from a study are caused by the treatment. Causal effect is created in an experiment when the results are replicated, there are comparison groups, and the other variables are controlled.

Sensory Diet

Sensory diets, or sensory integration therapies, are various procedures—some involving the child more actively or passively than others—where the interventionist creates activities within the child's routines that stimulate various gross motor, vestibular, and sensory systems with the goal of integrating the sensory information more efficiently, leading to improvements in attention, withstanding of sensory input, behaviour, and social skills (Case-Smith, Weaver, & Fristad, 2014). Sensory-based interventions, such as brushing skin, massaging, or bouncing, implemented when arousal is too high or low are additional components that can be incorporated (Case-Smith et al., 2014). These strategies have been developed in response to the reported sensory issues that individuals with ASD experience. Unfortunately, the research base has not been consistent in the use or definition of these treatments. There is more support for the use of sensory intervention therapies in the literature, with sensory-based interventions shown to be ineffective at times. Additional evidence is available since the *EBI Report* (Wong et al., 2014); however, further literature is needed with more participants to demonstrate the effectiveness of sensory diets.

Sensory Integration and Fine Motor Intervention

This intervention is based on a study by Pfeiffer, Koenig, Kinnealey, Sheppard, and Henderson (2011), in which sensory integration therapy, as described above, was used with a group who also received an intervention for fine motor skills, compared to a group who received only a fine motor intervention. Results demonstrated that both groups showed improvement in reaching personalized goals, although there were more significant effects for the group receiving sensory integration for fine motor difficulties. Much more research is needed to discern individual or combined effects.

Sentence-Combining Technique

Sentence-combining techniques involve teaching students to "combine two or more short, simple sentences to produce a single, more mature sentence" (Rousseau, Krantz, Poulson, Kitson, & McClannahan, 1994, p. 20). This is one of the most efficient methods for increasing students' use of longer sentences, clauses, and adjectives (Rousseau et al., 1994). Although this procedure is effective with children who are developing typically, little research is evident with those with disabilities; just one study was carried out specific to children with ASD.

Test-Taking Strategy Instruction

Test-taking strategy instruction is a manualized approach using intensive after-school training to teach test-taking skills to students (Songlee, Miller, Tincani, Sileo, & Perkins, 2008). It involves modelling the cognitive processes involved in using a mnemonic to take tests most effectively, then practicing in more controlled and then progressively more natural environments, with assistance from the instructor. Although the intervention is effective for students who are developing typically, and one study has demonstrated success with adolescents with ASD, additional research is needed.

Theory of Mind Training

Theory of Mind training has several different names and involves individuals putting themselves in another person's shoes, or developing an internal representation of themselves and those around them (Begeer et al., 2011). Other versions of the training have been called social cognition, mind reading, picture-in-the-head, or thought-bubble training (Begeer et al., 2011). Numerous training programs have been created that are carried out in a natural environment, with video training, and using complex scenarios where the individual needs to reason about what another person is thinking in a situation. In one current study, although conceptual understanding of Theory of Mind skills increased, more advanced understanding and generalization into the natural environment did not occur (Begeer et al., 2011). Additional evidence is needed.

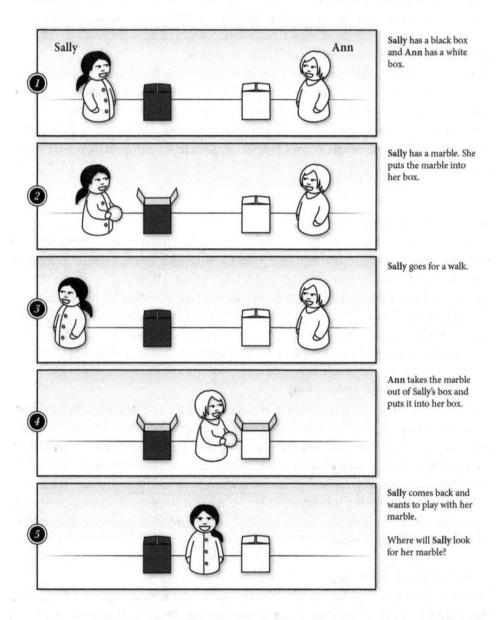

Figure 3.5: Sample Theory of Mind Task
Source: Byom & Mutlu, 2013, p. 3.

Toilet Training

Toilet training interventions for children with ASD and other disabilities have been available for many years, and one of the most popular is Azrin and Foxx's (1989) *Toilet Training in Less Than a Day*. Since then, additional studies have used a similar procedure for toilet training children with ASD, while changing the use of punishment from restitutional, in which the child cleans up the mess and engages in a long process of changing clothes after having an accident, to positive practice, in which the child engages in the desired behaviours after having an accident (e.g., sitting on the toilet and dressing) (LeBlanc, Carr, Crossett, Bennett, & Detweiler, 2005). A study completed by LeBlanc and colleagues (2005) used a modified version of Azrin and Fox's toilet training procedure that included "(a) a sitting schedule, (b) programmed consequences for successful urinations and self-initiations, (c) increased fluids, (d) communication training, (e) a urine sensor and alarm, and (f) positive practice for accidents" (p. 100). Two studies have demonstrated positive effects, although additional research is required (Wong et al., 2014).

Touch-Point Instruction

Touch-point instruction utilizes numbers that have touch-points on them to indicate the amount represented by each number. The TouchMath Program is a commercialized package to teach children math that uses the touch-points (Innovative Learning Concepts, 2013). Students count and touch the points on the numbers in sequences, while counting forward or backward for addition and subtraction and in sequences for multiplication or division (Innovative Learning Concepts, 2013). Research has demonstrated the effectiveness of the approach for students who are developing typically and has recently demonstrated its effectiveness for students with ASD. Additional research is needed for this population.

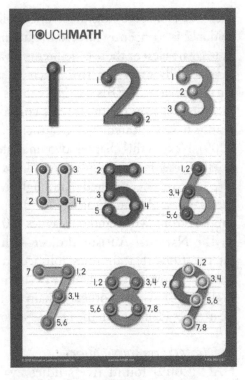

Figure 3.6: TouchMath Memory Cue Poster

Source: Innovative Learning Concepts, 2013.

Touch Therapy

Touch therapy includes treatments that utilize the contact of another's hands on one's body in a directed manner, such as massage therapy (Field et al., 1997). Field and colleagues (1997) examined the effects of stroking the child's body with moderate pressure from a therapist on attentiveness, on-task behaviour, touch aversion, and withdraw. Results have demonstrated positive effects, although additional studies are needed across additional subjects.

Read about it. Think about it. Write about it.

Which of the interventions with some support intrigues you the most? Research if additional evidence has accumulated for or against the treatment's effectiveness since the publication of the *EBI Report*.

Unsupported or Unestablished

Treatments that are considered unestablished, or have no support, are those where evidence is stringently limited by the small amount of literature in peer-reviewed journal articles, or there is no literature available. In addition, research in this area may actually show negative effects or no effectiveness (NAC, 2009). The most current review of EBIs for individuals with ASD (Wong et al., 2014) did not include a section on treatments considered ineffective. However, previous EBI reports have indicated these treatments in their review of the literature (e.g., NAC, 2009). Next in this chapter, two unestablished treatments from 2009 onwards are briefly presented, to increase awareness of these interventions and procedures in case they are encountered. Although five unestablished treatments were listed in the National Autism Project's 2009 report, three were later found to have some support from Wong and colleagues (2014).

The National Autism Project—Phase II (NAC, 2015) has identified 13 interventions that are unestablished in the literature. Some of these have been reviewed above and are identified as having some evidence in the *EBI Report* (Wong et al., 2014), whereas others remain on this list. See Box 3.2 for the unestablished treatments identified in the recent National Autism Project's (NAC, 2015) report.

Facilitated Communication

NAC (2009) found five studies evaluating the effectiveness of facilitated communication for individuals with ASD. This approach "involves having a facilitator support the hand or arm of an individual with limited communication skills, helping the individual express words, sentences, or complete thoughts by

Box 3.2: Unestablished Treatments

The following interventions have been identified as falling into the unestablished category of evidence:
- Animal-assisted therapy
- Auditory integration training
- Concept mapping
- Developmental, Individual-differences, and Relationship-based model (DIR) and the DIRFloortime® approach
- Facilitated communication
- Gluten-free/casein-free diet
- Movement-based intervention
- SENSE theatre intervention
- Sensory intervention package
- Shock therapy
- Social behavioural learning strategy
- Social cognition intervention
- Social thinking intervention

Source: NAC, 2015, p. 72.

using a keyboard of words or pictures or typing device" (NAC, 2009, p. 72). It is based on the belief that nonverbal individuals are able to communicate, if given the proper opportunities (American Psychological Association [APA], 1994). However, research has demonstrated that the communication the individuals typed on a keyboard was directed by the individual who was helping the individual to type (APA, 1994). The American Psychological Association (1994) has advised against the use of facilitated communication, as it threatens the human and civil rights of the individual by allowing others to potentially miscommunicate desires and wishes. Other professional organizations have issued similar statements (NAC, 2009).

Gluten- and Casein-Free Diet
This approach involves limiting an individual's dietary intake of gluten, casein, or both (NAC, 2009). The approach demonstrated some effectiveness initially in studies with scientific designs that were not strong, but further research has demonstrated no effects or potentially harmful effects to individuals. Therefore, additional research is needed to understand if diets of this nature are effective, or possibly harmful to individuals with ASD.

> **Read about it. Think about it. Write about it.**
>
> Explain how you would continue to work with an individual and their family who are engaged in an unestablished practice.

CONTROVERSY WITH EVIDENCE-BASED INTERVENTIONS

There is strong support for the use of EBIs, driven in part by situations in which children and others have been harmed or killed because of the implementation of a non-supported intervention or pseudoscience. In addition, the movement toward EBIs has encouraged research and made clinicians accountable for researching the literature appropriately to determine the effectiveness of an intervention before implementing it. However, there have also been drawbacks to this evidence-based movement; these have been highlighted in the literature. Prominent among them is that many are unsure of the meaning of "evidence-based interventions" and how to use the literature to find them (Gibbs & Gambrill, 2002). In fact, many research reviews show different results based on the different evaluation methodologies, as seen between the multiple EBI reports such as the National Standards Project (NAC, 2015) and the EPI report (Wong et al., 2014) for individuals with ASD (Gibbs & Gambrill, 2002; Mesibov & Shea, 2011). Discrepancies and differences in outcomes can be introduced by the way research evaluations and summaries are operationalized and by involving authors from different theoretical backgrounds (Mesibov & Shea, 2011). In addition, in comparison to literature bases for other populations or fields, the number of research articles on interventions for ASD remains smaller overall (Mesibov & Shea, 2011). In particular, many of these interventions were developed for preschoolers and children, and the literature remains sparse for adolescents and adults with ASD (Mesibov & Shea, 2011).

In addition, in the ASD research field, some of the research may gravitate naturally toward behaviours that lend themselves to easy and immediate measurement, and thus goals such as long-term success, quality of life, employment, and personal relationship outcomes may not be measured (Mesibov & Shea, 2011). A criticism of EBIs in other fields, such as social work and psychology, is the inherently manual-based treatment that has developed as a result, which favours a cookie-cutter approach that does not allow for personalized services for individuals, or for the personalized approach of the therapist (Gibbs & Gambrill, 2002). Research has repeatedly demonstrated that in traditional talk therapy, therapist factors (called common factors), which include the therapeutic alliance with a client, warmth, and empathy, have more of an impact on client outcome than the school of therapy the therapist is using (Lambert & Barley, 2001). Mesibov and Shea (2011) point out that more attention should be paid to this when examining ASD literature, as the relationship with the client as well as the experience and skills the therapist brings to the treatment are important to recognize. Individuals with ASD range across a spectrum and may include those with intellectual disabilities and those who have average to above-average intelligence: "for autism treatment manuals to be useful, the concept of a manual should be flexible enough to take into account individuals' patterns of cognitive and language skills, atypical interests, social relationship patterns, degree of rigidity and stereotyped behavior, co-morbid conditions, and variety of treatment settings and agents (e.g., parents, teachers)" (Mesibov & Shea, 2011, p. 120).

As a result of awareness of the EBI movement, public funds have been put toward strategies that are considered EBIs. In most cases this is a beneficial approach; however, at times, this can leave certain populations inadequately served, and fail to promote funding toward additional research to examine emerging strategies.

Read about it. Think about it. Write about it.

When working with a vulnerable population, such as individuals with ASD, do you feel that clinicians should strictly adhere to EBI guidelines? Why or why not? Are there situations where an intervention that is not an EBI can be used?

A LOOK BACK

Chapter 3, "Evidence-Based Interventions," focused on:
- An overview of evidence-based interventions (EBIs), including how to find evidence, the strength of the evidence, and comparing them to pseudoscience;
- The most recent project evaluating EBIs for ASD;
- An overview of the established treatments, promising/emerging treatments, and unsupported/unestablished treatments for ASD; and
- Brief overviews of each intervention with some support (promising/emerging treatments) based on the most recent review of EBIs for ASD.

A LOOK AHEAD

Chapter 4, "Communication-Based Interventions," focuses on:
- The receptive and expressive language difficulties that individuals with ASD face;

- An overview of functional communication, nine critical communication skills, and augmentative and alternative communication (AAC);
- Who is involved in the process and how to receive communication supports in Ontario; and
- Interventions to teach communication, including the picture exchange communication system (PECS), naturalistic interventions, pivotal response training (PRT), functional communication training (FCT), and technology-aided instruction.

ADDITIONAL RESOURCES

- A Parent's Guide to Evidence-Based Practice and Autism (National Autism Center, 2011):
  http://www.nationalautismcenter.org/resources/for-families/
- Autism Internet Modules: Bringing Research to Real Life (Autism Internet Modules, 2015):
  www.autisminternetmodules.org
- Autism Intervention Program Guideline Revision (Ontario Ministry of Children and Youth Services, 2011):
  www.children.gov.on.ca/htdocs/English/topics/specialneeds/autism/aip_guidelines.aspx#4
- Evidence-Based Practice and Autism in the Schools (National Autism Center, 2011):
  http://www.nationalautismcenter.org/resources/for-educators/
- *Evidence-Based Practices for Children and Adolescents with Autism Spectrum Disorder: Review of the Literature and Practice Guide* (Children's Mental Health Ontario, 2003):
  www.kidsmentalhealth.ca/documents/EBI_autism.pdf
- *Evidence-Based Practices for Children, Youth, and Young Adults with Autism Spectrum Disorder* (Wong et al., 2014):
  www.fpg.unc.edu/sites/fpg.unc.edu/files/resources/reports-and-policy-briefs/2014-EBI-Report.pdf
- National Standards Report (National Autism Center, 2009):
  www.mn.gov/mnddc/asd-employment/pdf/09-NSR-NAC.pdf National PD. autismpdc.fpg.unc.edu/content/structured-work-systems
- Resolution on facilitated communication by the American Psychological Association (American Psychological Association, 1994):
  www.apa.org/divisions/div33/fcpolicy.html

- The National Professional Development Center's Evidence-Based Practices (National Professional Development Center on Autism Spectrum Disorder, 2015): autismpdc.fpg.unc.edu/evidence-based-practices

REFERENCES

American Psychological Association. (1994). Resolution on facilitated communication by the American Psychological Association. Retrieved from www.apa.org/divisions/div33/fcpolicy.html

Azrin, N., & Foxx, R. M. (1989). *Toilet training in less than a day*. New York, NY: Pocket Books.

Barrett, S. (2010). Roy E. Kerry, M.D. charged with unprofessional conduct. Retrieved from www.casewatch.org/board/med/kerry/complaint.shtml

Baxter, A. J., & Krenzelok, E. P. (2008). Pediatric fatality secondary to EDTA chelation. *Clinical toxicology, 46*(10), 1083–1084.

Begeer, S., Gevers, C., Clifford, P., Verhoeve, M., Kat, K., Hoddenbach, E., & Boer, F. (2011). Theory of mind training in children with autism: A randomized controlled trial. *Journal of Autism and Developmental Disorders, 41*(8), 997–1006. doi: 10.1007/s10803-010-1121-9

Bennett, K., Reichow, B., & Wolery, M. (2011). Effects of structured teaching on the behavior of young children with disabilities. *Focus on Autism and Other Developmental Disabilities, 26*(3), 143–152. doi: 10.1177/1088357611405040

Byom, L. J., and Mutlu, B. (2013). Theory of mind: Mechanisms, methods, and new directions. *Frontiers in Human Neuroscience, 7*, 413. http://dx.doi.org/10.3389/fnhum.2013.00413

Carlson, B., McLaughlin, T., Derby, K. M., & Blecher, J. (2009). Teaching preschool children with autism and developmental delays to write. *Electronic Journal of Research in Educational Psychology, 7*(1), 225–238.

Carr, E. G. (1977). The motivation of self-injurious behavior: A review of some hypotheses. *Psychological Bulletin, 84*(4), 800.

Case-Smith, J., Weaver, L. L., & Fristad, M. A. (2014). A systematic review of sensory processing interventions for children with Autism Spectrum Disorder. *International Journal of Research and Practice, 19*(2), 133–148.

Cosby, E., McLaughlin, T. F., Derby, K. M., & Huewe, P. (2009). Using tracing and modeling with a Handwriting without Tears® worksheet to increase handwriting legibility for a preschool student with autism. *Open Social Science Journal, 2*, 67–69.

Delano, M. E. (2007). Use of strategy instruction to improve the story writing skills of a student with Asperger syndrome. *Focus on Autism and Other Developmental Disabilities, 22*(4), 252–258. doi: 10 .1177/10883576070220040701

Drager, K. D., Postal, V. J., Carrolus, L., Castellano, M., Gagliano, C., & Glynn, J. (2006). The effect of aided language modeling on symbol comprehension and production in 2 preschoolers with autism. *American Journal of Speech-Language Pathology, 15*(2), 112. doi:10.1044/1058-0360(2006/012)

Dugan, E., Kamps, D., Leonard, B., Watkins, N., Rheinberger, A., & Stackhaus, J. (1995). Effects of cooperative learning groups during social studies for students with autism and fourth-grade peers. *Journal of Applied Behavior Analysis, 28*(2), 175–188. doi:10.1901/jaba.1995.28-175

Edelson, S. M., Arin, D., Bauman, M., Lukas, S. E., Rudy, J. H., Sholar, M., & Rimland, B. (1999). Auditory Integration Training a double-blind study of behavioral and electrophysiological effects in people with autism. *Focus on Autism and Other Developmental Disabilities, 14*(2), 73–81.

Field, T., Lasko, D., Mundy, P., Henteleff, T., Kabat, S., Talpins, S., & Dowling, M. (1997). Brief report: Autistic children's attentiveness and responsivity improve after touch therapy. *Journal of Autism and Developmental Disorders, 27*(3), 333–338. doi:10.1023/A:1025858600220

Flores, M. M., & Ganz, J. B. (2007). Effectiveness of direct instruction for teaching statement inference, use of facts, and analogies to students with developmental disabilities and reading delays. *Focus on Autism and Other Developmental Disabilities, 22*(4), 244–251. doi:10.1177/10883576070220040601

Ganz, J. B., & Flores, M. M. (2009). The effectiveness of direct instruction for teaching language to children with Autism Spectrum Disorder: Identifying materials. *Journal of Autism and Developmental Disorders, 39*(1), 75–83. doi: 10.1007/s10803-008-0602-6

Gibbs, L., & Gambrill, E. (2002). Evidence-based practice: Counterarguments to objections. *Research on Social Work Practice, 12*(3), 452–476.

Gillespie-Lynch, K. (2013, May 1). Response to and initiation of joint attention: Overlapping but distinct roots of development in autism? *OA Autism, 1*(2), 13. Retrieved from www.oapublishinglondon.com/article/596

Green, G. (1996). Evaluating claims about treatments for autism. In C. Maurice, G. Green, & S. C. Luce (Eds.), *Behavioral intervention for young children with autism: A manual for parents and professionals* (pp. 15–28). Austin, TX: PRO-ED.

Herbert, J. D., Sharp, I. R., & Gaudiano, B. A. (2002). Separating fact from fiction in the etiology and treatment of autism: A scientific review of the evidence. *The scientific review of mental health practice, 1*(1), 23–43.

Ingersoll, B. (2010). Brief report: Pilot randomized controlled trial of reciprocal imitation training for teaching elicited and spontaneous imitation to children with autism. *Journal of Autism and Developmental Disorders, 40*(9), 1154–1160. doi:10.1007/s10803-010-0966-2

Innovative Learning Concepts. (2013). How it works: Math for all senses. Retrieved from https://www.oncoursesystems.com/school/webpage/12712431/1242281

Jennett, H., Hagopian, L. P., & Beaulieu, L. (2011). Analysis of heart rate and self-injury with and without restraint in an individual with autism. *Research in Autism Spectrum Disorder, 5*(3), 1110–1118.

Kane, K. (2007, August 22). Doctor who used chelation therapy charged in autistic boy's death. *Pittsburgh Post-Gazette*. Retrived from www.post-gazette.com/local/neighborhoods/2007/08/22/Doctor-who-used-chelation-therapy-charged-in-autistic-boy-s-death/stories/200708220294

Kane, K., & Linn, V. (2005, August, 25). Boy dies during autism treatment. *Pittsburgh Post-Gazette*. Retrieved from old.post-gazette.com/pg/05237/559756.stm

Kasari, C., Paparella, T., Freeman, S. N., & Jahromi, L. (2008). Language outcome in autism: Randomized comparison of joint attention and play interventions. *Journal of Consulting and Clinical Psychology, 76*, 125–137. doi:10.1037/0022-006X.76.1.125

Kern, P., & Aldridge, D. (2006). Using embedded music therapy interventions to support outdoor play of young children with autism in an inclusive community-based child care program. *Journal of Music Therapy, 43*(4), 270–294.

Lambert, M. J., & Barley, D. E. (2001). Research summary on the therapeutic relationship and psychotherapy outcome. *Psychotherapy: Theory, Research, Practice, Training, 38*(4), 357.

Lanovaz, M. J., Sladeczek, I. E., & Rapp, J. T. (2011). Effects of music on vocal stereotypy in children with autism. *Journal of Applied Behavior Analysis, 44*(3), 647–651. doi:10.1901/jaba.2011.44-647

LeBlanc, L. A., Carr, J. E., Crossett, S. E., Bennett, C. M., & Detweiler, D. D. (2005). Intensive outpatient behavioral treatment of primary urinary incontinence of children with autism.

Focus on Autism and Other Developmental Disabilities, 20(2), 98–105. doi:10.1177/1088357 6050200020601

Mayer, G. R., Sulzer-Azaroff, B., & Wallace, M. (2014). *Behavior analysis for lasting change* (3rd ed.). Cornwall-on-Houston, NY: Sloan Publishing.

McNeece, C. A., & Thyer, B. A. (2004). Evidence-based practice and social work. *Journal of evidence-based social work, 1*(1), 7–25.

Mesibov, G. B., & Shea, V. (2011). Evidence-based practices and autism. *Autism, 15*(1), 114–133.

National Autism Center. (2009). *National standards report.* Retrieved from mn.gov/mnddc/asd-employment/pdf/09-NSR-NAC.pdf

National Autism Center. (2015). Findings and conclusions, national standards project, phase 2. Retrieved from http://www.nationalautismcenter.org/national-standards-project/

National Institute for Direct Instruction. (2014). Basic philosophy of direct instruction. Retrieved from www.nifdi.org/what-is-di/basic-philosophy

Odom, S. L., Collet-Klingenberg, L., Rogers, S. J., & Hatton, D. D. (2010). Evidence-based practices in interventions for children and youth with Autism Spectrum Disorder. *Preventing school failure: Alternative education for children and youth, 54*(4), 275–282.

Ontario Ministry of Children and Youth Services. (2011). Autism intervention program guideline revision. Retrieved from www.children.gov.on.ca/htdocs/English/topics/specialneeds/autism/aip_guidelines.aspx#4

Ontario Ministry of Education. (2007). Policy/program memorandum No. 140. Retrieved from www.edu.gov.on.ca/extra/eng/ppm/140.html

Pfeiffer, B. A., Koenig, K., Kinnealey, M., Sheppard, M., & Henderson, L. (2011). Effectiveness of sensory integration interventions in children with Autism Spectrum Disorder: A pilot study. *The American Journal of Occupational Therapy, 65*(1), 76–85. doi:10.5014/ajot.2011.09205

Reichow, B., & Wolery, M. (2009). Comprehensive synthesis of early intensive behavioral interventions for young children with autism based on the UCLA young autism project model. *Journal of autism and developmental disorders, 39*(1), 23–41.

Riviere, V., Becquet, M., Peltret, E., Facon, B., & Darcheville, J. C. (2011). Increasing compliance with medical examination requests directed to children with autism: Effects of a high-probability request procedure. *Journal of Applied Behavior Analysis, 44*(1), 193–197.

Rockwell, S. B., Griffin, C. C., & Jones, H. A. (2011). Schema-based strategy instruction in mathematics and the word problem-solving performance of a student with autism. *Focus on Autism and Other Developmental Disabilities, 26*(2), 87–95. doi:10.1177/1088357611405039

Romano, J. P., & Roll, D. (2000). Expanding the utility of behavioral momentum for youth with developmental disabilities. *Behavioral Interventions, 15*(2), 99–111. doi:10.1002/(SICI)1099-078X(200004/06)15:2<99::AID-BIN48>3.0.CO;2-K

Rousseau, M. K., Krantz, P. J., Poulson, C. L., Kitson, M. E., & McClannahan, L. E. (1994). Sentence combining as a technique for increasing adjective use in writing by students with autism. *Research in Developmental Disabilities, 15*(1), 19–37. doi:10.1016/0891-4222(94)90036-1

Ruble, L. A., Dalrymple, N. J., & McGrew, J. H. (2010). The effects of consultation on Individualized Education Program outcomes for young children with autism: The collaborative model for promoting competence and success. *Journal of Early Intervention, 32*(4), 286–301. doi:10.1177/1053815110382973

Shabani, D. B., & Fisher, W. W. (2006). Stimulus fading and differential reinforcement for the treatment of needle phobia in a youth with autism. *Journal of Applied Behavior Analysis, 39*(4), 449–452. doi:10.1901/jaba.2006.30-05

Simpson, R. L. (2005). Evidence-based practices and students with Autism Spectrum Disorder. *Focus on Autism and Other Developmental Disabilities, 20*(3), 140–149.

Songlee, D., Miller, S. P., Tincani, M., Sileo, N. M., & Perkins, P. G. (2008). Effects of test-taking strategy instruction on high-functioning adolescents with Autism Spectrum Disorder. *Focus on Autism and Other Developmental Disabilities, 23*(4), 217–228. doi:10.1177/1088357608324714

Thames Valley Children's Center & Greater Essex County District School Board. (2008). *Structured learning environment work tasks: A guide for the elementary educator* (2nd ed.). London, ON: Author. Retrieved from http://www.ncdsb.net/education/student_services/work_task/ch1-2%20intro.pdf

Wong, C., Odom, S. L., Hume, K. Cox, A. W., Fettig, A., Kucharczyk, S., ... Schultz, T. R. (2014). *Evidence-based practices for children, youth, and young adults with Autism Spectrum Disorder.* Chapel Hill: The University of North Carolina, Frank Porter Graham Child Development Institute, Autism Evidence-Based Practice Review Group.

CHAPTER 4

COMMUNICATION-BASED INTERVENTIONS

As previously indicated, the diagnostic criteria for autism spectrum disorder (ASD) includes social communication and social interaction deficits (American Psychiatric Association [APA], 2013). Chapter 4 is focused on providing information on effective, evidence-based intervention strategies that aim to assist, improve, or enhance communication skills in individuals with ASD.

DEFINITION

Within a diagnosis of ASD, clinicians are required to indicate if the individual also has an accompanying language disorder, which includes the number of verbal words individuals emit and how often they speak (APA, 2013). The

Diagnostic and Statistical Manual-5 (DSM-5) indicates that there is often an overlap between the communication challenges that individuals with ASD face and their challenges with social interactions, and thus, the two characteristics that were once separate are now combined in one diagnostic criterion (APA, 2013). Some individuals who have verbal language struggle to combine it with nonverbal features, such as tone, intonation, volume control, and hand gestures, making social interaction difficult or awkward at times (APA, 2013). In this sense, language abilities vary greatly across the autism spectrum. The range can extend from being completely nonverbal, through using speech non-functionally, to being able to speak in complex sentences with amazing vocabulary, but still struggling to use this communication fluently in conversation (APA, 2013). Under the *DSM-5*'s severity scale for ASD (see chapter 2), someone classified as a level-three learner may not have intelligible speech, or may use it only to request certain items, and use echoing as her or his primary mechanism for language (APA, 2013).

> **Intonation:** Intonation involves the changing rhythm of speech, whereby the pitch and tone of language rises and falls to convey pragmatic meaning within the sentence (Levis, 1999).

Interventions for individuals who are at level three on the severity scale will often require language programs that draw on alternative methods of communication besides verbal speech. It is estimated that half of individuals with a diagnosis of ASD do not acquire speech or only acquire a small amount of speech (Ganz et al., 2012; Jahr, 2001). It is critical that this language delay is identified early, as childhood is often a crucial time for language development (Bennett et al., 2014). In many cases, individuals who are at level three in severity need to be taught the function of communication and how to use it. In essence, they are learning that when they *approach* someone with an *action* they get an *outcome* (Frost & Bondy, 2002). Typically developing children learn this as young as six months, when they are smiling, babbling, and pointing to get what they want from their caregivers (Frost & Bondy, 2002). However, because ASD also involves a deficit in social skills, individuals often do not naturally use joint attention to look at the reactions of others and pick up the social cues for how others use this information. What is often involved is teaching

> **Joint Attention:** Joint attention is an individual's ability to follow another's attention and share the attention of others by actively engaging with the same item or pointing to items in order to share the item or event (e.g., a plane in the sky passing overhead) (Kasari, Paparella, Freeman, & Jahromi, 2008).

children how to communicate, the same way typically developing young children pick this up naturally from their environment. Often it involves using a type of communication (sign, speech, pictures, or devices) that is given to another person to receive an outcome. This chapter will explore how this is done in various approaches and with different options for communication.

Individuals who are at level two in social communication according to the *DSM-5*'s severity scale (APA, 2013) may require some training on how to communicate, but these interventions will usually focus more on using speech appropriately. This may involve training individuals on how to use inflections, including tone, pitch, and intonation, appropriately when talking to others, or how to appropriately initiate and end a conversation. When working with individuals with ASD, a characteristic sign is often how they start or end conversations. Usually social greetings are started with, "How are you?" or a comment on the weather. Conversations are usually ended with a social nicety such as "Thank you" or "It was nice talking to you." Individuals with ASD may approach a stranger at a social gathering and rather abruptly say, "What is your favourite colour and where do you live?" Starting a conversation this way and asking for private social information of this nature can make many people uncomfortable. Thus, interventions targeting language may overlap with strategies also used for social skills and repetitive and restricted patterns of behaviour. These are certainly interconnected.

A Canadian study examined 330 children aged two to four who had been recently diagnosed with ASD (Bennett et al., 2014). Three groups were included: those who were diagnosed with ASD only, those who were diagnosed with ASD and a language impairment (LI), and those with ASD and an intellectual disability (ID). At baseline, the individuals with ASD and an LI were more socially impaired than those with ASD only, and those with ASD and an ID were more socially impaired than both groups. One year later, those with language deficits improved, similarly to those with no language impairment.

Intellectual Disability: "An intellectual disability (also commonly referred to as a developmental disability, among other terms) is, simply stated, a disability that significantly affects one's ability to learn and use information. It is a disability that is present during childhood and continues throughout one's life. A person who has an intellectual disability is capable of participating effectively in all aspects of daily life, but sometimes requires more assistance than others in learning a task, adapting to changes in tasks and routines, and addressing the many barriers to participation that result from the complexity of our society" (Community Living Ontario, 2015, para. 1).

However, those with an ID continued to fall behind the other groups in terms of their social development. The study showed that the majority of children who had a language deficit at the time of diagnosis no longer had the LI one year later. However, these children continued to struggle socially, and thus these early difficulties with language may also influence social ability.

Receptive Language

Another area of need for those with ASD involves receptive language skills (Kover, McDuffie, Hagerman, & Abbeduto, 2013). The manner in which children understand language versus the use of expressive language is a distinction that does not receive much attention in the *DSM-5*. In typically developing children, the preschool period is when most language development occurs; children can acquire up to 10,000 English words by the age of six (Sénéchal, 1997). Much of this comes from picking up language in the natural environment, not from direct teaching. Usually, a child's ability to understand language is much greater than his or her ability to expressively communicate (Kover et al., 2013).

Receptive Language: Receptive language is the ability to understand spoken words, vocabulary, and syntax. This is often demonstrated when a person follows directions (Kover et al., 2013).

In children with ASD, Kover and colleagues (2013) found that receptive language acquisition was delayed for overall development compared to typically developing children. A child's receptive language ability was related to her or his nonverbal ability and expressive language ability. Unlike typically developing children, when expressive language began to develop

Expressive Language: Expressive language is the ability to express oneself with language (Kover et al., 2013). This can include methods of communication other than verbal speech, such as sign language or pictures.

for individuals with ASD, receptive language did not always increase as well. The authors suggested that individuals with ASD develop receptive language 20 percent slower than they develop expressive language. Hudry and colleagues (2010) found that receptive language was more impaired than expressive language in a study of 152 preschoolers with autism. This highlights the need for both receptive and expressive language interventions for individuals with ASD. In many early intervention programs in Ontario and beyond, both expressive and receptive language are taught separately, both in direct and naturalistic teaching.

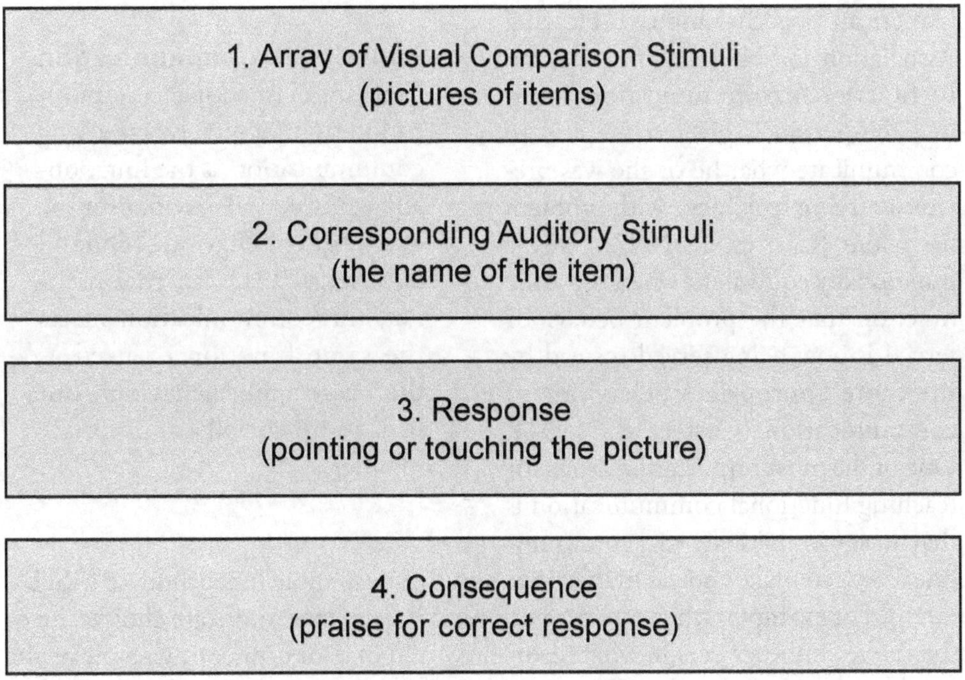

---
1. Array of Visual Comparison Stimuli
(pictures of items)

---

2. Corresponding Auditory Stimuli
(the name of the item)

---

3. Response
(pointing or touching the picture)

---

4. Consequence
(praise for correct response)

Figure 4.1: Receptive Language Skills
Source: Adapted from Grow, 2011.

WHAT IS FUNCTIONAL COMMUNICATION?

Communicating with others is a critical part of everyday life. This can involve asking for what one needs, listening to a friend, or pointing to what one is referring to. "Communication involves behaviour (defined in form by the community) directed to another person who in turn provides related direct or social rewards" (Frost & Bondy, 2002, p. 24). Speech is one of the most common methods of communication, and what most people think of as communication, but for many children with ASD, different methods are used to communicate. Similarly, just because someone talks does not mean that she or he is communicating, as communication needs to be directed toward someone else (Frost & Bondy, 2002). Children with autism often demonstrate echolalia, where they repeat what is said or what they may have heard in their environment (e.g., through TV and movies), either immediately afterward or after some time has passed—this is not typically considered communication. The goal of communication is functional communication. When expressing oneself functionally, the person is able to communicate without "resorting to problem behaviour or experiencing communication breakdown"

(American Speech-Language-Hearing Association [ASHA], 2015, para. 9). In functional communication training, the person is given a method to communicate what he or she was previously trying to achieve with problem behaviour (Carr et al., 1997). This is functionally equivalent when the same function that the problem behaviour served is now being served instead by the more appropriate behaviour of communication (Carr et al., 1997). One of the most important reasons for teaching functional communication is that when individuals can communicate, they can make choices in their lives and engage in more independence (ASHA, 2015). For example, when a person can functionally communicate choices, he or she can tell another person what he or she would like for dinner or what he or she would like to wear that day. When people can communicate what they would like to order at a restaurant, they no longer need to rely on someone else ordering, or can go to the restaurant on their own.

Functional Communication Training: Functional communication training involves teaching communication as the functionally equivalent behaviour for the challenging behaviour (Durand & Carr, 1991). In this manner, the communication meets the same function or need as the challenging behaviour, but in a more socially appropriate manner.

When working with individuals with ASD, it is important to note that all individuals can learn to communicate, and this does not have to involve speech (ASHA, 2015). Communication can involve multiple modalities, and choosing a modality that is right for the individual is crucial. This assessment may involve the work of a speech-language therapist in combination with an occupational therapist to determine the communication and motor planning skills the individual has in order to find an alternative form of communication. For example, an individual who has poor fine motor skills would most likely not engage in sign language. Another person may not have use of her or his arms, so eye gaze is used to determine what she or he is communicating, via a communication board. As Frost and Bondy (2002) indicate, the primary goal is always teaching a person to communicate, no matter what type of modality they use; speech is a secondary priority. Being able to speak and understand only the caregiver is not functional communication.

Read about it. Think about it. Write about it.

Explain how you would begin to assess if a person is capable of functional communication.

Box 4.1: A Collaborative Approach to Communication

There is a need for augmentative and alternative communication (AAC) system providers to collaborate with autism services, as approximately half of the children who have autism may fail to develop functional speech and language skills. If both AAC and autism service providers work together to share knowledge and information, all staff can benefit from increased access to resources and knowledge.

Thames Valley Children's Centre (TVCC) Interdisciplinary Approach
Knowing that children who have autism often enrol in both AAC and autism services, TVCC developed an interest in aligning these two services in order to enhance the possibility of positive outcomes for children with autism. Staff members from both services would participate in joint consultations in order to coordinate their service delivery during a 16-month initiative.

This knowledge exchange framework included:

1. Allowing stakeholders from both services to identify priority needs and plan for their joint collaboration
2. Implementing a plan for priority goals
3. Evaluating and sustaining ongoing collaboration

Priority goals included:

- Increased knowledge and training
- Relationship building and service delivery alignment
- Joint consultation and assessment

Evaluation of collaboration:

- Fifty-four Service Providers (42 from the autism program and 12 from the AAC program) shared feedback through focus groups and a questionnaire.
- Participants shared their opinions on the success of the 16-month collaboration project.

Key Findings

- Knowledge and training activities allowed service providers from both programs to increase their knowledge of one another's roles and goals when working with children who have autism.

- Service providers commented that they felt they had improved relationships with the other provider and noted an increase in trust and rapport.
- The collaborative service delivery activities increased the benefits that clients experienced and additionally increased consistent practice between both service providers.

Comments for sustainability:

- Participants noted that they would benefit from joint training and continued check-ins.
- Participants also commented that they would benefit from a knowledge exchange professional who would be accessible for questions.

Overall learning:

- Time, space, and support are essential for collaboration to occur. All parties involved must understand the goals and share a common communication system that includes trust and value of one another's perspectives.
- Shared vision, a concrete plan, leadership support, ongoing knowledge exchange, and understanding the unique roles of each provider contributed to the overall success of the collaboration.

Source: McDougall & Servais, 2012.

Nine Critical Communication Skills

The picture exchange communication system (PECS) approach talks about nine critical communication skills that need to be the focus of communication, regardless of the modality used. "They are critical, because, if the student cannot calmly and effectively engage in each skill, then the student will most likely try other means to obtain the same outcome" (Frost & Bondy, 2002, p. 32). Often these other means may involve difficult or challenging behaviours. These nine skills are broken into two categories: expressive language (productive skills) and receptive language (receptive skills) (see Table 4.1). By learning these skills, individuals will get many of their needs met across the day, thus decreasing the likelihood of challenging behaviours.

Table 4.1: Nine Critical Communication Skills

Productive skills	Description	Receptive Skills	Description
1. Asking for reinforcers	This is one of the first steps of communication training and is highly reinforcing to the individual because it provides access to the desired item. It also provides access to things that are required in daily living.	6. Responding to "wait"	At times, the learner may not get to have what he or she requests immediately, or it is not available (e.g., dinner is being warmed up). Learning to wait and knowing that the desired item will come will help to decrease problematic behaviours.
2. Asking for help	Asking for assistance from others is especially important for those with ASD, as there are times they may need assistance in school, at home, and in the community. This will also help decrease frustration when they cannot do something on their own.	7. Responding to functional directions	Following directions can help with learning routines, avoiding danger, and getting what the individual wants.
3. Asking for a break	This enables individuals to appropriately escape a task when they may need a break. This is especially important for learners with ASD, who may not understand the socially appropriate way to do this. This can also decrease the learner's frustration when engaged in a difficult task.	8. Responding to transitional cues	Since individuals with ASD often have difficulty transitioning, understanding when a transition will occur and having advanced notice will help make it smooth. Using visuals, transition objects, or words, the learner can understand when a transition is occurring.

| 4. Rejecting | When asked "Do you want ____?", the individual is able to respond, "No." If he or she can do this in a socially appropriate way and does not get upset when given something or asked to do something he or she doesn't like or want, this will be appreciated much more by those around them. | | |
| 5. Affirming | When asked, "Do you want ____?", the individual can respond, "Yes." This allows others to know what the individual likes and allows him or her to calmly request an item instead of using an alternative challenging behaviour. | 9. Following a schedule | This will help learners understand the day's events and their expectations, and assist them with upcoming transitions. This is often done with visual supports/pictures in the environment, because they are constant and not fleeting, like verbal language. |

Source: Adapted from Frost & Bondy, 2002.

> **Read about it. Think about it. Write about it.**
>
> Brainstorm how you could teach each of the nine critical communication skills to an individual who is nonverbal.

AUGMENTATIVE AND ALTERNATIVE COMMUNICATION STRATEGIES

As mentioned earlier, communication does not have to involve speech, and some individuals must rely on augmentative and alternative communication (AAC) strategies in order to communicate. These involve using modalities other than speech to communicate. This can include using sign language, pictures, or an iPad with a communication board app. A major misconception persists that utilizing alternative communication devices inhibits speech development (ASHA, 2015; Frost & Bondy, 2002). Research has shown directly the opposite; many types of AAC actually promote the development of speech (ASHA, 2015).

The use of AAC strategies for individuals with ASD was found to have strong effects in increasing communication skills in individual studies (Ganz et al., 2012). However, in the *National Standards Project* (National Autism Center, 2015), it was found to be an emerging intervention. It is important to note that AAC has a long history of success with individuals with multiple disabilities; however, some differing results may arise due to the inclusion criteria for the studies and if individuals with ASD were the participants in the studies.

AAC has also had an effect on enhancing social skills, decreasing challenging behaviours, and increasing academic skills, although there is less research in this area (Ganz et al., 2012). In their review, Ganz and colleagues (2012) found that the use of PECS and speech-generating devices had

Augmentative and Alternative Communication Devices: Augmentative and alternative communication (AAC) is "the term used to describe methods of communication which can be used to add to the more usual methods of speech and writing when these methods are impaired. AAC includes unaided systems such as signing and gesture, as well as aided techniques ranging from picture charts to the most sophisticated computer technology. AAC can be a way to help someone understand, as well as a means of expression" (Ontario Ministry of Health and Long Term Care, 2011, p. 9).

the largest effects, with only small effects seen with other picture-based systems. Table 4.2 explains some of the different AAC modalities and the strengths and weaknesses of each.

Table 4.2: Communication Modalities for Augmentative and Alternative Communication

Modality	Pros	Cons
Speech	• Quick method to communicate message • Most common method of communicating for typically developing individuals • Does not require additional materials; available to the learner at all times	• Different languages can create barriers to communicating with other cultures • Cannot manipulate speech sounds to imitate when learning • May have negative associations for people trying to teach using verbal language and not being successful or accessing reinforcement • Many people with ASD may not have strong vocal cords due to not babbling or not imitating speech • Can take weeks or months to imitate basic sounds
Gestures	• Partially universal way of communicating • Many babies start with gestures to get what they want	• Not very accurate • One gesture can mean multiple things
Sign language	• If a person can imitate motor behaviours, they can learn sign • Easier to imitate hand movements than sounds	• Not everyone knows sign language • Difficult for those with motor planning/fine motor difficulties

Sign language con't	• Many signs are similar to the function in the environment (i.e., ball is signed with the shape of a ball) • Research demonstrates increases in speech associated with use of sign language • Does not require additional materials; available to the learner at all times	• Sign programs don't have full verbal repertoires • Requires caregivers and others close to the student to learn sign • Does not generalize well into the natural environment
Pictures	• People do not need to know another "language" to understand the learner • Research demonstrates increases in speech associated with the use of pictures to communicate • Inexpensive	• Can require much material preparation • If a new symbol is needed, it needs to be created • Difficult to portray some verbs with pictures • Requires carrying of boards or binders • Requires students to scan pictures • Same muscle movements associated with each word
a. Symbol/ picture boards	• One board usually made with multiple pictures over time • Can be used in combination with other high-tech systems • Can use universal items on the board, such as letters, to make sentences	• Requires matching to sample before they can be used to communicate • May be ambiguous if learner cannot point to a specific picture and uses open hand • Listeners need to be trained on how to use boards

b. PECS	• Focuses first on "how" to communicate before "what" to communicate • Involves direct interaction with listener through exchange of the picture	• Binder can get large and difficult to scan for pictures • Can take extra time to search for pictures, make sentence strips, and provide to a partner
Writing	• Can use sentences to communicate exactly what is meant • Requires few materials	• Difficult for those with motor planning difficulties • Must learn to spell as well • Slower method to communicate (unless using keyboard) • Not transferable across different languages
Speech-generating device	• Pictures are instantly available on devices by searching their databases, taking photos, using the Internet, etc. • The device speaks messages so others can easily understand • Increases amount, complexity, and clarity of speech the learner can communicate • Increases speed to deliver messages with programmed shortcuts • Can program touch functions to accommodate for motor planning difficulties	• Requires carrying of the device • Can pose technical difficulties, including no power, update requirements, broken devices, etc. • Requires fine motor and other skills to manipulate (i.e., swiping on an iPad) • Can be expensive

Sources: Frost & Bondy, 2002; Sundberg, 1990; Speech-Language Audiology Canada (SAC), 2014.

MOTIVATION TO COMMUNICATE

At times, it is suggested that a person with ASD has no motivation to communicate. It may seem like this because the person is able to get his or her wants and needs met without communicating (e.g., gets his or her own food, screeches to get the TV on, etc.). People in his or her environment may be very familiar with the individual's gestures and needs, so that the person does not need to communicate in a formal way (ASHA, 2015). Before starting communication interventions, it is important to understand what is reinforcing for the individual by completing a preference assessment (ASHA, 2015; Attainment Family, 2011). Making a list of the things the individual likes or accesses in her or his day will help to determine some of the first words to teach.

WHOM TO INVOLVE WHEN TEACHING LANGUAGE

Teaching language is a team effort. Often when we think of language development, we immediately think of speech-language pathologists, but in fact, in Ontario, the team is usually much larger (SAC, 2014). For individuals with ASD, who often present challenges other than just language impairments, such as cognitive, social, and motor difficulties, an interprofessional team is a must (SAC, 2014). In addition, the number of speech-language pathologists who have specific training in or experience with AAC is low compared to the incidence rate of the disorder (SAC, 2014). The use of a communication system should be based on the strengths and needs of the individual, and multiple people around the table can help support this.

An occupational therapist is often part of the team, as this professional

Speech-Language Pathologists: "Speech-language pathologists screen, assess, identify and treat speech, language, voice, fluency (stuttering), swallowing and feeding problems for all age groups in addition to advocating for the prevention of these disorders" (SAC, n.d., para. 5).

Occupational Therapists: "Occupational therapists use a systematic approach based on evidence and professional reasoning to enable individuals, groups and communities to develop the means and opportunities to identify, engage in and improve their function in the occupations of life. The process involves assessment, intervention and evaluation of the client related to occupational performance in self-care, work, study, volunteerism and leisure" (Canadian Association of Occupational Therapists, 2015, para. 4).

can assist in deciding what fine motor or motor planning considerations must be involved in choosing the method of communication, including any aids that may need to be prescribed (Ontario Ministry of Health and Long Term Care, 2011). Communication disorder assistants work under the direct supervision of a speech-language pathologist and carry out her or his goals (Communication Disorders Assistant Association of Canada [CDAAC], 2011). Behaviour analysts are also often part of this team in Ontario, as they are often trained in AAC strategies such as PECS and can provide detailed methods on how to teach communication to individuals with ASD and more severe cognitive delays by breaking language down into its verbal operants. Together this team guides the implementation and follow-through of the appropriate communication intervention.

EVIDENCE-BASED INTERVENTIONS

The interventions covered in this chapter are all considered evidence-based interventions according to the guidelines set by the Autism Evidence-Based Review Group (Wong et al., 2014). Because there are some discrepancies between this review and the *National Standards Project*'s (NAC, 2015) review, including the grouping of multiple interventions together, it will be noted when there is differing information. Each intervention focuses on teaching communication skills, but may have some overlap with other domains in the ASD diagnosis, most

Communication Disorder Assistants: "A Communication Disorder Assistant (CDA) is someone who works with a speech-language pathologist (SLP) or audiologist (AUD) to provide intervention to individuals with difficulties in the area of communication. CDAs do not work independently from an SLP or AUD. CDAs are trained to work in the areas of speech, language, augmentative communication and hearing with individuals of any age" (Communication Disorders Assistant Association of Canada, n.d., para. 1).

Behaviour Analyst: Behaviour analysts are clinicians who carry out work in applied behaviour analysis. A certified practitioner is called a board-certified behaviour analyst (BCBA). "The BCBA conducts descriptive and systematic behavioral assessments, including functional analyses, and provides behavior analytic interpretations of the results. The BCBA designs and supervises behavior analytic interventions. The BCBA is able to effectively develop and implement appropriate assessment and intervention methods for use in unfamiliar situations and for a range of cases" (Behavior Analyst Certification Board, n.d., para. 1). There are 339 BCBAs in Ontario and 24 at the doctoral level.

Box 4.2: The Ontario Assistive Devices Program

The Ontario Assistive Devices Program (ADP) is funded by the Ministry of Health and Long-Term Care for individuals in Ontario who are living with long-term physical challenges (Ontario Ministry of Health and Long-Term Care, 2014). The goal of the program is to help individuals achieve independence with assistive devices. There are over 8,000 pieces of equipment that are funded under the program, including wheelchairs, diabetes equipment, communication devices, and feeding supplies.

For the purpose of this chapter, AAC devices are covered under this program. In order to access AAC devices, individuals must go through authorized program providers, who are regulated health professionals registered with the ADP. These authorizers assess the need of the individual and recommend the particular device he or she needs to communicate most effectively, leading to the most independence. People accessing the program for the first time need to get a note indicating the communication need from a doctor or nurse practitioner. The equipment also needs to be purchased from vendors who are registered with the ADP. In most cases, the client will also need to pay for a portion of the device, although private insurance may cover these costs at times. When a high-technology speech-generating device is needed, a communication clinic must assess and approve the device. There is also an option to lease these high-technology devices from communication clinics.

The types of communication aides covered by the program include:

- electrolarynges
- communication boards
- mounting systems for communication aids
- teletypewriters
- voice amplifiers
- voice output communication aides
- voice prostheses
- writing aids

Source: Ontario Ministry of Health and Long-Term Care, 2014.

Note: A list of approved vendors for communication devices in Ontario can be found on the ADP website. To apply for the program by getting an assessment from an ADP registered authorizer, call 1-800-268-6021 to get a list of authorizers.

notably social skills, and may be appropriate to assist with other interventions (e.g., challenging behaviour). For instance, increasing an individual's functional communication ability will decrease challenging behaviours, as long as the individual can now communicate her or his wants and needs and it meets the same reinforcement as the challenging behaviour (Carr et al., 1997).

PECS

Frost and Bondy developed the Picture Exchange Communication System (PECS) in 1985 as a result of other modalities of communication not working for individuals with more severe forms of ASD and other social communication disorders (Frost & Bondy, 2002). Many of the children originally worked with were nonverbal and did not use functional communication. Since then, the system has been used with a variety of children to make speech more complex or assist with articulation. PECS has six sequential phases, teaching with the principles of applied behaviour analysis. PECS is considered an emerging intervention in the *National Standards Project's* review (NAC, 2015).

Picture Exchange Communication Systems (PECS): "Children using the Picture Exchange Communication System (PECS) learn to communicate first with single pictures, but later learn to combine pictures to learn a variety of grammatical structures, semantic relationships, and communicative functions" (Frost & Bondy, 2002, p. 47).

PECS is distinguished from other picture-based AAC strategies in that it uses picture symbols that are actually exchanged from the learner with ASD to the listener. In this manner, it teaches children how to communicate first, and the actual messages second (Frost & Bondy, 2002). The physical exchange of giving the picture symbol to another person mirrors the movement of the vocal message toward the communicative partner. The pictures are stored in a binder and, through various phases, are strategically placed on the front of the binder; as children learn to discriminate between the pictures, they are placed within the binder. Eventually the individual will flip through his or her binder, choose the symbol(s) he or she is communicating, place them on his or her communication strip, and hand the sentence to the communicative partner. See Table 4.3 for the phases of PECS.

One of the most significant misconceptions is that all laminated pictures with Velcro are PECS. It is important to note that picture symbols can be used for expressive language (as in the method of PECS), where the learner with ASD communicates to the listener, and in receptive language, where the communication

Table 4.3: The Six Phases of PECS

PECS Phase	Description
Phase I How to Communicate	This phase begins with two people: a communicative partner, and a physical prompter who sits behind the student. One picture is on the table. The communicative partner has something the child wants. The physical prompter prompts the learner from behind to pass the picture symbol to the communicative partner. The communicative partner provides the learner with what she or he requested. The physical prompt is faded. Terminal objective: "Upon seeing a 'highly preferred' item, the student will pick up a picture of the item, reach toward the communicative partner, and release the picture into the trainer's hand" (Frost & Bondy, 2002, p. 67).
Phase II Distance and Persistence	During this phase, the learner learns how to remove the picture from the front of their communication binder, travel to give the picture to the communicative partner, travel to go and get their binder, and use the picture for a variety of reinforcers in a variety of environments and activities. Terminal objective: "The student goes to his/her communication board, pulls the picture off, goes to the trainer, gets the trainer's attention, and releases the picture into the trainer's hand" (Frost & Bond, 2002, p. 93).
Phase III Picture Discrimination	Phase IIIa The learner learns to discriminate between and request one of two pictures on the front of their binder: a preferred item, and a distractor item that serves no interest to the learner (i.e., a sock or Kleenex). Phase IIIb The learner again requests one of two pictures on the front of the binder; however, both items are preferred. Terminal objective: "The student requests desired items by going to a communication book, selecting the appropriate picture from an array, going to a communication partner, and giving the picture" (Frost & Bondy, 2002, p. 123).

Phase IV Sentence Structure	The learner makes sentences using an "I want" symbol and eventually adds multiple items and attributes on the sentence strip. Terminal objective: "The student requests present and non-present items using a multi-word phrase by going to the book, picking up a picture/symbol of "I want," putting it on a sentence strip, picking out the picture of what is wanted, putting it on the sentence strip, removing the strip from the communication board, approaching the communicative partner, and giving the sentence strip to him" (Frost & Bondy, 2002, p. 159).
Phase V Responding to "What do you want?"	This phase focuses on learners answering the question, "What do you want?" Terminal objective: "The student spontaneously requests a variety of items and answers the question, 'What do you want?'" (Frost & Bondy, 2002, p. 209)
Phase VI Commenting	During this phase, learners first learn how to answer multiple questions, and then learn to comment in response to something in the environment. Terminal objective: "The student answers 'What do you want?' 'What do you see?' 'What do you have?' 'What do you hear?' and 'What is it?' and spontaneously requests and comments" (Frost & Bondy, 2002, p. 223).

Sources: Bondy & Frost, 1994; Frost & Bondy, 2002.

partner, teacher, or instructor communicates his or her message or expectations to the learner with ASD. PECS is an expressive language system, and the learner's PECS binder is not designed for others to communicate to her or him. Alternatively, when a visual schedule is used to communicate to the learner, this is a visual schedule with individual picture symbols.

For a detailed overview of the approach and each phase, see the National Professional Development Center on the ASD website for Intervention Steps: autismpdc.fpg.unc.edu/sites/autismpdc.fpg.unc.edu/files/PECS_Steps.pdf

There are numerous studies supporting the effectiveness of PECS, with four single-case research studies and two group designs in *Evidence-Based Practices for Children, Youth, and Young Adults with Autism Spectrum Disorder* (herein referred as the *EBI Report*) (Wong, 2013b; Wong et al., 2014). The *National Standards*

Project—Phase II report found that this was an emerging intervention; however, further details are not provided to explain the reasons for this discrepancy. Dogoe, Banda, and Lock (2010) found that three children with autism were able to acquire PECS and generalized the skill by making requests to others. Other research has demonstrated that PECS increases corresponding speech initiations and responses to communication. Carr and Felce (2007) found that 5 out of 24 children increased their communication acts, with no children decreasing in speech in comparison to the control group.

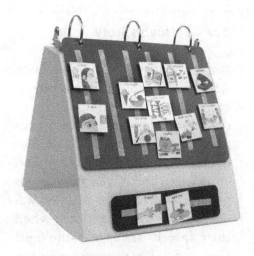

Figure 4.2: PECS Binder
Source: PECS-Canada, 2015.

Additional support was found when four individuals decreased their spoken words in the control group (Carr & Felce, 2007).

Read about it. Think about it. Write about it.

Go to YouTube and watch videos of individuals using PECS. What were your initial impressions? What are the benefits that you saw in the video? The drawbacks?

Discrete-Trial Training

Discrete-trial training (DTT) is a method of instruction in which there is usually one instructor with one learner, and single trials are usually done en masse, called massed trials (Wong et al., 2014). Each discrete trial is made of three components: 1) the instructor's instruction or discriminative stimulus; 2) the learner's response or lack of response; and 3) the instructor's response (either positive reinforcement for a correct answer or

Discrete Trial Training: "A behaviorally based type of teaching that breaks functional tasks into their smallest component behaviors and teaches/shapes these behaviors by providing a clearly delineated Stimulus-Response-Consequence contingency" (Gulick & Kitchen, 2007, p. 191).

Box 4.3: Noah's Story

When Noah was diagnosed with ASD at two and a half, his parents can remember him trying to communicate. He had no words and wanted to communicate, but instead was getting frustrated and crying on the kitchen floor as his parents tried to guess what he was asking for. At that time, when their speech-language pathologist suggested PECS, they were willing to try anything. He had lots of sounds, but they were not functional, and he did not babble like most children who are typically developing. Within weeks of starting PECS, Noah was making huge strides. He was passing pictures of what he wanted, and the frustration and crying lessened as he became able to communicate.

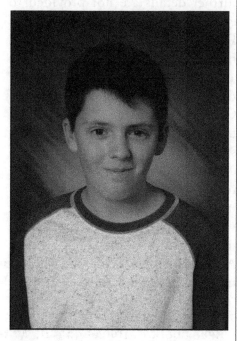

Figure 4.3: Noah

His speech-language pathologist said he was one of the quickest PECS learners she had seen. He soared through the phases, and his parents were thrilled. His mom remembers that the biggest change happened with the adults, who learned to make communication temptations throughout the house. They put things out of reach or in containers with snap locks so that he would need to request the item with his PECS. When intensive behaviour intervention started at age three, the number of opportunities to use his communication system throughout the day skyrocketed, and Noah became proficient. His mom says when going to bed at night she dreamt of the sound of Velcro as the sentence strip came off of his PECS book and was handed to whomever was in his sight: "He was so good at giving his sentence strip to all of our family members, and really picked up on generalizing it well."

His mom says she worried that he would become reliant on his PECS and not develop vocal communication: "I couldn't understand how it could increase speech, but I trusted the system." What came next was fascinating. Noah began to talk. He started to say "cookie," and sometimes he got many cookies a day because his caregivers were so excited that he was talking and requesting. They remember sitting in the garage in the car turning the lights on and off as he said the words, and stopping and going while driving as he requested with words! The words continued to come, and when he hit kindergarten he was still using his PECS book, but was gaining more and more words. His mom remembers it being such a positive experience for their family, as it was portable, inexpensive, and easy to do. She has kept his PECS book to this day to remember the change that it brought to the family.

Today Noah is a Grade 8 student who is looking forward to high school. Although he doesn't remember using PECS, he remembers his IBI team fondly. He is fully verbal, carrying on a conversation as any adolescent boy would. When asked what he is excited for, he tells me about his upcoming summer plans at Camp Kodiak, near Parry Sound, Ontario, a camp designed to build self-esteem, confidence, and social skills in campers (Camp Kodiak, n.d.). He speaks of his future plans as well, saying he isn't sure which university he will go to in Ontario, but thinks he may even attend Queen's University in Kingston. He said he is also curious to travel the world, hoping to potentially get a job in travel or working with animals. From a learner who struggled with communication, to utilizing an AAC device, Noah has truly overcome communication challenges in his life!

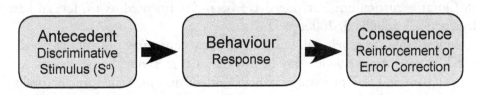

Figure 4.4: Three-Term Contingency

error correction for an incorrect answer) (Lovaas Institute, 2007). This is ultimately the three-term contingency that Skinner described in his operant conditioning of the antecedent, behaviour, and consequence (Skinner, 1948). The trial is often completed quickly to ensure that the least amount of time occurs between each of these variables. Repetition of this sequence occurs consistently for individuals who may need basic structure to learn language and other skills while breaking the skill down.

Using DTT for individuals with ASD and other developmental disabilities is beneficial because: 1) the instruction is learned with a consistent discriminative stimulus each time; 2) the consequence is immediate after the learner's response, letting him or her know if the response was accurate (differing from traditional work, where it may be marked after a number of questions or days); 3) it is consistent for each learning trial and prevents the learner from becoming confused with large amounts of unknown language when beginning to learn; and 4) it allows for easy data collection that demonstrates whether progress is being made (Lovaas, 2003). Because individuals with ASD may have shorter attention spans, are not as socially motivated to learn due to deficits in social skills, have difficulty with abstract concepts, and may have cognitive delays, these short units, or trials, of teaching are very appropriate (de Rivera, 2008). Although DTT training methods are not universally accepted or used, and are criticized for possibly not producing generalization of the skills to the natural environment, DTT is often a first step to teach learners "how to learn" and attain basic receptive and expressive language skills in order to go on and develop more complex language and social skills (Lovaas, 2003).

Discrete trial training is done to teach many different skills, including language, and has been shown to be effective for teaching preschoolers (ages 3–5) and elementary-aged children (age 6–11) with ASD "social, communication, behavior, joint attention, school-readiness, academic, adaptive, and vocational skills" (Fleury, 2013, para. 4). In most early intervention and intensive behaviour intervention programs in Ontario, language is a major component of teaching DTT. "Some specific instructional programs within our school systems also employ DTI/ DTT methodology. These programs are not widespread nor are they mandated in Ontario curriculum but they have been documented as evidenced-based instruction" (Lindbald, 2006, p. 7).

In Ontario, the provincially funded IBI programs carry out varying levels of DTT as part of their wide array of instructional methods. Some programs are more reliant on DTT procedures, whereas others may focus on more naturalistic teaching methodologies. For example, the Toronto Partnership for Autism Services began using this DTT approach, but has since moved to a natural language paradigm, in which language is taught in natural settings when the individual initiates interaction with an item (de Rivera, 2008). The method of teaching can also vary within each program across different types of learners and depending on what skills are being taught. Currently, the Ontario IBI program is called the Autism Intervention Program and is mandated to be based on the principles of ABA, not necessarily on specific types of teaching procedures, such as DTT; it can be done individually or in small groups, and is customized for the individual to gain independence (Ontario Ministry of Children and Youth Services, 2011).

Discrete trial training is considered an evidence-based intervention in the *EBI Report*, with 13 single-case research studies demonstrating its effectiveness for individuals ages 3 to 11 with ASD, and is grouped under behavioural interventions in the *National Standards Project*'s report (NAC, 2015; Wong et al., 2014). Smith (2001) indicates that research is still needed to determine what amount of DTT and natural teaching strategies are effective for individuals with ASD. One of the

Table 4.4: Some Advantages and Disadvantages of DTT

Advantages of DTT	Disadvantages of DTT
• Allows for numerous training trials	• Requires additional procedures to promote generalization
• Easy for many different staff to use	• Prompts to respond often not present in natural settings
• Good way to develop specific language skills	• Primarily a teacher-directed activity
• Ease of use in a classroom setting	• Immediate and powerful reinforcers often not available outside of the training session
• Instructional stimuli and detailed curriculum provided to staff	• The drill nature of the training may generate rote responding
• Target responses are known and easily identified	• Nonfunctional nature of the training may generate escape and avoidance behaviors
• Contrived consequence is often readily available and easy to deliver	• The interaction between the speaker and the listener is very different from that observed by typical speakers and listeners
• Data collection is relatively straightforward	
• Progressive steps in the curriculum clearly delineated	
• Progress or lack thereof is measurable	
• May help to establish "ready to learn" behaviors (e.g., attend to teacher, expectation of reinforcement for correct response, ability to make discriminations, learns to sit and "work," acquires an increased tolerance of demands)	

Source: Steege, Mace, Perry, & Longnecker, 2007, p. 96.

downfalls is the specific training required for instructors to become proficient in this type of intervention (Smith, 2001). In one study, undergraduate students were able to increase skills in carrying out DTT procedures after an eight-hour training; however, even with practice and feedback during implementation, much variability continued to occur across individuals, demonstrating the continued training and feedback that is needed (Downs & Downs, 2013). In Ontario, in response to the training needed for individuals to work in IBI programs, the

Autism and Behavioural Graduate Certificate Program was created in 2005 with the Ministry of Training, Colleges, and Universities for individuals interested in the field (Ontario Ministry of Children & Youth Services, 2006).

Naturalistic Interventions

Naturalistic interventions are a group of interventions based on ABA principles, also called milieu teaching, incidental teaching, natural environment training, and natural language paradigm. In contrast to DTT procedures, naturalistic interventions wait for appropriate situations to naturally arrive in the environment or set the stage for them in the natural environment in order to teach the skill. The goal is that generalization is targeted from the beginning, rather than facing difficulties with generalization after the skill is learned in a highly structured manner such as DTT (Smith, 2001). Like DTT, naturalistic interventions can be used to teach any skill, although there is a large body of literature that focuses on teaching language skills by letting the learner have an intent to communicate, providing effective teaching by modelling and prompting, and then reinforcing when the learner completes the communication attempt successfully (Hancock & Kaiser, 2002).

> **Naturalistic Interventions:** Naturalistic interventions include "a variety of strategies that closely resemble typical interactions and occur in natural settings, routines and activities" (Odom, Collet-Klingenberg, Rogers, & Hatton, 2010, p. 278).

For example, when an individual is playing with a train on the ground, he is showing motivation to play with the train. One of the trains is out of reach. As he goes to get it, the teacher holds it up and waits for a predetermined time delay for him to say the word "train." If he does not say it, the teacher says the sound "t," and if he says "train," the teacher naturally reinforces him by giving him the train (Charlop-Christy & Carpenter, 2000). Clinicians and researchers often turn to naturalistic interventions because they have greater generalization; however, it may take longer for the individual to learn the skill because the instruction may not be as consistent during each trial, or the trials may not appear as frequently in the naturally occurring settings (Charlop-Christy & Carpenter, 2000).

> **Time Delay:** "The addition of a brief period of time between the [discriminative stimulus], and the prompt [which] challenges the child to eventually respond *before* the prompt is delivered—providing the instructor with a very effective prompt-fading method" (Gulick & Kitchen, 2007, p. 207).

Table 4.5: Differences between Analog and Naturalistic Conditions

	Analog	Naturalistic
Stimulus items	• Chosen by clinician • Pictures/photographs containing target sounds	• Chosen by child • Objects and toys containing target sounds • Selection of items of high interest to child
Steps	• Begin with sounds in isolation; drill until mastered • Sounds presented sequentially in words, phrases, and sentences; drill until mastered at each level	• Begin with word production of item • Productions are immediately embedded in words, phrases, and sentences in naturalistic conversational play interactions until mastered
Interaction	• Clinician models sound production • Direct feedback (e.g., motor placement cues)	• Clinician models word following child attempts • Clinician and child naturally (play) interact with stimulus items
Response-reinforcer contingency	• Child verbally reinforced for production of correct responses in a shaping paradigm, with successive approximations reinforced, and feedback provided for motor placement	• A broad shaping contingency employed so that both correct responses and verbal attempts are reinforced, and includes a correct model of the target sound
Consequences	• Social reinforcers, desired objects, and edible reinforcers	• Social reinforcers, and natural reinforcers (e.g., opportunity to play with stimulus item)

Source: Koegel et al., 1998, p. 244.

Box 4.4: Sabotaging the Environment, or Communication Temptations

An easy way to teach language in a naturalistic approach is by adapting the environment so individuals need to request items. This can be done in any situation in the school, home, or community, and it is desirable because it is based on naturally occurring situations. When trying to increase language, parents or teachers may say, "He gets everything on his own, so he doesn't really need to ask for it." Although there is always a goal of balancing independence and language, when language is the goal, sometimes the environment needs to be sabotaged to give the individual the opportunity to practice language targets as much as possible. In this situation, the access to the item that the person wants or needs to do a routine (e.g., a lunch bag to eat lunch, sugar for coffee) is contingent upon her or him asking for the item (Mancil, 2009). This not only increases the desire to communicate, but can also assist with increasing spontaneity, and makes it fun for the individual (Leaf & McEachin, 1999).

The environment can be changed by, for example, putting the lunch bag out of reach, or putting the sugar in a container that the person cannot open on his or her own. Prompts are provided when needed, and the goal is to fade these prompts (Mancil, 2009). The item is then given when it is requested. The goal is not to make the learner upset or mad, and diligence must be taken to provide a little frustration without annoying the learner or leading her or him to experience a communication failure (Teach Me to Talk, 2008). Depending on the type of communication modality, the student can use words, exchange pictures, or use his or her speech generating device. When working on language, articulation can be a separate goal, and the behaviour can be shaped (Leaf & McEachin, 1999). In order for the child to succeed in communication, the teacher is urged to be thoughtful when using these techniques. Techniques such as being right there to help the learner and not changing things in a way that will cause detrimental influences (for instance, changing the environment so that the learner cannot get out to recess on time to play with friends) are encouraged. Teach Me to Talk (2008) provides five strategies to create slight frustration to help learners communicate, without creating failure:

1. Approach the situation with a fun attitude, rather than thinking, "I am going to make you ask for this or else!"
2. Hold out for your intended word, sign, or gesture only three to five times.
3. If the child gives you a word or an attempt that is acceptable, but not perfect, reward the effort.
4. Don't overuse sabotage so that she feels like she shouldn't even try.
5. Use true withholding only for words or signs the learners can already say or do on their own.

Research studies have demonstrated that this is an effective intervention for ages 0 to 11, and it was found to be effective for teaching social, communication, behaviour, joint attention, play, and academic skills (Wong, 2013a; Wong et al., 2014). This is also an EBI in *National Standards Project—Phase II* (NAC, 2015). Hancock & Kaiser (2002) demonstrated that four individuals with ASD were able to increase their targeted communication skills after a natural teaching procedure, and this increase was retained six months later. Three of the children generalized this increase in language skill to the home environment. Koegel, Camarata, Koegel, Ben-Tall, and Smith (1998) found that when comparing a naturalistic intervention with a more structured approach of discrete trial training, both conditions demonstrated increases in the pronunciation of speech; however, the naturalistic intervention demonstrated more functional speech improvement. Charlop-Christy and Carpenter (2000) found that a modified incidental teaching approach, combining aspects of naturalistic interventions and DTT, produced better outcomes and generalization for incidental speech in a home environment.

> **Read about it. Think about it. Write about it.**
>
> What are the most difficult aspects of implementing naturalistic interventions? How can you overcome these barriers?

Pivotal Response Training

Pivotal response training is an ABA-based naturalistic intervention that focuses on teaching pivotal behaviours in order to enhance the communication, complexity of communication, play, and social skills of individuals with ASD (Wong, 2013c). The training is based on the idea that teaching key pivotal skills to individuals with ASD helps them learn foundational skills that can then facilitate the generalization and learning of other skills in the environment (Koegel, Koegel, & Brookman, 2003; Wong, 2013c). These skills have a significant impact on other areas and can often influence and effect change in untargeted skills (Verschuur, Didden, Lang, Sigafoos, & Huskens, 2014). The intervention is taught in natural, inclusive settings and involves parents as a large component to increase independence and self-learning for the individual (Koegel et al., 2003). The four pivotal skills that are taught in the approach are: (a) motivation; (b) self-initiation; (c) self-management; and (d) responding to multiple cues (Verschuur et al., 2014). One example of using the approach to teach self-initiation involves teaching "Wh" questions in the natural environment.

This approach is effective for learners aged 0 to 14, as outlined in the *EBI Report* and the *National Standards Project* (NAC, 2015; Wong, 2013c). In a review of the research, most studies examining pivotal skills looked at self-initiation, showing

---

Box 4.5: Teaching "What Is It?"

Choose items that are highly motivating to the learner with ASD and put them in a paper bag. Shake the bag to get the learner's attention.

1. When the child looks to the bag, the instructor prompts the child to say, "What is it?"
2. The child says, "What is it?"
3. The instructor opens the bag and pulls out the item.
4. The instructor says, "It's a (name of toy)."
5. The child is prompted to label the item as well.

Source: Adapted from Koegel et al., 2003.

---

that this intervention was successful in teaching collateral skills such as language and communication, social skills, and play, and helped decrease challenging behaviours (Verschuur et al., 2014). The research to date is inconclusive on the question of whether other skills, such as academic, life, and cognitive skills, improve as a result of teaching these pivotal skills (Verschuur et al., 2014).

Functional Communication Training

Functional communication training (FCT) involves teaching an individual to effectively and appropriately communicate to replace challenging behaviour that serves the same function (Carr & Durand, 1985; Fettig, 2013). It is thought that individuals who have less sophisticated communication skills use challenging behaviours instead of communication to attain reinforcers (Carr et al., 1997). By teaching the individual to communicate how to gain access to these reinforcers with FCT, the new, more appropriate behaviour still meets the same function, and the problem behaviour decreases or is eliminated (Carr et al., 1997). For example, if the individual is falling to the floor and screaming during math period, when he is required to concentrate for a long period of time, it may be that he is trying to escape the math. By learning to ask for a break when he gets overwhelmed, he has learned an appropriate way to communicate.

Usually FCT begins with a functional assessment to determine the function of the problem behaviour (escape, attention, tangible, or sensory), and a communication skill is then identified that will serve this same function (Fettig, 2013). The communication skill is taught and reinforcement is provided with this new skill. In contrast, the problem behaviour is put on extinction, meaning the individual is

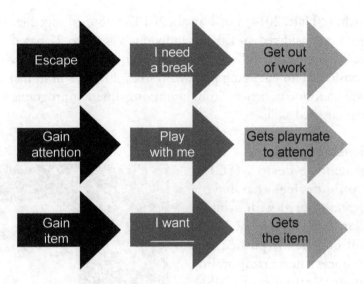

Figure 4.5: Functional Communication Training.
Source: Autism Classroom News, n.d.

no longer reinforced for the problem behaviour (Carr et al., 1997; Fettig, 2013).

Functional communication training is considered an evidence-based intervention, with 12 single-case research studies demonstrating its effectiveness in the *EBI Report*, and is listed under behavioural interventions in the *National Standards Project* (Fettig, 2013; NAC, 2015). "FCT can be used effectively to address social, communication, behavior, play, school-readiness, and adaptive outcomes" (Fettig, 2013, para. 4). In one study, FCT was effective in reducing problem behaviour for five participants, and it was found that when reinforcement for new communicative acts was decreased or thinned, problem behaviour came back (Volkert, Lerman, Call, & Trosclair-Lasserre, 2009).

Technology-Aided Instruction

Technology-aided instructions are a class of interventions that rely on different technologies as the primary teaching mechanisms for individuals with ASD to learn new skills (Odom, 2013). This can include learning social skills, using devices to communicate, learning academic and vocational skills, increasing joint attention, and decreasing problem behaviours (Odom, 2013). Technology in this context is defined as an "electronic item/equipment, application, or virtual network that is used to intentionally increase, maintain, and/or improve daily living, work/productivity, and recreation/leisure capabilities of adolescents with Autism Spectrum Disorder" (Odom et al., 2014, p. 2). Because of the popularity and cost-effectiveness of devices such as iPads and smartphones, technology is more widely available to classrooms and individual families than ever before

(Hall, Maich, & Hatt, 2014; Lorah et al., 2013). Grouped together, this class of interventions is considered an EBI for individuals age 3 to 22 based on 9 group designs and 11 single-case studies (Odom, 2013). In the *National Standards Project,* this was considered an emerging practice (NAC, 2015). Still in its infancy, this research will continue to benefit from examining different programs and devices for different targeted skills.

Speech-Generating Devices

Speech-generating devices (SGDs) are electronic devices that have a communication board with symbols or letters on a visual display. When the symbol or letter is pushed, the device produces the corresponding speech output (Sigafoos et al., 2011). The advancement of mobile devices and low-cost, user-friendly technology has allowed families to purchase these on the iPad (SAC, 2014). For instance, the iPad supports numerous purchasable apps that are SGDs, such

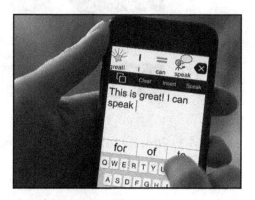

Figure 4.6: Proloquo2Go
Source: AssistiveWare, 2014.

as Proloquo2Go (AssistiveWare, 2014). Although the cost-effectiveness of the apps has allowed more children access, the limitation is that speech-language pathologists and other professionals are not always involved in helping decide which device is appropriate for each child based on his or her skills (SAC, 2014).

SGDs are effective communication devices as the production of speech helps individuals with ASD communicate more naturally to listeners, and helps others to understand the speech output by the computer without requiring additional knowledge, like sign language (Sigafoos et al., 2011). In addition, symbols can be programmed so that they produce a proper sentence (such as, "Could you please pass the butter?" [Sigafoos et al., 2011]) The use of SGDs for communicating and thus increasing social skills is an EBI in the *EBI Report,* and is a subcategory in the AAC intervention in the *National Standards Project,* which is considered an emerging intervention (NAC, 2015; Odom, 2013).

Technology for Other Skills

Technology and computers have also been successful in teaching "social, communication, behavior, joint attention, cognitive, school-readiness, academic, motor, adaptive, and vocational skills" (Odom, 2013, para. 4). For instance, computer software that allows individuals to learn how to differentiate between faces was successful in enhancing facial recognition (Faja, Aylward, Bernier, & Dawson, 2007). Another study demonstrated that watching an animated children's TV series could increase emotional understanding and emotion recognition in a group of children with ASD (Golan et al., 2010). In addition, the independent completion of tasks and routines increased with the use of digital assistants, computer programming, and iPads (Hall, Maich, & Hatt, 2014; Mechling, Gast, & Cronin, 2006; Mechling, Gast, & Seid, 2009; Mechling & Savidge, 2011). The field of utilizing technology to teach skills continues to build for individuals with ASD, with support appearing regularly in the literature.

> **Read about it. Think about it. Write about it.**
>
> Research two different technology-based instructional aides used with individuals with ASD. Describe how they are beneficial and the research to support them.

A LOOK BACK

Chapter 4, "Communication-Based Interventions," focused on:
- The receptive and expressive language difficulties that individuals with ASD face;
- An overview of functional communication, nine critical communication skills, and augmentative and alternative communication (AAC);
- Who is involved in the process and how to receive communication supports in Ontario; and
- Interventions to teach communication, including Picture Exchange Communication System (PECS), naturalistic interventions, pivotal response training (PRT), functional communication training (FCT), and technology-aided instruction.

A LOOK AHEAD

Chapter 5, "Social Skills Interventions," focuses on:
- The social skill characteristics of individuals with ASD, including skill and performance deficits and types of social skills;
- How to assess social skills and teach them in the natural versus contrived environment; and
- Strategies to teach social skills, including cognitive behavioural interventions, modelling, video modelling, peer-mediated instruction, prompting, scripting, social narrative, social skills training, and structured play groups.

ADDITIONAL RESOURCES

- Augmentative & Alternative Communication Applications (Garcia, 2012):
  http://autismontario.novosolutions.net/default.asp?id=83&Lang=1&SID=
- Communication Access for People Who Have Communication Disabilities (Ontario Ministry of Community and Social Services, 2009):
  http://www.mcss.gov.on.ca/documents/en/mcss/accessibility/Developing Standards/Communication_Access_ENG_no_ack.pdf
- Discrete Trial Training (Educate Autism, 2015):
  http://www.educateautism.com/applied-behaviour-analysis/discrete-trial-training.html
- Evidence-Based Practices Module Brief (National Professional Development Center for ASD, 2013):
  http://autismpdc.fpg.unc.edu/node/19
- Fact Sheets for Evidence-Based Practices (National Professional Development Center for ASD, 2013):
  http://autismpdc.fpg.unc.edu/evidence-based-practices
- Functional Communication Training (Grand Valley State University, n.d.):
  https://www.gvsu.edu/cms3/assets/.../functional_communication.docx
- Koegel Autism: Pivotal Response Treatment (PRT) Training and Services:
  http://www.autismprthelp.com/about-prt.php
- Communication aides: Policy and administration manual: Assistive devices program (Ontario Ministry of Health and Long Term Care, 2011):
  www.health.gov.on.ca/en/pro/programs/adp/information_technology/docs/communication_aids_manual.pdf
- Picture Exchange Communication System (PECS) (PECS Canada, 2015):
  http://autismpdc.fpg.unc.edu/node/19
- PECS Canada: Downloads:
  http://www.pecs-canada.com/downloads.php
- PECS Canada: Research:
  http://www.pecs-canada.com/research.php
- Proloquo2Go:
  http://www.assistiveware.com/product/proloquo2go
- Proloquo2Go e-Learning Videos:
  http://www.assistiveware.com/e-learning
- SAC position paper on the role of speech-language pathologists with respect to augmentative and alternative communication (Speech-Language Audiology Canada, 2014):
  sac-oac.ca/sites/default/files/resources/AAC_PP_EN.pdf

REFERENCES

American Psychiatric Association. (2013). *Diagnostic and statistical manual: DSM-5* (5th ed.). Washington, DC: Author.

American Speech-Language-Hearing Association. (2015). Communication services and supports for individuals with severe disabilities: FAQs. Retrieved from www.asha.org/NJC/faqs-comm-dev.htm

AssistiveWare. (2014). Proloquo2Go. www.assistiveware.com/product/proloquo2go

Attainment Family. (2011). Teaching communication skills to children with autism. Retrieved from www.attainmentfamily.com/category/parent-resources

Autism Classroom News. (n.d.). Functional communication training: Why it's more than just "Use Your Words." Retrieved from www.autismclassroomnews.com/2014/09/functional-communication-training-why.html

Behavior Analyst Certification Board. (n.d.). About BACB credentials. Retrieved from www.bacb.com/index.php?page=4

Bennett, T. A., Szatmari, P., Georgiades, K., Hanna, S., Janus, M., Georgiades, S., ... Thompson, A. (2014). Language impairment and early social competence in preschoolers with Autism Spectrum Disorder: A comparison of DSM-5 profiles. *Journal of Autism and Developmental Disorders, 44*(11), 1–12. doi: 10.1007/s10803-014-2138-2

Bondy, A. S., & Frost, L. A. (1994). The picture exchange communication system. *Focus on Autism and Other Developmental Disabilities, 9*(3), 1–19.

Camp Kodiak. (n.d.). Camp Kodiak: A place to grow. Retrieved from http://www.campkodiak.com

Canadian Association of Occupational Therapists. (2015). What is occupational therapy? Retrieved from www.caot.ca/default.asp?pageID=3824

Carr, E. G., & Durand, V. M. (1985). Reducing behavior problems through functional communication training. *Journal of Applied Behavior Analysis, 18*(2), 111–126.

Carr, D., & Felce, J. (2007). Brief report: Increase in production of spoken words in some children with autism after PECS teaching to phase III. *Journal of Autism and Developmental Disorders, 37*(4), 780–787.

Carr, E. G., Levin, L., McConnachie, G., Carlson, J. I., Kemp, D. C., & Smith, C. E. (1997). *Communication-based intervention for problem behavior: A user's guide for producing positive change.* Baltimore, MD: Paul H. Brookes.

Charlop-Christy, M. H., & Carpenter, M. H. (2000). Modified incidental teaching sessions: A procedure for parents to increase spontaneous speech in their children with autism. *Journal of Positive Behavior Interventions, 2*(2), 98–112.

Communication Disorders Assistant Association of Canada. (n.d.). Frequently asked questions. Retrieved from http://www.cdaac.ca/faq.htm

Communication Disorders Assistant Association of Canada. (2011). Scope of practice of a communicative disorders assistant. Retrieved from www.cdaac.ca/scope-of-practice-documents.htm

Community Living Ontario. (2015). What is an intellectual disability? Retrieved from www.communitylivingontario.ca/about-us/what-intellectual-disability

de Rivera, C. (2008). The use of intensive behavioural intervention for children with autism. *Journal on Developmental Disabilities, 14*(2), 1–15.

Dogoe, M. S., Banda, D. R., & Lock, R. H. (2010). Acquisition and generalization of the Picture Exchange Communication System behaviors across settings, persons, and stimulus classes with three students with autism. *Education and Training in Autism and Development Disabilities*, *45*(2), 216–229.

Downs, A., & Downs, R. C. (2013). Training new instructors to implement discrete trial teaching strategies with children with autism in a community-based intervention program. *Focus on Autism and Other Developmental Disabilities*, *28*(4), 212–221.

Durand, V. M., & Carr, E. G. (1991). Functional communication training to reduce challenging behavior: Maintenance and application in new settings. *Journal of Applied Behavior Analysis*, *24*(2), 251–264.

Faja, S., Aylward, E., Bernier, R., & Dawson, G. (2007). Becoming a face expert: A computerized face-training program for high-functioning individuals with Autism Spectrum Disorder. *Developmental neuropsychology*, *33*(1), 1–24.

Fettig, A. (2013). *Functional communication training (FCT) fact sheet*. Chapel Hill: The University of North Carolina, Frank Porter Graham Child Development Institute, The National Professional Development Center on Autism Spectrum Disorder.

Fleury, V. P. (2013). *Discrete trial teaching (DTT) fact sheet*. Chapel Hill: The University of North Carolina, Frank Porter Graham Child Development Institute, The National Professional Development Center on Autism Spectrum Disorder.

Frost, L., & Bondy, A. (2002). *The picture exchange communication system: Training manual* (2nd ed.). Etobikoe, ON: Pyramid.

Ganz, J. B., Earles-Vollrath, T. L., Heath, A. K., Parker, R. I., Rispoli, M. J., & Duran, J. B. (2012). A meta-analysis of single case research studies on aided augmentative and alternative communication systems with individuals with Autism Spectrum Disorder. *Journal of autism and developmental disorders*, *42*(1), 60–74.

Golan, O., Ashwin, E., Granader, Y., McClintock, S., Day, K., Leggett, V., & Baron-Cohen, S. (2010). Enhancing emotion recognition in children with autism spectrum conditions: An intervention using animated vehicles with real emotional faces. *Journal of autism and developmental disorders*, *40*(3), 269–279.

Grow, L. (2011, October 14). *Teaching receptive language skills to young children with asd: past, present, and future*. Presented at UBC Centre for Interdisciplinary Research and Collaboration in Autism. Retrieved from http://circa.educ.ubc.ca/sites/circa.educ.ubc.ca/files/Laura%20 Grow%20CIRCA%20presentation%20Oct%2014_0.pdf

Gulick, R. F., & Kitchen, T. P. (2007). *Effective instruction for children with autism: An applied behavior analytic approach*. Erie, PA: The Dr. Gertrude A. Barber National Institute.

Hall, C., Maich, K., & Hatt, A. (2014). Using a photographic electronic activity schedule to decrease latency in transition time for a nine-year-old girl with an autism spectrum disorder. *DADD Online Journal*, *1*(1), 91–102.

Hancock, T. B., & Kaiser, A. P. (2002). The effects of trainer-implemented enhanced milieu teaching on the social communication of children with autism. *Topics in Early Childhood Special Education*, *22*(1), 39–54.

Hudry, K., Leadbitter, K., Temple, K., Slonims, V., McConachie, H., Aldred, C., ... Charman, T. (2010). Preschoolers with autism show greater impairment in receptive compared with expressive language abilities. *International Journal of Language & Communication Disorders*, *45*(6), 681–690.

Jahr, E. (2001). Teaching children with autism to answer novel wh-questions by utilizing a multiple exemplar strategy. *Research in Developmental Disabilities*, *22*(5), 407–423. doi:10.1016/S0891-4222(01)00081-6

Kasari, C., Paparella, T., Freeman, S. N., & Jahromi, L. (2008). Language outcome in autism: Randomized comparison of joint attention and play interventions. *Journal of Consulting and Clinical Psychology, 76*, 125–137. doi:10.1037/0022-006X.76.1.125

Koegel, R. L., Camarata, S., Koegel, L. K., Ben-Tall, A., & Smith, A. E. (1998). Increasing speech intelligibility in children with autism. *Journal of Autism and Developmental Disorders, 28*(3), 241-251.

Koegel, R. L., Koegel, L. K., & Brookman, L. I. (2003). Empirically supported pivotal response interventions for children with autism. In A. E. Kazdin (Ed.), *Evidence-based psychotherapies for children and adolescents: Evidence-based psychotherapies for children and adolescents* (pp. 341–357). New York, NY: Guilford Press.

Kover, S. T., McDuffie, A. S., Hagerman, R. J., & Abbeduto, L. (2013). Receptive vocabulary in boys with autism spectrum disorder: Cross-sectional developmental trajectories. *Journal of Autism and Developmental Disorders, 43*(11), 2696–2709. doi:10.1007/s10803-013-1823-x

Leaf, R., & McEachin, J. (1999). *A work in progress: Behavior management strategies and a curriculum for intensive behavioral treatment of autism.* New York, NY: DRL Books.

Levis, J. M. (1999). Intonation in theory and practice. *TESOL Quarterly, 33*(1), 37–63. doi:10.2307/3588190

Lindbald. (2006). ABA in schools: Essential or optional? Retrieved from www.autismontario. com/Client/ASO/ABA.nsf/object/ABA+in+School+full+article+edited/$file/ABA+in+School+full+article+edited.pdf

Lorah, E. R., Tincani, M., Dodge, J., Gilroy, S., Hickey, A., & Hantula, D. (2013). Evaluating picture exchange and the iPad™ as a speech generating device to teach communication to young children with autism. *Journal of Developmental and Physical Disabilities, 25*(6), 637–649.

Lovaas Institute. (2007). Why discrete trials work. Retrieved from www.lovaas.com/meetingpoint-2007-09-article-04.php

Lovaas, O. I. (2003). *Teaching individuals with developmental delays: Basic intervention techniques.* Austin, TX: PRO-ED.

Mancil, G. R. (2009). Milieu therapy as a communication intervention: A review of the literature related to children with autism spectrum disorder. *Education and Training in Developmental Disabilities, 44*(1), 105.

McDougall, S., & Servais, M. (2012). AAC and autism service providers collaborating for communication: An evaluation of a knowledge exchange framework. *Facts To Go, 8*(3). London, ON: Thames Valley Children's Centre.

Mechling, L. C., Gast, D. L., & Cronin, B. A. (2006). The effects of presenting high-preference items, paired with choice, via computer-based video programming on task completion of students with autism. *Focus on Autism and Other Developmental Disabilities, 21*(1), 7–13. doi: 10.1177/10883576060210010201

Mechling, L. C., Gast, D. L., & Seid, N. H. (2009). Using a personal digital assistant to increase independent task completion by students with autism spectrum disorder. *Journal of Autism and Developmental Disorders, 39*(10), 1420–1434. doi:10.1007/s10803-009-0761-0

Mechling, L. C., & Savidge, E. J. (2011). Using a personal digital assistant to increase completion of novel tasks and independent transitioning by students with autism spectrum disorder. *Journal of Autism and Developmental Disorders, 41*(6), 687–704. doi:10.1007/s10803-010-1088-6

National Autism Center. (2015). Findings and conclusions, national standards project, phase 2. Retrieved from http://www.nationalautismcenter.org/national-standards-project/

Odom, S. L. (2013). *Technology-aided instruction and intervention (TAII) fact sheet.* Chapel Hill: The University of North Carolina, Frank Porter Graham Child Development Institute, The National Professional Development Center on Autism Spectrum Disorder.

Odom, S. L., Collet-Klingenberg, L., Rogers, S. J., & Hatton, D. D. (2010). Evidence-based practices in interventions for children and youth with Autism Spectrum Disorder. *Preventing School Failure: Alternative Education for Children and Youth, 54*(4), 275–282.

Odom, S. L., Thompson, J. L., Hedges, S., Boyd, B. A., Dykstra, J. R., Duda, M. A., ... Bord, A. (2014). Technology-aided interventions and instruction for adolescents with autism spectrum disorder. *Journal of Autism and Developmental Disorders, 45*(12), 1–15.

Ontario Ministry of Children & Youth Services. (2006). McGuinty government committed to helping children and youth with autism [Press release]. Retrieved from news.ontario.ca/archive/en/2006/07/07/McGuinty-Government-Committed-to-Helping-Children-and-Youth-with-Autism.html

Ontario Ministry of Children & Youth Services. (2011). Autism intervention program guidelines. Retrieved from www.children.gov.on.ca/htdocs/English/topics/specialneeds /autism/aip_guidelines.aspx

Ontario Ministry of Health and Long-Term Care. (2011). Communication aides: Policy and administration manual: Assistive devices program. Retrieved from www.health.gov.on.ca/en/pro/programs/adp/information_technology/docs/communication_aids_manual.pdf

Ontario Ministry of Health and Long-Term Care. (2014). Assistive devices. Retrieved from http://www.health.gov.on.ca/en/public/programs/adp/

PECS-Canada. (2015). Large communication book. Retrieved from www.pecs-canada.com/catalog/product_info.php?cPath=24&products_id=52

Prizant, B. M. (1983). Echolalia in autism: Assessment and intervention. *Seminars in Speech and Language, 4*(1), 63–77.

Sénéchal, M. (1997). The differential effect of storybook reading on preschoolers' acquisition of expressive and receptive vocabulary. *Journal of Child Language, 24*(01), 123–138.

Sigafoos, J., Wermink, H., Didden, R., Green, V. A., Schlosser, R. W., O'Reilly, M. F., & Lancioni, G. E. (2011). Effects of varying lengths of synthetic speech output on augmented requesting and natural speech production in an adolescent with Klinefelter syndrome. *Augmentative and Alternative Communication, 27*(3), 163–171.

Skinner, B. F. (1948). Verbal behavior. Retrieved from http://store.behavior.org/resources/595.pdf

Smith, T. (2001). Discrete trial training in the treatment of autism. *Focus on Autism and Other Developmental Disabilities, 16*(2), 86–92.

Speech-Langauge Audiology Canada. (n.d.). Info sheet. Retrieved from sac-oac.ca/sites/default/files/resources/SLPs_Who%20we%20are_info%20sheet.pdf

Speech-Language Audiology Canada. (2014). SAC position paper on the role of speech-language pathologists with respect to augmentative and alternative communication. Retrieved from sac-oac.ca/sites/default/files/resources/AAC_PP_EN.pdf

Steege, M. W., Mace, F. C., Perry, L., & Longenecker, H. (2007). Applied behavior analysis: Beyond discrete trial teaching. *Psychology in the Schools, 44*(1), 91–99.

Sundberg, M. L. (1990). Teaching verbal behavior to the developmentally disabled. Retrieved from www.marksundberg.com/files/3-Teaching_Verbal_Behavior_to_the_Developmentally_Disabled.pdf

Teach Me to Talk. (2008). A little frustration can go a long way .....Using sabotage and withholding effectively to entice your toddler to talk. Retrieved from teachmetotalk.com/2008/04/20/a-little-frustration-can-go-a-long-way-using-sabotage-and-withholding-effectively-to-entice-your-toddler-to-talk/

Verschuur, R., Didden, R., Lang, R., Sigafoos, J., & Huskens, B. (2014). Pivotal response treatment for children with Autism Spectrum Disorder: A systematic review. *Review Journal of Autism and Developmental Disorders, 1*(1), 34–61.

Volkert, V. M., Lerman, D. C., Call, N. A., & Trosclair-Lasserre, N. (2009). An evaluation of resurgence during treatment with functional communication training. *Journal of Applied Behavior Analysis, 42*(1), 145–160. doi:10.1901/jaba.2009.42-145

Wong, C. (2013a). *Naturalistic intervention (NI) fact sheet.* Chapel Hill: The University of North Carolina, Frank Porter Graham Child Development Institute, The National Professional Development Center on Autism Spectrum Disorder.

Wong, C. (2013b). *Picture Exchange Communication System (PECS) fact sheet.* Chapel Hill: The University of North Carolina, Frank Porter Graham Child Development Institute, The National Professional Development Center on Autism Spectrum Disorder.

Wong, C. (2013c). *Pivotal response training (PRT) fact sheet.* Chapel Hill: The University of North Carolina, Frank Porter Graham Child Development Institute, The National Professional Development Center on Autism Spectrum Disorder.

Wong, C., Odom, S. L., Hume, K. Cox, A. W., Fettig, A., Kucharczyk, S., ... Schultz, T. R. (2014). *Evidence-based practices for children, youth, and young adults with Autism Spectrum Disorder.* Chapel Hill: The University of North Carolina, Frank Porter Graham Child Development Institute, Autism Evidence-Based Practice Review Group.

CHAPTER 5

SOCIAL SKILLS INTERVENTIONS

As noted before, a diagnosis of autism spectrum disorder (ASD) requires significant difficulties in social communication and social interaction skills (American Psychiatric Association [APA], 2013). Chapter 5 starts by explaining what social skills are and how to assess them in individuals with ASD. The chapter then provides effective, evidence-based interventions (EBIs) to enhance and support individuals with ASD in learning social skills to interact appropriately and effectively with others.

DEFINITION

A diagnosis of ASD involves a deficit in social skills, which is termed *social communication* in the *Diagnostic and Statistical Manual, 5th Edition (DSM-5)* (APA, 2013). These deficits may include difficulties interacting with others, understanding and emitting appropriate nonverbal communication in social interactions, and understanding social relationships (APA, 2013). Many of these social skills deficits go hand-in-hand with communication deficits, and thus many of the interventions explained in this chapter will focus not only on social behaviour but also on social communication. Ultimately, however, the goal is to interact with others and understand social situations.

There are many social skills required across an individual's day. Thus, social skills training can involve a wide variety of skills that can be onerous to teach. These skills can range from nonverbal skills, such as using body posture to demonstrate interest in what the other person is saying, to ending conversations appropriately, to theory of mind (understanding what another person is thinking). As mentioned in the *DSM-5*, there are wide varieties in and severities of social skills difficulties that range anywhere from appearing not interested in interaction to interacting incorrectly with others (APA, 2013). Therefore, it is necessary to choose the type of social intervention based on the individual's skill level and level of functional communication.

WHAT ARE SOCIAL SKILLS?

Almost anything that involves interacting with other people can be classified as a social skill. In some situations, people have even gone as far as classifying hygiene as a social skill. For example, people are not going to want to interact with someone who smells, and smelling clean is therefore a prerequisite for social interactions. However, is it a social skill or a functional living skill? In the same sense, learning to communicate could be classified as social, as the primary purpose of communication is to interact with others. However, the development of language is usually somewhat separated from social skills. Overall, the point is that almost any skill can be classified as a social skill, as long as it involves interacting with others.

Performance Deficit versus Skill Deficit

Before starting to teach skills to learners with ASD, it is important to verify whether the person has not acquired the skill or simply has difficulty demonstrating the skill in certain social situations. Anxiety from past failures in social situations or difficulties reading the situation can be a significant detriment to interacting. This is called a performance deficit. In these situations, the individual knows how to perform the skill, but has difficulty performing it in natural settings with others (Bellini, 2009). A skill acquisition deficit, on the other hand, is when the individual needs to be taught a specific social skill that she or he has not learned (Bellini, 2009). For example, when initiating a conversation with others, the high school student with ASD abruptly walks up to a group of peers, not acknowledging what they are discussing, and starts talking about his favourite topic—*The Tonight Show*.

> **Performance Deficit:** A performance deficit "refers to a skill or behaviour that is present, but not demonstrated or performed" (Bellini, 2006, p. 100).

> **Skill Acquisition Deficit:** A skill acquisition deficit "refers to the absence of a particular skill or behaviour" (Bellini, 2006, p. 99).

He had never been taught how to approach a group and join a conversation. This is a skill deficit. In contrast, if the individual is able to join in conversations with close family members but not with peers, this would be a performance deficit.

Types of Social Skills

Six common social skill categories that individuals with ASD struggle with are: 1) social initiation; 2) reciprocity and interaction termination; 3) nonverbal communication; 4) social cognition; 5) perspective taking and self-awareness; and 6) social anxiety (Bellini, 2006). When planning to teach social skills, it is important that the meaning of each social skill is broken down to understand why the skill is being taught and what the goal is. Also, in most social

> **Hidden Curriculum:** The hidden curriculum "includes skills, actions, modes of dress, and so on, that most people know and take for granted ... This unspoken curriculum is the one that causes challenges, and indeed, grief for those with AS[D]" (Smith-Myles & Simpson, 2001, p. 280).

situations there are *many* skills to teach, and thus breaking it down and teaching each component systematically will be more effective than trying to teach *all* of the skills.

> **Read about it. Think about it. Write about it.**
>
> Take each of the six social skills listed above and research a way that you could teach the skill to an individual with ASD.

Table 5.1: Types of Social Skills

Type	Description
Nonverbal	Often foundation to understanding others' cues that do not involve verbal speech that can provide much meaning. This can include body posture, movements, facial expressions, and combinations of these.
Social initiation	Includes the start of a social interaction with another. Can involve those who initiate incorrectly and frequently and those who don't at all.
Social reciprocity	Back and forth of conversation, and the reading of cues that signal an end to the conversation. Ending the conversation also involves appropriate body movements and language.
Social cognition	Involves problem solving social situations, understanding the hidden curriculum, considering theory of mind, and joint attention.
Perspective taking and self-awareness	Failure to consider others' interests, hygiene, and space.
Social anxiety	Fear of social situations and anticipating problems that can occur. Can be performance or social interaction fears.

Source: Bellini, 2006.

ASSESSING SOCIAL SKILLS

Before beginning any social skills program, it is important to understand the person's current skill set and identify important areas of focus. An easy way to start is to observe the learner in interactions with others in his or her environment, including adults and peers. Observe typically developing peers in a similar setting to determine what the age-appropriate skill is.

Another way to examine social skills is with social skill measures, which are questionnaires completed by others or by oneself. For an overall understanding of an individual's social skills, Scott Bellini's *Social Skill Profile* is a 49-item questionnaire that assesses social skill difficulties characteristic of ASD (Bellini, 2006). It is completed by caregivers or parents and can be used to understand areas of strength and areas for growth. Another resource for identifying social skills, especially in young learners and preschoolers, is McKinnon and Krempa's

NFER NELSON

Social Worries Questionnaire –
PUPIL

Date:	Name:	Sex:
Class:	School:	Age:

Please put a circle around the rating which best describes you *over the past four weeks*.
Please answer all questions.

('Avoid' means to try to get out of doing something.)

		Not true	Sometimes true	Mostly true
1	I avoid or get worried about going to parties	Not true	Sometimes true	Mostly true
2	I avoid or get worried about using the telephone	Not true	Sometimes true	Mostly true
3	I avoid or get worried about meeting new people	Not true	Sometimes true	Mostly true
4	I avoid or get worried about presenting work to the class	Not true	Sometimes true	Mostly true
5	I avoid or get worried about attending clubs or sports activities	Not true	Sometimes true	Mostly true
6	I avoid or get worried about asking a group of kids if I can join in	Not true	Sometimes true	Mostly true
7	I avoid or get worried about talking in front of a group of adults	Not true	Sometimes true	Mostly true
8	I avoid or get worried about going shopping alone	Not true	Sometimes true	Mostly true
9	I avoid or get worried about standing up for myself with other kids	Not true	Sometimes true	Mostly true
10	I avoid or get worried about entering a room full of people	Not true	Sometimes true	Mostly true
11	I avoid or get worried about using public toilets or bathrooms	Not true	Sometimes true	Mostly true
12	I avoid or get worried about eating in public	Not true	Sometimes true	Mostly true
13	I avoid or get worried about taking tests at school	Not true	Sometimes true	Mostly true

SOCIAL SKILLS TRAINING

Figure 5.1: Social Worries Questionnaire
Source: Spence, 1995, p. 24.

(2002) *Social Skills Checklist*, which has three levels of social skill development. Lastly, *Social Skills Training* by Susan Spence (1995) includes a Social Worries Questionnaire that examines social anxiety and performance deficits (see Figure 5.1). There is also an assessment to determine the individual's ability to understand body posture and facial cues (Spence, 1995).

LEARNING IN THE SOCIAL CONTEXT

There are advantages and disadvantages to inclusion for students with ASD when considering social skills teaching. When looking at the social context and the fact that individuals with ASD struggle to learn social skills, there are definite advantages to having peer models who demonstrate age-appropriate social behaviour (White, Keonig, & Scahill, 2007). If children with ASD are all put in the same classroom, the difficulty is that they will all have social skill difficulties inherent with ASD. Therefore, there are few models to demonstrate the socially appropriate behaviour and help the child with ASD to learn this behaviour. Although ASD classrooms allow for consistent teaching goals, and staff training is concentrated and highly skilled, the lack of social skill models leaves a major gap in teaching.

In addition to having models for social skill instruction, skills taught by peers are age-appropriate (White et al., 2007). When adults teach social skills, as much as they try to make them age-appropriate, there may be situations where they inadvertently teach skills or language inappropriate to the student's age or out of touch with current trends (Thames Valley Children's Centre, 2010). For example, in a classroom, an adult may teach the word "cool" as a descriptor for clothing. When peers start snickering in the background, one soon finds out that "cool" is really not that cool. The term used by peers, instead, is "sick." By having peers be models, the social skills will be much more age-appropriate.

When reviewing social skills strategies implemented in schools, Bellini, Peters, Benner, and Hopf (2007) found that inclusive interventions were more effective than "pull-out" approaches, where the individual was taken out of the general educational setting. In this method, generalization is practiced from the beginning, rather than teaching the skill and planning or hoping for generalization. In Ontario, there are many models of education and recreation, both inclusive and segregated. In most cases, Catholic boards of education tend to have more inclusive settings for education, whereas public boards of education have more options for placement that range from segregated classrooms to fully inclusive settings. Recreation environments are the same. There are both fully inclusive settings, where individuals with disabilities are included with same-age typically developing peers at camps and day camps, and camps designed specifically for those with ASD and other related disabilities.

> **Read about it. Think about it. Write about it.**
>
> What environment do you feel would be most suited to teaching social skills to individuals with ASD? Does your opinion change when considering children, youth, or adults?

EVIDENCE-BASED INTERVENTIONS

The strategies presented in this chapter are considered evidence-based interventions (EBIs) according to the Evidence-Based Review Group, herein referred to as the *EBI Report* (Wong et al., 2014). Most of the strategies in this chapter focus on skills needed to interact appropriately in social situations. Nonetheless, like other chapters focusing on interventions, many of these interventions will also assist with other areas, including communication in social situations, cognitive processing, and functional living skills.

Cognitive Behavioural Interventions

Cognitive behaviour interventions, or cognitive behaviour therapy (CBT), are a form of intervention that believes that behaviour is caused by various patterns of cognitive processes or thoughts (Brock, 2013). These thought patterns can be dysfunctional or irrational, and thus cause a person to become anxious or angry. Although estimates vary, anxiety is thought to affect 11 to 84 percent of individuals with ASD (Lang, Regester, Lauderdale, Ashbaugh, & Haring, 2010). For example, a high-school student with ASD believes that she will never interact appropriately with her peers because she doesn't understand social situations. When she comes in contact with her peers, this dysfunctional belief causes her anxiety, and she then avoids the situation. Much of the literature around CBT has examined how to assist individuals with anxiety and anger. For a step-by-step guide to using CBT strategies with people on the spectrum, reference Tony Attwood's books, *Exploring Feelings: Anxiety* and *Exploring Feelings: Anger* (Attwood, 2004a, 2004b).

Cognitive Behaviour Therapy: Cognitive behaviour therapy is "an effective treatment to change the way a person thinks about and responds to emotions such as anxiety, sadness, and anger. CBT focuses on the maturity, complexity, subtlety, and vocabulary of emotions, and dysfunctional or illogical thinking and incorrect assumptions" (Attwood, 2007, p. 151).

CBT was originally developed as a talk therapy approach for typically developing adults with anxiety and depression (Beck, 2011). It is still widely used today and enhances both a person's introspection and ability to self-monitor feelings and emotions (Lang et al., 2010). However, because individuals with ASD have difficulty engaging in introspection and understanding theory of mind, or other people's perspectives, modifications to the approach are needed (Lang et al., 2010). Attwood (2006) suggests adapting CBT to make strategies more concrete and easy to understand for people with ASD by making an emotions scrapbook, identifying tools that can assist in restructuring thoughts with an emotional toolbox, and using a special-interest tool to relate to the person's interests, among other ideas. For additional modifications to CBT, see Table 5.2.

CBT is considered an evidence-based intervention according to the *EBI Report* based on three group designs and one single-case study, and was found to be effective for individuals aged 6 to 18 for "social, communication, behavior, cognitive, adaptive, and mental health outcomes" (Brock, 2013, para. 4). It has been classified as effective for individuals under 22 and unestablished for those 22 and older in the *National Standards Report—Phase II* (National Autisim Center [NAC], 2015). In a recent review of the research, it was demonstrated that CBT

Table 5.2: CBT Modifications

Treatment components	Modifications	Examples
Sessions 1–4: *Building Rapport and Focusing on Recognizing Thoughts and Feelings*	1. Use of visual aids 2. Decrease of verbal demands 3. Role playing	1. Weekly Agenda, coping plan chart 2. "Feeling Frightened" to "Feelings" 3. Feeling charades
Sessions 5–7: *Development and Implementation of the Coping Plan Using Social Stories*	4. Inclusion of special interests 5. Use of visual social stories	4. Videogame characters affect recognition, coping plan situations 5. Use of illustrated social stories (Wood & McLeod, 2008)
Sessions 8–11: *Relaxation Techniques and Inclusion of Parents in Therapy*	6. Inclusion of parents in therapy 7. Physical play activities	6. "Simon Says" relaxation game 7. Coping plan scavenger hunt

Source: Aimes & Weiss, 2013, p. 65.

was effective for individuals with Asperger's disorder, but not necessarily other subtypes of ASD (Lang et al., 2010). Asperger's disorder appeared in the *Diagnostic and Statistical Manual-IV* and included average intelligence and normal language development (APA, 2000). Adapting CBT and using many applied behaviour analysis (ABA) principles seems to be common in the literature, but questions remain as to whether CBT or ABA components are causing the changes (Lang et al., 2010). In one study in Ontario, a nine-year-old boy with ASD and mild intellectual delays completed group CBT for anxiety and aggression (Aimes & Weiss, 2013). With adaptations to the CBT protocol, some anecdotal changes were made, but no measures demonstrated qualitative changes. It is thought that group homogeneity may influence outcomes, as well as additional adaptations for those who have verbal delays (Aimes & Weiss, 2013).

Modelling

Modelling involves the demonstration of a behaviour that acts as a prompt for the individual to imitate (Cox, 2013a; Mayer, Sulzer-Azaroff, & Wallace, 2014). This is an ABA strategy that is often used in combination with many other strategies in interventions. Modelling is important for individuals with ASD, as imitation of others' behaviour is often not automatically

> **Modelling:** Modelling "is the demonstration of a behaviour. People learn many behaviours, both appropriate and inappropriate, by imitating a model" (Alberto & Troutman, 2013, p. 14).

developed in this population. Teaching an individual with ASD to imitate opens up a large number of other skills that can be learned, as there are many complex behaviours in the environment demonstrated by both adults and peers he or she can learn that are hard to teach in other manners (Lovaas, 2003; Mayer et al., 2014). For example, someone who has learned how to imitate can imitate someone doing a routine such as brushing hair, emptying the dishwasher, or learning a job skill. It is thought that it is so effective because the nuances involved in some actions and routines cannot be communicated verbally (Mayer et al., 2014).

When teaching imitation, a nonverbal progression is often followed (Lovaas, 2003). This usually begins with gross motor imitation with objects and proceeds to gross motor imitation without objects, fine motor imitations, imitation of facial motions and expressions, and imitation of multi-step behaviours (Lovaas, 2003). (Examples of each of these can be found in Table 5.3.). Modelling can be used to teach a wide variety of skills and was found to be an EBI for "social, communication, joint attention, play, school-readiness, academic, and vocational skills" (Cox, 2013a). Modelling met the EBI criteria with one group research design and four single-case research studies and was found to be effective for ages 0 to 22 (Cox, 2013a). It is also evidence-based in the *National Autism Project—Phase II* (NAC, 2015). Through modelling, individuals with ASD have learned empathy skills (Schrandt, Townsend, & Poulson, 2009), employment-related work and social skills (Rigsby-Eldredge & McLaughlin, 1992), and social imitation with eye contact (Landa, Holman, O'Neill, & Stuart, 2011), among other skills.

Table 5.3: Examples of Imitation

Type of imitation (in order to be taught)	Examples
1. Gross motor imitations with objects	Shaking tambourine
	Pretend reading a book
	Putting on a hat
2. Gross motor imitations without objects	Clapping hands
	Slapping things
	Waving bye-bye
3. Fine motor imitations	Pointing to eyes
	Drumming on table with fingers
	Putting tips of index fingers together
4. Imitation of facial movements and expressions	Smacking lips
	Nodding head "yes"
	Making angry, happy, sad faces

Source: Lovaas, 2003.

Read about it. Think about it. Write about it.

What are some skills you could teach adults to imitate in order to increase the skills they can perform in their everyday lives?

Box 5.1: A Therapist's Journey of Teaching Imitation
By Brianna Anderson, BSc, ABS, Instructor Therapist, Private Practice

Before teaching complex functional skills to my clients, I always aim to determine which preliminary imitation targets are necessary in order for them to be successful at learning the broader skill. For instance, it would prove to be quite challenging to teach an individual how to put on a baseball hat before she or he is able to imitate touching her or his head. What may seem like a straightforward skill to you or me might look like a confusing jumble of unrecognizable instructions for an individual with ASD or a developmental disability if he or she hasn't been taught basic imitation skills. Even the most basic of tasks we do on a daily basis can be divided into smaller constituents. By teaching the smaller imitation targets first, I have found that my clients are more successful at picking up more complex skills.

Many of the targets I teach within an imitation program help create a foundation for the development of other imitation and functional skills. There are a handful of key imitation skills underpinning a variety of functional skills; therefore, I will often begin by teaching similar imitation targets to all of my clients. Some of the most rudimentary imitation targets, such as "touch head," "clap," "touch table," or "stomp feet," serve as preliminary skills for a host of other functional targets. For example, by successfully teaching my clients how to imitate "touch head," I can begin teaching more complex functional skills, such as putting on a hat, brushing hair, putting on glasses, and so on.

Furthermore, I have also observed in my practice that teaching basic imitation targets in an environment with minimal distractions, such as at a table or individual workspace, and fewer peripheral demands has helped my clients become more successful. It can be difficult for many individuals with ASD and other developmental disabilities to attend to one simple imitation target with added distractions from the natural environment. By breaking down these skills into simpler parts and teaching them in a location where they are able to fully attend, I have found it to be much easier to teach these skills in the natural environment in the future.

Video Modelling

Video modelling involves videotaping a model and having the individual with ASD watch it to acquire a visual model of the desired skill (Plavnick, 2013). In 2011, Autism Ontario completed a literature review of the social skill interventions and found video modelling to be the only EBI at that time. In one study, video modelling led to a quicker attainment of skills for four out of five children with ASD than live modelling (Charlop-Christy & Freeman, 2000). Video modelling is thought to be effective because it helps focus what the learner needs to concentrate on with the lens of the camera, without distractions from multiple stimuli in the environment (Charlop-Christy & Freeman, 2000). It may also be motivating to watch the behaviour on a screen because of the lack of intrinsic motivation that children with ASD often show toward social situations, versus the often reinforcing quality of TV shows and movies, and it may provide a different working environment from the traditional table (Charlop-Christy & Freeman, 2000).

As well, with video modelling, different perspectives that you would like an individual to focus on can be highlighted onscreen (McCoy & Hermansen, 2007). For example, when teaching a person to be the cashier at a grocery store during play, and an area of focus is looking up from the register at the customer when asking "How are you?", this can be zoomed in on. Similarly, if the key is putting a bowl in the sink after breakfast, this can be highlighted or focused on. There are various types of video modelling, as described in Table 5.4, in terms of how the video is edited and who the models are (Cox, 2013a; McCoy & Hermansen, 2007). The difficulty with video modelling is the generalization to untrained tasks, because some of the cues (discriminative stimuli) in the environment will have changed (Mayer et al., 2014). Video modelling has remained popular due to the efficiency of the approach and the fact that it often plays into the interests of individuals with ASD (McCoy & Hermansen, 2007). With technology becoming more widespread and available in all settings, the use of smartphones and tablets can facilitate quick usage of video modelling that can be adapted and watched instantaneously. Van Laarhoven, Kos, Pehlke, Johnson, and Burgin (2014) found that the iPad was an effective tool to teach vocational skills to four young adults with video modelling, with three of the four having more skill acquisition with video modelling and performance feedback.

Video modelling was found to be an effective EBI based on 31 single-case studies and one group design for individuals ages 0 to 22, and "can be used effectively to address social, communication, behavior, joint attention, play, cognitive, school-readiness, academic, motor, adaptive, and vocational skills" (Plavnick, 2013, para. 4). It is also considered evidence-based according to the *National Standards Project—Phase II* (NAC, 2015). All types of video modelling have been shown to be effective, regardless of who the model is in the video (McCoy & Hermansen, 2007), except in mixed-method approaches, which are not clearly effective in teaching target skills. In addition, when comparing different types of video modelling, results have varied somewhat from study to study, with some citing that peers were more effective models and others demonstrating that the model did not matter.

Table 5.4: Types of Video Modelling

Type		Description
Basic video modelling	Adult models	An adult, who can be familiar or unfamiliar, is the model for the video.
	Peer models	Peers model the skills for the video. Usually same-age and -gender. Can be familiar or unfamiliar.
Video self-modelling		The individual themselves engages in the optimal target behaviour. Edits and cuts are completed to see the entire skill being carried out and to remove adult prompts.
Point-of-view video modelling		The video angle is from the perspective of the individual completing the task. (i.e., own hands or feet are visible).
Video prompting		Involves breaking the target skill into steps and including pauses in the video after each step. This allows the individual to attempt each step before moving on to the subsequent step.
Mixed methods		Uses videos of multiple components of the above types of video modelling.

Sources: Mayer et al., 2014; McCoy & Hermansen, 2007; Plavnick, 2013.

Read about it. Think about it. Write about it.

Think of an individual you have worked with in the past. Think about a skill you could teach him or her with video modelling. What type of video modelling would you use? List the steps you would proceed through.

Peer-Mediated Interventions

Peer-mediated interventions are a method of teaching social skills whereby peers are used to assist in modelling and teaching the appropriate social, communication, academic, or behavioural response in various situations (Laushey & Heflin, 2000; McConnell, 2002). This approach is differentiated from an adult-mediated approach, where the adult works directly with children with ASD to improve social skills that they will then apply to interactions with their peers, and expands on ecological models, where research has demonstrated that placing a student with ASD with their peers alone in an inclusive setting with no training does not support the interactions between the individual and her or his peers (Laushey & Heflin, 2000; McConnell, 2002). A peer-mediated approach involves training peers who will then teach social skills to the group or the individual with ASD (DiSalvo & Oswald, 2002). The most significant limitation of a peer-mediated approach is the lack of generalization to untrained peers (McConnell, 2002).

A number of different peer-mediated approaches have been developed to focus on different skills and different peer roles (Utley & Mortweet, 1997). See the various approaches in Table 5.5. There are both advantages and disadvantages to utilizing peer-mediated instructional approaches compared to adult-mediated approaches. One of the most significant benefits of peer approaches is that peers are highly available in many inclusive classrooms and community centres (often more than adults), and once the peers are trained, less reliance on the adult is required. In addition, adult-mediated approaches rely on the adult teaching the social skill, and thus may not impart social skills appropriate to the age of the peer group (Thames Valley Children's Centre, 2010). When peers are teaching the skill, they are using the vocabulary and slang that is appropriate for inclusion within the peer group. See Table 5.6 for the benefits and drawbacks of teacher (adult)-mediated versus peer-mediated approaches.

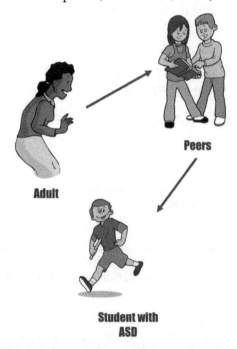

Peers

Adult

Student with
ASD

Figure 5.2: Peer-Mediated Instruction

Table 5.5: Types of Peer-Mediated Interventions

Type	Description
Peer modelling	Instructional method whereby the environment is manipulated so that peers model the appropriate skills for a less-skilled child to imitate. This is often a component of many peer-mediated trainings. Also called peer-proximity, peer-pairing, and filmed modelling interventions.
Peer initiation training	A commonly used and researched method in which peers are trained to initiate and maintain social communicative acts from the child with ASD.
Peer monitoring	Peers are put in supervisory roles where they assist children with ASD in discriminating between appropriate and inappropriate behaviours. This is carried out during transitions across the school day and when individuals are engaging in off-task behaviours.
Peer network strategies	Another highly popular approach that trains peers to engage in social and language skills and involves inclusion strategies whereby peers prompt, model, and reinforce the individual with ASD in natural settings and small groups.
Peer tutoring approaches	Peers are given a tutor role whereby the peer instructs the individual one-on-one in academic and social skills through "practice, repetition, and clarification of concepts" (Utely & Mortweet, 1997, p. 12).
Group-oriented contingencies	These strategies are based on the fact that in inclusive settings, peers are strong models for behaviour. The peers deliver reinforcement when the reinforcement is based on the whole group's behaviour.

Source: Adapted from Utley & Mortweet, 1997.

Table 5.6: Comparison of Social Skills Training

<u>Continuum of School-Based Social Intervention Components</u>
Recommended Evidence-Based Practices

Typically referred to as	**Reverse-mainstreaming**	**Social skill training/groups**	**Peer-mediated interventions**
Focus of treatment	Focus child's social skills	Focus child and some peer skills	Reciprocal social interactions
Setting	Self-contained classrooms	Partial inclusion	Fully included with supports/ pull-out
Peer availability	Limited	Sometimes	Most of the time
Opportunities for societal practice	Need to be created	Created with some available	Available daily
Adult involvement	High	Moderate	Mainly up front
Generalization of skills	High level of adult input	Moderate level of adult input	Less adult input needed
Administrative support needed	Low	Low-to-moderate	High
Feasibility and scheduling issues	Fewer	Some	More

Source: Thiemann, 2006.

The strategy was found to be effective for preschoolers to high school students (ages 3 to 18) with ASD in teaching academic tasks, joint attention, social skills, language, play, and school-readiness skills (Fettig, 2013a; NAC, 2015). Research has demonstrated that peer-mediated intervention is one of the most robust, comprehensive approaches to teaching social communication skills (McConnell, 2002). Research has also shown an increase in social communication skills in individuals with ASD in preschool settings (Laushey & Heflin, 2000), small groups (Thiemann & Goldstein, 2004), recess interventions (Mason et al., 2014; McFadden, Kamps, & Heitzman-Powell, 2014), and community group settings such as camps (Maich, Hall, van Rhijn, & Quinlan, 2015).

Read about it. Think about it. Write about it.

List the benefits of peer-mediated intervention for individuals who are typically developing. How could this be implemented with adults? Would it benefit adults who are typically developing as well?

Prompting

Prompting is used to assist a learner in acquiring skills with the insertion of a verbal, physical, or environmental manipulation before or as the learner is completing the skill (Cox, 2013b). The prompt can consist of a verbal reminder, the first sound of the word you want a child to say, or pointing to the correct answer (Mayer et al., 2014). These can be thought of as reminders; when the antecedent, instruction, or discriminative stimulus fails to produce the correct behaviour, a prompt is added (Mayer et al., 2014). Prompts are very important in teaching students with ASD, and when tracked and faded properly, they can teach many new skills. However, the difficulty with prompts is that individuals can become dependent on them, and thus they can interfere with independence. In these instances, the person is reinforced not for doing the skill, but for being prompted (Lovaas, 2003). For example, an individual may wait to clear the dishes until you tell her or him to, because she or he has become dependent on the verbal prompt. Alternatively, an individual may wait for your gesture to perform a routine such as lining up.

Prompt Dependency: Prompt dependency is when a prompt is needed for a behaviour to occur, and the behaviour does not occur on its own without the prompt (Gulick & Kitchen, 2007).

The most effective prompting strategies involve planning the prompt fading from the beginning. This is accomplished by continuing with the same instruction (descriptive stimulus) and fading the prompt, to make it weaker, until there is just the instruction and no prompt (Lovaas, 2003). To identify which prompt to start with, find out at which level the individual can complete the behaviour, starting with the most natural (least intrusive) and moving to the most artificial (most intrusive) (Mayer et al., 2014). Moving from least to most intrusive, stop when the individual can complete the skill with the least amount of assistance and start there (Mayer et al., 2014). Gradually fade the prompts, making them more and more natural until the learner can do it on his or her own. Two common types of prompt hierarchies are least-to-most and most-to-least. See Table 5.7 for examples of common prompts and Figures 5.3 and 5.4 for explanations of prompt hierarchies.

Table 5.7: Types of Prompts

Prompt	Topography/Method	Common Application	Prerequisites	Limitations
Positional prompt	Placing target object closer to the student	Receptive selection (point/touch/give) tasks	Basic attending skills	Not applicable when drill involves verbal responses
Proximity prompt	Positioning the instructor's body closer to or farther from the student	Receptive pronoun drills ("touch my nose")	Student must be able to verbally imitate	Limited to pronoun or possession drills
Voice inflection prompt	Magnifying or reducing the volume of the instructor's voice for a specific word	Magnification— Receptive selection (point/touch/give) tasks Reduction—Preventing echolalia	Basic attending skills	None encountered
Gestural (tap/point)	Tapping or pointing to target object	Discrimination tasks Visual performance tasks	Basic attending skills	Highly imitative students may mimic the tap/point
Gestural (hand placement)	Placing the instructor's outstretched hand nearer to the target object	Receptive selection (giving) tasks	Basic attending skills	None encountered
Gestural (blocking)	Shielding the non-target object or otherwise blocking access to it	Receptive selection (point/touch/give) tasks	Basic attending skills	None encountered

	Description	Tasks	Prerequisite skills	Limitations
Gestural (eye gaze or head nod)	Directing instructor's eye gaze or nodding head toward the target object	Receptive selection (point/touch/give tasks)	Well-developed attending skills	Requires student to be aware of subtle body cues
Highlighting	Placing brightly colored paper or other marking on or in close proximity to the target object or location	Receptive selection (point/touch/give) tasks Receptive placement tasks (prepositions)	Basic attending skills	None encountered
Size	Increasing the size of the target object relative to the non-target object	Receptive selection (point/touch/give) tasks	Basic attending skills	None encountered
Templates	Placing paper templates on the table to indicate specific locations for placement of objects	Sequencing and seriation tasks	Basic attending skills	None encountered
Dotted line prompt	Providing dotted line or lightly drawn figures as guides for the student to complete a written or drawn response	Graphic imitation (drawing/copying/writing) skills	Basic attending skills Correct grasp of writing implement	None encountered

Source: Gulick & Kitchen, 2007, p. 114 & 115.

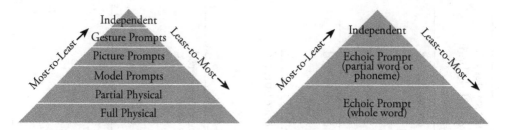

Figure 5.3: Prompt Hierarchy for Responses with Motor Movements

Figure 5.4: Prompt Hierarchy for Verbal Responses

Table 5.8: Least-to-Most versus Most-to-Least Prompting

	Least-to-most prompting	Most-to-least prompting
Description	• Start with the least amount of support as needed and move up to more prompts if needed. Usually a predetermined amount of time is waited before responding (e.g., 3–5 seconds).	• Start with the prompt that will ensure the learner gets the correct response and move to lesser and lesser prompts as the learner masters each prompt level.
Benefits	• Learner does not get prompt dependent. • Learner may acquire the skill faster (in less teaching trials).	• Learner will achieve success/reinforcement from the start. • Gradual fading ensures the task is not too difficult.
Drawbacks	• The student may practice errors. • May be difficult to attain new skills with fewer prompts.	• The student may proceed through unnecessary learning steps when he or she is ready for a less intrusive prompt. • The learner may get complacent or prompt dependent.

Sources: Mayer et al., 2014; Mims, n.d.

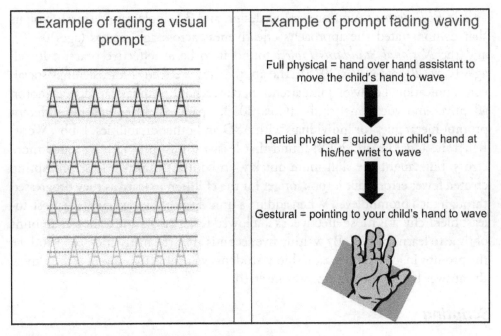

Figure 5.5: Examples of Prompt Hierarchies
Source: ErinoakKids, 2012, p. 2.

Box 5.2: Rules for Prompting

- Avoid unintentional prompts such as positioning of materials, voice inflection, facial expressions and not changing the order of concepts or instructions.
- If it is not possible to prompt simultaneously with the instruction, prompt IMMEDIATELY following the instruction.
- Reinforce unprompted responses more than prompted responses.
- Do not allow your child to fail repeatedly.
- Fade prompts gradually.
- Make the prompts less intrusive (e.g., move from full physical to partial physical).
- As prompts are faded, remember to reinforce more independent responses.
- Provide more/longer access to reinforcers for unprompted skill responses.

Source: ErinoakKids, 2012, p. 2.

The *EBP Report* found one group design and 32 single-case research designs that demonstrated the approach's effectiveness across age groups (ages 0–22), and the *National Standards Project* found it to be an effective practice for all ages (Cox, 2013a; NAC, 2015). The approach was effective for teaching "social, communication, behavior, joint attention, play, school-readiness, academic, motor, adaptive, and vocational skills" (Cox, 2013b, para. 4). In comparing different prompt hierarchies for individuals with ASD and other disabilities, Libby, Weiss, Bancroft, and Ahearn (2008) found that least-to-most prompting created more errors, but taught the skill more quickly. In contrast, most-to-least prompting created fewer errors, but it took longer for the children to learn as they progressed through each prompt level. When adding a time delay of five seconds, the most-to-least hierarchy was most effective, as it allowed fewer errors and a shorter amount of time to learn the skill. By waiting five seconds after the instruction to introduce the prompt in a most-to-least fashion, students were able to respond if they knew the answer before the prompt was inserted.

Scripting

"Scripting (SC) involves presenting learners with a verbal and/or written description about a specific skill or situation that serves as a model for the learner" (Fleury, 2013, para. 1). Initiating social communication skills such as reciprocal conversations and turn taking is often difficult for individuals with ASD, and imitating speech is therefore an effective way to model the language appropriate for these various situations (Ganz, Kaylor, Bourgeois, & Hadden, 2008). It is thought that allowing

---

Box 5.3: Sample Reading Script

Good reading, [name].
[Name], do you like to read?
Do you want to read?
Wow that's good!
I'll get a book.
You get a book.
I'm using [name of book].
This is fun!
Let's read some more.
[Name], what do you want to do?

Source: Thiemann & Goldstein, 2001.

individuals to anticipate the next socially acceptable response in the conversation and practice it multiple times will assist with learning the skills (Fleury, 2013). The goal is to provide the script and then systematically fade it so that they no longer need it to carry out the social communication interaction independently (Pollard, Betz, & Higbee, 2012). Scripting procedures are usually used with modelling, prompting, and reinforcement (Fleury, 2013; Ganz et al., 2008).

Scripting was considered an evidence-based intervention based on eight single-case research studies and one group design for learners aged 3 to 18 in the *EBI Report* and the *National Standards Project—Phase II* (Fleury, 2013). It is effective in teaching "social, communication, joint attention, play, cognitive, school-readiness, and vocational skills" (Fleury, 2013, para. 4). In the peer-mediated literature, text cues assisted individuals in increasing the amount of speech used with peers (Thiemann & Goldstein, 2001;

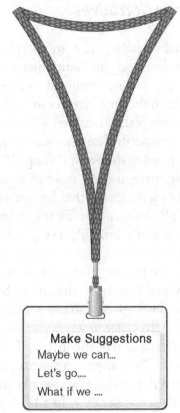

Make Suggestions
Maybe we can...
Let's go....
What if we ....

Figure 5.6: Sample Text Cues for Games and Recess

Source: Adapted from Thiemann, 2006.

Thiemann, 2006). In some situations, this gain was not maintained when the text cues were removed, leading to questions as to whether the children had learned the behaviour after it was initially taught with the scripts. Ganz and colleagues (2008) found similar results, that scripts increased communication skills and decreased repetitive speech; however, this failed to generalize when the scripts were no longer present. A major area for additional research involves how to effectively fade the scripts so that individuals can communicate without them in natural conversations with peers.

Read about it. Think about it. Write about it.

Write a script for the steps in ordering a meal at McDonald's.

Social Narratives

Social narratives are written explanations of social behaviour and social situations that detail certain components of a situation and what communication to use (Wong, 2013), "designed to meet the specific needs and academic level of the student, they use pictures for early readers, or plain text for experienced readers" (Thames Valley Children's Centre, 2009, p. 35). They are often individualized for the specific learner, including the learner's name and picture, and are often short and to the point (Wong, 2013). The narratives are usually written from the perspective of the learner so that the story can match the feelings, behaviours, and experiences of that learner and describe workings of a social situation that are often confusing for the individual with ASD and how the learner should respond in a desirable way (Gray, 1995; Wong, 2013). Because individuals with ASD often find social situations confusing, the social narrative is intended to describe the situation, rather than just tell the individual what to do.

Social Stories, trademarked by Carol Gray, have traditionally been used to describe a specific manner in which a social narrative is constructed (Gray, 1995). In order to write a social story, the types of sentences used must follow a formula so that the intent of the story is to describe rather than direct (Gray, 1995). The largest misconception with Social Stories is that any written material that describes what a child should do is automatically a Social Story, which is not the case. In addition, social narratives are meant to be read when the child is quiet and calm, not as a punishment for a challenging behaviour or social mistakes. The purpose of the intervention is to teach the student the appropriate skills and apply them when the situation occurs. For other tips on writing social narratives, see Table 5.9.

Social narratives are often used to describe difficult situations or prepare for a transition. Letting an individual know what is coming will help to decrease her or his anxiety. For example, as part of the mandate for managing transitions in Ontario (Ontario Ministry of Education, 2002), social narratives are often prepared at the end of each year to help the students know what they will face next year when entering the new classroom or school. They are also used to teach different social skills, such as how to initiate a conversation, end a conversation, understand another's perspective, be a good friend, or be a good sport when losing a game, and many other situations in which the hidden curriculum is often ambiguous for those with ASD.

In the past, social narratives have been combined with other intervention strategies, making it difficult to discern whether it was the social narrative or the other treatment interventions causing the effect (Chan & O'Reilly, 2008). However, in the newest *EBI Report* and the *National Standards Project—Phase II,*

Table 5.9: Social Narrative Tips

DOs	DON'Ts
• Write what you would like the learner to do.	• Write what you do not want the learner to do (i.e., pick, bite, punch).
• Describe more than direct.	• List the behaviours a person must engage in, rather than describe what is happening and why in a social situation.
• Make the story positive (i.e., "You can do it!").	• Make the story negative or punishment-based.
• Take the perspective of the child to guide your decision on what is important to write about in that situation.	• Make the story generic so that it is long and doesn't focus on the skills or understanding the specific learner needs.
• Read the story often, with multiple caregivers, at times when the individual is calm.	• Read it when the individual is upset, emotional, or for punishment after an event.

Sources: Gray, 1995; Thames Valley Children's Centre, 2009.

social narratives met the criteria for an EBI, effective for learners ages 3 to 18 in the latter review (NAC, 2015; Wong, 2013). Research has also supported the use of social narratives presented on computers, although generalization did not occur for all participants (Sansosti & Powell-Smith, 2008). This method is effective for "social, communication, behavior, joint attention, play, school-readiness, academic, and adaptive skills" (Wong, 2013, para. 4); however, one meta-analysis found that it was more effective for decreasing challenging behaviours than for social skills teaching (Kokina & Kern, 2010).

Read about it. Think about it. Write about it.

Write a social narrative for a social situation that you have seen someone struggle with in the past.

Box 5.4: Social Narrative Example

My Turn to Be Special Helper for Calendar Time

We start each morning with calendar time. There are 12 different calendars: January, February, March, April, May, June, July, August, September, October, November, and December, one for every month. I will get a turn once every month to be the special helper during calendar time.

Everyone in the class will get a turn to be the special helper for calendar time. When it is my turn, I will stand up in front of the circle, on the small blue carpet beside Mrs. MacIsaac.

My teacher will give me a number that is called the date. It has a Velcro spot on the back and will stick to the empty spots on the calendar when I put it on. I will put the number on the calendar after yesterday's date. If I don't know where it goes, Mrs. MacIsaac will show me. It is okay to ask for help.

Mrs. MacIsaac will ask me what day of the week it is. She wants to know if it is Monday, Tuesday, Wednesday, Thursday, or Friday. If I don't know I can use my finger to follow the column to the top. I will see the day of the week.

After my class sings the days of the week, I can sit down in my spot between Marcy and Daniel. My turn will be over until the next calendar month. It is fun to be the special helper.

Source: Thames Valley Children's Centre, 2009, p. 36.

Social Skills Training

Social skills training involves the systematic teaching of social skills required to interact with peers (Fettig, 2013b). This is primarily done in an adult-mediated approach, where the adult teaches the skills and then the learner applies the skills with peers in a natural setting (McConnell, 2002). Peers can be used to facilitate these approaches, but the key is that skills are taught initially by the adult. "Most social skills meetings include instruction on basic concepts, role-playing or practice, and feedback to help learners acquire and practice communication, play, or social skills to promote positive interactions with peers" (Fettig, 2013b, para. 1). The type of intervention for social skills training can vary significantly in the procedures used.

For example, Lego-based therapy is a method in which individuals work in dyads or triads to build Lego and solve a problem while communicating together (Green, 2013). It is based on the premise that the structured, sequential nature of the Lego system as a play tool is attractive to individuals with ASD because of the characteristics of their disorder (Owens, Granader, Humphrey, Baron-Cohen, 2008). Three studies have demonstrated that Lego-based therapy is effective in increasing social skills and decreasing challenging behaviours compared with no treatment (LeGoff, 2004; LeGoff & Sherman, 2006; Owens et al., 2008). Social skills training is considered an evidence-based intervention based on eight single-subject research studies and seven group design studies for learners ages 0 to 22 (Fettig, 2013b; NAC, 2015).

Structured Play Group

Structured play groups teach within the natural environment by physically arranging the environment to assist with play, guiding the child within these environments while taking advantage of child-led initiations (Wolfberg & Schuler, 1993). They utilize small groups with typically developing peers, with the adult leading the group through defined themes while using prompting and scaffolding to assist the learner in attaining play goals (Odom, 2013). The integrated play group is one method of teaching in this format and is based on eight underlying principles (Wolfberg & Schuler, 1993). First, they are conducted in natural settings with typically developing peers, so that peers who have more age-appropriate social skills are available to model and interact with. Second, the play environment is spatially designed, so that each play space is organized and allows for the most optimal play. Third, play toys are chosen carefully based on structure, complexity, and interactive potential—all areas demonstrated to be important in play for individuals with ASD. Fourth, due to the desire for sameness and routine in individuals with ASD, a consistent routine and schedule for play is maintained. Fifth, play groups are appropriately balanced with familiar and unfamiliar peers. Sixth, the learner's initiations within the play are identified as areas of competence and developmental level, or Zone of Proximal

> **Zone of Proximal Development (ZPD):** The Zone of Proximal Developement is "the distance between the actual developmental level as determined by independent problem solving, and the level of potential development as determined through problem solving under adult guidance or in collaboration with more capable peers" (Vygotsky, 1978, p. 86).

Box 5.5: Lego Therapy Principles

Building in Pairs

- The "engineer" gives verbal descriptions of the pieces needed and directions for assembling them.
- The "builder" follows his directions, collects and puts the pieces together.
- There is much checking back and forth between the plan and the creation.
- Roles are then switched so they both have a chance to be "engineer" and "builder."

Groups of Three

- The "engineer" describes the instructions.
- The "supplier" finds the correct pieces.
- The "builder" puts the pieces together.
- After a time, they swap roles.

Lego Club Rules

- Build things together!
- If you break it you have to fix it or ask for help to fix it.
- If someone else is using it, don't take it—ask first.
- Use indoor voices—no yelling.
- Keep your hands and feet to yourself.
- Use polite words.
- Clean up and put things back where they came from.
- Don't put Lego bricks in your mouth.

The Therapist's Role

The therapist's role is not to point out specific social problems or give solutions to social difficulties, rather to highlight the presence of a problem and help children to come up with their own solutions.

Solutions that children have come up with are practiced until they can do it, and the therapist can remind children of strategies in the future if similar difficulties arise.

Source: Green, 2013, p. 6, 7, 9, 10.

Development, and the amount of support given is matched to this level. Seventh, the adult engages in guided participation, where they support rather than guide the learner in developing play skills. Lastly, the learner participates in the whole group experience of the play, even if her or his level of participation is less than that of peers. Extensions of the integrated play group have also been completed with teen social groups, which focus on popular culture, games, and sports instead of toys (Wolfberg, Bottema-Beutel, & DeWitt, 2012).

Research into structured play groups has found them to be EBIs based on two group and two single-case designs for learners ages 6 to 11 (Odom, 2013), and they are included in peer EBIs in the *National Standards Project—Phase II*. Research into integrated play groups found that children were more able to engage in collaborative social play and functional play with toys, and this was generalized outside of the play group, with accompanying language gains (Wolfberg & Schuler, 1993).

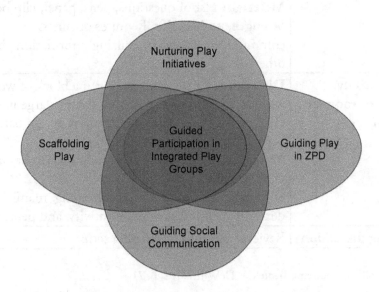

Figure 5.7: Guided Participation in Integrated Play Groups
Source: Wolfberg, Bottema-Beutel, & DeWitt, 2012, p. 62.

Table 5.10: Sample Teen Social Group Schedule

Opening script	**Purpose of the meeting:** Learn how to collaborate with people with different abilities, backgrounds, and interests. **Things to think about during the meeting:** How have life experiences been different for each group member? How have these experiences shaped and been shaped by different abilities and interests?
Group check-in	**Participant-led ice breaker:** Have each individual meet the person on his or her left and introduce the person to the whole group. Have the individual present his or her name, age, and the important information to know about the person.
Main activity: Get to know ya	**Directions:** As a group, participants answer a list of questions involving experiences and personalities of each group member **Materials:** List of questions, pens, paper, clip board **Strengths to identify:** Requires openness, communication, and organizing information about others
Brief activity: Plenty of room at the top	**Directions:** Participants are given a block of wood with a nail in it, and twenty additional large nails. The challenge is to see how many nails they can balance on the head of the nail in the block of wood. **Materials:** Wood block with nail in it, twenty large decking nails **Strengths to identify:** Visual thinking, manual dexterity, communication, creativity, and perseverance
Closing discussion	Review questions in opening script

Source: Wolfberg, Bottema-Beutel, & DeWitt, 2012, p. 71.

Parent-Implemented Interventions

In parent-implemented interventions, the parents of a child with ASD apply part of or the entire intervention after training (Schultz, 2013). Parents are often trained as a method to generalize skills that the child has learned in a more restrictive setting and apply them to his or her everyday life. This method could be applied to any of these interventions, as long as parents are trained one-on-one or in a group on how to implement the specific strategy (Schultz, 2013). This intervention is placed in the social skills chapter because parents are often trained in these strategies so that social skills can be incorporated into their natural settings as quickly as possible.

This is considered an EBI based on 12 single-case studies and eight group designs (Schultz, 2013), and is also included as an EBI in the *National Standards Project—Phase II*. Research has found it to be effective for individuals with ASD ages 0 to 11 for "social, communication, behavior, joint attention, play, cognitive, school-readiness, academic, and adaptive skills" (Schultz, 2013, para. 4). In one study, mothers were successfully trained to teach their children to verbally initiate during play (Reagon & Higbee, 2009). The mothers were trained through instructions, modelling, prompting, and providing feedback while role-playing with the researcher.

A LOOK BACK

Chapter 5, "Social Skills Interventions," focused on:
- The social skill characteristics of individuals with ASD, including skill and performance deficits and types of social skills;
- How to assess social skills and teach them in the natural versus contrived environment; and
- Evidence-based interventions to teach social skills, including cognitive behavioural interventions, modelling, video modelling, peer-mediated instruction, prompting, scripting, social narratives, social skills training, structured play groups, and parent-implemented intervention.

A LOOK AHEAD

Chapter 6, "Behaviour-Based Interventions," focuses on:
- The repetitive and restricted patterns of behaviour that individuals with ASD exhibit;
- How these patterns of behaviour differ from other diagnoses, such as obsessive-compulsive disorder (OCD); and

- Evidence-based interventions to work with repetitive and restricted behaviours, including antecedent-based interventions, differential reinforcement, exercise, extinction, functional behaviour assessment, response interruption/redirection, self-management, task analysis, time delay, visual supports, and reinforcement.

ADDITIONAL RESOURCES

- Applied Behaviour Analysis (ErinOakKids, 2015):
  http://www.erinoakkids.ca/Resources/Autism/Applied-Behaviour-Analysis.aspx
- CBT publications by Jonathan Weiss (York University):
  http://www.researchgate.net/profile/Jonathan_Weiss2/publications
- Classroom Supports: Social Narratives (Kansas Technical Assistance Network, 2015):
  http://www.kansasasd.com/socialnarratives.php
- Do It Yourself: Video Modeling (University of Kansas, 2015):
  http://www.specialconnections.ku.edu/~kucrl/cgi-bin/drupal/?q=node/221
- Including Children with Autism in Social and Imaginary Play with Typical Peers (Wolfberg, Bottema-Beutel, & DeWitt, 2012):
  http://www.journalofplay.org/sites/www.journalofplay.org/files/pdf-articles/5-1-article-including-children-with-autism.pdf
- Making (and Keeping) Friends: A Model for Social Skills Instruction (Bellini, 2009):
  http://www.iidc.indiana.edu/?pageId=488
- Peer-Mediated Interventions (Texas Statewide Leadership for Autism, 2013):
  http://www.txautism.net/uploads/target/PeerMediated.pdf
- PEERS Social Skills Program (UC Regents, 2011):
  http://www.semel.ucla.edu/peers
- Social Worries Questionnaire—Spence Children's Anxiety Website (Spence, 2005):
  www.scaswebsite.com
- Social Matters (Autism Ontario, 2011):
  http://www.autismontario.com/Client/ASO/AO.nsf/object/Social Matters/$file/Social+Matters.pdf
- Social Narratives and Resources (ErinOakKids, 2015):
  http://www.erinoakkids.ca/Resources/Autism/Social-Narratives.aspx
- Tony Attwood (CBT Reseracher and Practitioner) (Attwood, 2015):
  http://www.tonyattwood.com.au
- Watch Me Learn (Watch Me Learn, 2015):
  http://www.watchmelearn.com

REFERENCES

Aimes, M., & Weiss, J. (2013). Cognitive behavioural therapy for a child with autism spectrum disorder and verbal impairment: A case study. *Journal of Developmental Disabilities, 19*(1), 61–69.

Alberto, P. A., & Troutman, A. C. (2013). *Applied behavior analysis for teachers* (9th ed.). Upper Saddle River, NJ: Pearson.

American Psychiatric Association. (2000). *Diagnostic and statistical manual: DSM IV-R* (4th ed.). Washington, DC: Author.

American Psychiatric Association. (2013). *Diagnostic and statistical manual: DSM-5* (5th ed.). Washington, DC: Author.

Attwood, A. (2006). *The complete guide to Asperger's syndrome.* London, UK: Jessica Kingsley Publishers.

Attwood, T. (2004a). *Exploring feelings (anger).* Arlington, TX: Future Horizons.

Attwood, T. (2004b). *Exploring feelings (anxiety).* Arlington, TX: Future Horizons.

Attwood, T. (2007). *The complete guide to Asperger's syndrome.* Jessica Kingsley Publishers: London.

Autism Ontario. (2011). Social matters: Improving social skills interventions for Ontarians with autism spectrum disorder. Retrieved from www.autismontario.com/Client/ASO/AO.nsf/object/SocialMatters/$file/Social+Matters.pdf

Beck, J. S. (2011). *Cognitive behavior therapy: Basics and beyond.* New York, NY: Guilford Press.

Bellini, S. (2006). *Building social relationships: A systematic approach to teaching social interaction skills to children and adolescents with autism spectrum disorder and other social difficulties.* Shawnee Mission, KS: Autism Asperger Publishing Company.

Bellini, S. (2009). Making (and keeping) friends: A model for social skills interaction. *The Reporter, 8*(3), 1–10. Retrieved from www.iidc.indiana.edu/?pageId=488#sthash.b51FR3Mh.dpuf

Bellini, S., Peters, J. K., Benner, L., & Hopf, A. (2007). A meta-analysis of school-based social skills interventions for children with autism spectrum disorder. *Remedial and Special Education, 28*(3), 153-162.

Brock, M. E. (2013). *Cognitive behavioral intervention (CBI) fact sheet.* Chapel Hill: The University of North Carolina, Frank Porter Graham Child Development Institute, The National Professional Development Center on Autism Spectrum Disorder.

Chan, J. M., & O'Reilly, M. F. (2008). A Social Stories™ intervention package for students with autism in inclusive classroom settings. *Journal of Applied Behavior Analysis, 41*(3), 405–409.

Charlop-Christy, M. H., Le, L., & Freeman, K. A. (2000). A comparison of video modeling with in vivo modeling for teaching children with autism. *Journal of Autism and Developmental Disorders, 30*(6), 537–552.

Cox, A. W. (2013a). *Modeling fact sheet.* Chapel Hill: The University of North Carolina, Frank Porter Graham Child Development Institute, The National Professional Development Center on Autism Spectrum Disorder.

Cox, A. W. (2013b). *Prompting (PP) fact sheet.* Chapel Hill: The University of North Carolina, Frank Porter Graham Child Development Institute, The National Professional Development Center on Autism Spectrum Disorder.

DiSalvo, C. A., & Oswald, D. P. (2002). Peer-mediated interventions to increase the social interaction of children with autism consideration of peer expectancies. *Focus on Autism and Other Developmental Disabilities, 17*(4), 198–207.

ErinoakKids. (2012). *Prompting and fading.* Retrieved from www.erinoakkids.ca/getattachment/Resources/Autism/Applied-Behaviour-Analysis/ABA-for-Families-Prompting-and-Fading.pdf.aspx

Fettig, A. (2013a). *Peer-mediated instruction and intervention (PMII) fact sheet.* Chapel Hill: The University of North Carolina, Frank Porter Graham Child Development Institute, The National Professional Development Center on Autism Spectrum Disorder.

Fettig, A. (2013b). *Social skills training (SST) fact sheet.* Chapel Hill: The University of North Carolina, Frank Porter Graham Child Development Institute, The National Professional Development Center on Autism Spectrum Disorder.

Fleury, V. P. (2013). *Scripting (SC) fact sheet.* Chapel Hill: The University of North Carolina, Frank Porter Graham Child Development Institute, The National Professional Development Center on Autism Spectrum Disorder.

Ganz, J. B., Kaylor, M., Bourgeois, B., & Hadden, K. (2008). The impact of social scripts and visual cues on verbal communication in three children with autism spectrum disorder. *Focus on Autism and Other Developmental Disabilities, 23*(2), 79–94.

Gray, C. (1995). Teaching children with autism to "read" social situations. In K. A. Quill (Ed.), *Teaching children with autism: Strategies to enhance communication and socialization* (pp. 219–241). New York, NY: Delmar.

Green. (2013). *LEGO Therapy: An overview.* Paper presented at University of Warwick. Coventry, UK. Retrieved from www2.warwick.ac.uk/fac/sci/dcs/schools/cpd/legovent2013/programme/lego_therapy_-_compressed.ppt

Gulick, R. F., & Kitchen, T. P. (2007). *Effective instruction for children with autism: An applied behavior analytic approach.* Erie, PA: The Dr. Gertrude A. Barber National Institute.

Kokina, A., & Kern, L. (2010). Social Story interventions for students with autism spectrum disorder: A meta-analysis. *Journal of Autism and Developmental Disorders, 40*(7), 812–826.

Landa, R. J., Holman, K. C., O'Neill, A. H., & Stuart, E. A. (2011). Intervention targeting development of socially synchronous engagement in toddlers with autism spectrum disorder: A randomized controlled trial. *Journal of Child Psychology and Psychiatry, 52*(1), 13–21. doi:10.1111/j.1469-7610.2010.02288.x

Lang, R., Regester, A., Lauderdale, S., Ashbaugh, K., & Haring, A. (2010). Treatment of anxiety in autism spectrum disorder using cognitive behaviour therapy: A systematic review. *Developmental Neurorehabilitation, 13*(1), 53–63.

Laushey, K. M., & Heflin, L. J. (2000). Enhancing social skills of kindergarten children with autism through the training of multiple peers as tutors. *Journal of Autism and Developmental Disorders, 30*, 183–193.

LeGoff, D. B. (2004). Use of LEGO as a therapeutic medium for improving social competence. *Journal of Autism and Developmental Disorders, 34*(5), 557–571.

LeGoff, D. B., & Sherman, M. (2006). Long-term outcome of social skills intervention based on interactive LEGO play. *Autism, 10*(4), 317–329. doi:10.1177/1362361306064403

Libby, M. E., Weiss, J. S., Bancroft, S., & Ahearn, W. H. (2008). A comparison of most-to-least and least-to-most prompting on the acquisition of solitary play skills. *Behavior Analysis in Practice, 1*(1), 37.

Lovaas, O. I. (2003). *Teaching individuals with developmental disabilities: Basic intervention techniques.* Austin, TX: Pro-Ed.

Maich, K., Hall, C., van Rhijn, T., & Quinlan, L. (2015). Developing social skills of summer campers with autism spectrum disorder: A case study of camps on TRACKS implementation in an inclusive day-camp setting. *Exceptionality Education International, 25*(2), 27–41.

Mason, R., Kamps, D., Turcotte, A., Cox, S., Feldmiller, S., & Miller, T. (2014). Peer mediation to increase communication and interaction at recess for students with autism spectrum disorder. *Research in Autism Spectrum Disorder, 8*(3), 334–344. doi:10.1016/j.rasd.2013.12.014

Mayer, G. R., Sulzer-Azaroff, B., & Wallace, M. (2014). *Behavior analysis for lasting change* (3rd ed.). Cornwall-on-Houston, NY: Sloan Publishing.

McConnell, S. R. (2002). Interventions to facilitate social interaction for young children with autism: Review of available research and recommendations for educational intervention and future research. *Journal of Autism and Developmental Disorders, 32*(5), 351–372.

McCoy, K., & Hermansen, E. (2007). Video modeling for individuals with autism: A review of model types and effects. *Education and Treatment of Children, 30*(4), 183–213.

McFadden, B., Kamps, D., & Heitzman-Powell, L. (2014). Social communication effects of peer-mediated recess intervention for children with autism. *Research in Autism Spectrum Disorder, 8*(12), 1699–1712.

McKinnon, K., & Krempa, J. L. (2002). *Social skills solutions: A hands-on manual for teaching social skills to children with autism.* New York, NY: DRL Books.

Mims, P. (n.d.). Prompting systems. Retrieved from mast.ecu.edu/modules/ps/concept/

National Autism Center. (2015). Findings and conclusions, national standards project, phase 2. Retrieved from http://www.nationalautismcenter.org/national-standards-project/

Odom, S. L. (2013). *Structured play groups (SPG) fact sheet.* Chapel Hill: The University of North Carolina, Frank Porter Graham Child Development Institute, The National Professional Development Center on Autism Spectrum Disorder.

Ontario Ministry of Education. (2002). Transition planning: A resource guide. Retrieved from www.edu.gov.on.ca/eng/general/elemsec/speced/transiti/transition.html

Owens, G., Granader, Y., Humphrey, A. S., & Baron-Cohen, S. (2008). LEGO therapy and the Social Use of Language Programme: An evaluation of two social skills interventions. *Journal of Autism and Developmental Disorders, 38*, 1944–1957.

Plavnick, J. B. (2013). A practical strategy for teaching a child with autism to attend to and imitate a portable video model. *Research and Practice for Persons with Severe Disabilities, 37*(4), 263–270.

Pollard, J. S., Betz, A. M., & Higbee, T. S. (2012). Script fading to promote unscripted bids for joint attention in children with autism. *Journal of Applied Behavior Analysis, 45*(2), 387–393.

Reagon, K. A., & Higbee, T. S. (2009). Parent-implemented script fading to promote play-based verbal initiations in children with autism. *Journal of Applied Behavior Analysis, 42*(3), 659–664. doi:10.1901/ jaba.2009.42-659

Rigsby-Eldredge, M., & McLaughlin, T. F. (1992). The effects of modeling and praise on self-initiated behavior across settings with two adolescent students with autism. *Journal of Developmental and Physical Disabilities, 4*(3), 205–218. doi:10.1007/BF01046965

Sansosti, F. J., & Powell-Smith, K. A. (2008). Using computer-presented social stories and video models to increase the social communication skills of children with high-functioning autism spectrum disorder. *Journal of Positive Behavior Interventions, 10*(3), 162–178.

Schrandt, J. A., Townsend, D. B., & Poulson, C. L. (2009). Teaching empathy skills to children with autism. *Journal of Applied Behavior Analysis, 42*(1), 17–32. doi:10.1901/jaba.2009.42-17

Schultz, T. R. (2013). *Parent-implemented intervention (PII) fact sheet.* Chapel Hill: The University of North Carolina, Frank Porter Graham Child Development Institute, The National Professional Development Center on Autism Spectrum Disorder.

Smith-Myles, B. S., & Simpson, R. L. (2001). Understanding the hidden curriculum: An essential social skill for children and youth with Asperger syndrome. *Intervention in School and Clinic, 36*(5), 279–286.

Spence, S. H. (1995). *Social skills training: Enhancing social competence with children and adolescents.* London, UK: NFER-Nelson. Retrevied from http://www.scaswebsite.com/1_54_.html

Thames Valley Children's Centre. (2009). *Asperger's syndrome: A guide for educators.* London, ON: Author.

Thames Valley Children's Centre. (2010). *PEER Pals.* London, ON: Author.

Thiemann, K. (2006, April). *Comprehensive social communication interventions for elementary students with ASD*. Paper presented at ASD-School Support Program 2nd Annual Conference, Niagara Falls, ON.

Thiemann, K. S., & Goldstein, H. (2001). Social stories, written text cues, and video feedback: Effects on social communication of children with autism. *Journal of Applied Behavior Analysis, 34*(4), 425–446.

Thiemann, K. S., & Goldstein, H. (2004). Effects of peer training and written text cueing on social communication of school-age children with pervasive developmental disorder. *Journal of Speech, Language, and Hearing Research, 47*, 126–144. doi:10.1044/1092-4388(2004/012)

Utley, C. A., & Mortweet, S. L. (1997). Peer-mediated instruction and interventions. *Focus on Exceptional Children, 29*(5), 1–23.

Van Laarhoven, T., Kos, D., Pehlke, K., Johnson, J. W., & Burgin, X. (2014). Comparison of video modeling and video feedback to increase employment-related social skills of learners with developmental disabilities. *DADD Online Journal, 1*(1), 69–90.

Vygotsky, L. S. (1978). Interaction between learning and development (M. Lopez-Morillas, Trans.). In M. Cole, V. John-Steiner, S. Scribner, & E. Souberman (Eds.), *Mind in society: The development of higher psychological processes* (pp. 79–91). Cambridge, MA: Harvard University Press.

White, S. W., Keonig, K., & Scahill, L. (2007). Social skills development in children with autism spectrum disorder: A review of the intervention research. *Journal of autism and developmental disorders, 37*(10), 1858–1868.

Wolfberg, P., Bottema-Beutel, K., & DeWitt, M. (2012). Including children with autism in social and imaginary play with typical peers: Integrated play groups model. *American Journal of Play, 5*(1), 55–80.

Wolfberg, P. J., & Schuler, A. L. (1993). Integrated play groups: A model for promoting the social and cognitive dimensions of play in children with autism. *Journal of Autism and Developmental Disorders, 23*(3), 467–489.

Wong, C. (2013). *Social narratives (SN) fact sheet*. Chapel Hill: The University of North Carolina, Frank Porter Graham Child Development Institute, The National Professional Development Center on Autism Spectrum Disorder.

Wong, C., Odom, S. L., Hume, K. Cox, A. W., Fettig, A., Kucharczyk, S., ... Schultz, T. R. (2014). *Evidence-based practices for children, youth, and young adults with autism spectrum disorder*. Chapel Hill: The University of North Carolina, Frank Porter Graham Child Development Institute, Autism Evidence-Based Practice Review Group. Retrieved from autismpdc.fpg.unc.edu/sites/autismpdc.fpg.unc.edu/files/2014-EBIReport.Pdf

BEHAVIOUR-BASED INTERVENTIONS

As repetitive and restricted patterns of behaviour are a core characteristic of autism spectrum disorder (ASD), this chapter is dedicated to interventions that are often applied, sometimes in combination, to limit the intrusion of these challenging behaviours in the daily life of an individual with ASD. The chapter reviews some common characteristics of this category of behaviours in relation to interventions and differentiates these behaviours and interventions from those of other similar disorders.

DEFINITION

Repetitive and restricted patterns of behaviour are included as part of the *Diagnostic and Statistical Manual of Mental Disorders-5 (DSM-5)* as one criteria for a diagnosis of ASD (American Psychiatric Association [APA, 2013]). There are various types of behaviours indicated, and the amount and manner in which they are exhibited varies significantly from individual to individual (Leekam, Prior, & Uljarevic, 2011). In addition, some behaviours, such as repetitive movements and hyper- or hyporeactivity to sensory input, are considered to occur more often in those who are lower functioning, whereas adherence to routines with a resistance to change and restricted, intense interests seem to be higher-order processes (Leekam et al., 2011). The type of intervention will therefore depend on the type of repetitive and restricted behaviour and the functioning level of the individual. For instance, an intervention for a sensory-based reaction will be much different from an intervention for an insistence on sameness in routine causing a student to scream and hit others when something changes.

Many interventions used for these behaviours are common applied behaviour analysis (ABA) strategies used in intervention categories in chapters 4 and 5 as well. They are highlighted here because they can be used to reduce behaviours targeted for change or to increase other skills. One of the common misconceptions is that the repetitive and restricted behaviour criterion in the *DSM-5* is synonymous with challenging behaviour. This is not the case, although at times trying to engage in these repetitive behaviours and restricted interests can dominate an individual's focus, causing challenging behaviours to occur when they cannot engage in them. Research has demonstrated that there are fewer rates of these behaviours in adulthood as compared to childhood, and higher rates of stereotypic motor and self-injurious behaviours occur in those with an intellectual disability and lower nonverbal IQ scores (Leekam et al., 2011; Richler, Huerta, Bishop, & Lord, 2010). Looking at the same individuals over time, it was found that sensorimotor repetitive behaviours remained somewhat constant, whereas the insistence on sameness worsened (Richler et al., 2010). In addition to ABA interventions, pharmacological interventions have also been widely used to treat repetitive and restricted patterns of behaviours, although they are outside the scope of this chapter (Leekam et al., 2011).

DIFFERENTIATING FROM OTHER DISABILITY AREAS

The repetitive and restricted patterns of behaviour seen in ASD have also been seen in other disorders, including "Tourette Syndrome, Fragile X, Rett's Disorder, Parkinson's Disease, Obsessive Compulsive Disorder, Down's Syndrome, dementia, deafness, blindness, schizophrenia, and intellectual disabilities" (Leekam et al., 2011, p. 566). Most research has demonstrated, however, that the frequency and range of behaviours that individuals with ASD display are much higher and broader than other clinical populations (Leekam et al., 2011). In addition, the functioning level of the individual seems to determine the frequency of behaviours, with lower-functioning individuals experiencing a higher amount (Leekam et al., 2011).

ASD is sometimes informally connected with obsessive-compulsive disorder (OCD) because of similarities such as repetitive behaviours and hoarding. In one study, it was demonstrated that 20 percent of those with OCD were also labelled as having autism-like traits, which included lower socialization scores as compared to other subjects with OCD (Bejerot, Nylander, & Lindström, 2001). Bejerot (2007) proposes that a subtype of OCD with ASD behaviours should be available, as there are individuals with OCD who have ASD-like characteristics. In addition, research has demonstrated that family members of those with ASD are more likely to have OCD and OCD characteristics (Berjerot et al., 2001; Ruta, Mugno, D'Arrigo, Vitiello, & Mazzone, 2010). Numerous studies have demonstrated that the exhibited behaviour types differ between individuals with ASD and those with OCD. Ruta and colleagues (2010) found that those with ASD displayed more ordering and hoarding behaviours, whereas those with OCD showed more contamination compulsions and aggressive obsessions with checking. In general, the obsessions and compulsions of those with ASD tend to be less sophisticated and fewer in frequency overall than those with OCD (Zandt, Prior, & Kyrios, 2007).

EVIDENCE-BASED INTERVENTIONS

This chapter primarily covers ABA strategies that have been found to be effective in the *EBI Report* (Wong et al., 2014). In addition, these same strategies have been found effective and grouped under behavioural interventions in the *National Standards Project—Phase II* (NAC, 2015). As mentioned earlier, these strategies can be used across many of the different communication, social, and repetitive and restricted behaviour categories, but are placed in this section because they are interventions focusing on reducing challenging behaviour and building behaviour skills.

Antecedent-Based Interventions

Antecedent-based interventions, manipulations, or control procedures change or remove antecedents to problem behaviours in the social and physical environments, rather than focusing on consequence-based interventions, which may be perceived as punitive. Because they are proactive and may circumvent the onset of problem behaviours before they occur, they are often emphasized in program planning (Kern & Clemens, 2007; Miltenberger, 2012). For example, if a student does not enjoy solving math problems but loves looking at snakes, snakes can be included with math problems (e.g., counting snakes), or snakes can be used on that student's math sheet as decorative figures. An antecedent strategy like this can be utilized for individual interventions or on a class-wide basis. In order to develop appropriate strategies, "information is obtained about environmental events that appear to set the occasion for problematic behavior as well as those that are associated with desirable behavior. Modifications are then introduced so that events occurring before problems are either eliminated or changed in some way such that they no longer trigger the prior problems" (Kern & Clemens, 2007, p. 65).

Antecedent-Based Interventions: Antecedent-based interventions "help prevent the triggers of inappropriate behavior. When the groundwork is put in place in the form of preventative measures that take into consideration the reasons for such behaviour ... tools are provided for the student to enable him/her to avoid the use of these behaviors as a form of communication" (Moyes, 2002, p. 55).

Antecedent strategies have been shown to be effective for children from toddlerhood to young adulthood, through the findings of 32 single-case designs in the *EBI Report* (Hume, 2013; Wong et al., 2014).

Adcock and Cuvo (2009), for example, effectively utilized antecedent strategies (i.e., interspersing previously learned tasks with new tasks) to promote academic learning as part of an intervention package for three pre-adolescent students with ASD in inclusive classrooms. Hume (2013) found that six types of antecedent strategies are commonly used:

1. Modifying educational activities, materials, or schedules (e.g., incorporating student interest);
2. Incorporating student choice in educational activities and materials;
3. Preparing students ahead of time for upcoming activities (e.g., priming);
4. Varying the format, level of difficulty, or order of instruction during educational activities (e.g., varying high and low demand requests);
5. Enriching the environment to provide additional cues or access to additional materials (e.g., visual cues, access to sensory stimuli); and,
6. Modifying prompting and reinforcement schedules and delivery (e.g., varying access to reinforcement prior to educational activities) (adapted from Hume, 2013, p. 49).

The following example focuses on the first strategy: incorporating students' interests or incorporating special interests into everyday routines when attending specifically to students with what are often termed restricted areas of interest. Incorporating strong and unique interests into everyday routines can be an important strategy to motivate students who have a strong area of restricted interest, also typically termed a special interest or special area of interest, focusing on the positives of restricted interests rather than viewing them as deficits (Mancil & Pearl, 2008).

Winter-Messiers (2007) terms these "special interest areas (SIA)" (p. 140), and applies this term specifically to individuals with Asperger's syndrome (AS):

Restricted Interests: Special interests, or restricted interests, can be defined as "topics or objects individuals with ASD pursue with intensity and focus. Sometimes they are called circumscribed interests, obsessions, compulsions, special interests, or narrow interests" (Mancil & Pearl, 2008, p. 3).

> The families of children and youth with AS are well aware of these all-consuming special interests. Attwood (2003) stated that SIAs seem "to be a dominant characteristic, occurring in over 90% of children and adults with AS" (p. 127). SIA can include such diverse fascinations as deep fat fryers, the passenger list of the Titanic, waist measurements (Klin, Volkmar, & Sparrow, 2000), the livery of Great Western trains (Tantam, 1991), Rommel's desert wars, paper bags (Gillberg, 1991), light and darkness (Kanner, 1973), toilet brushes (Attwood, 1998), globes and maps (Myles & Simpson, 2003), yellow pencils, oil paintings of trains (Attwood, 2003), photocopiers (Myles & Adreon, 2001), the World War II propeller plane Hawker Hurricane (J. W. Messiers, personal communication, August 20, 2006), industrial fans, elevators, dust, or shoes.

Areas of special interest may also result in an area—or areas—of special skills, allowing a practical application of that passion and knowledge. Vital, Ronald, Wallace, and Happé (2009) have synonymously termed these "savant skills," "islets of ability" (p. 1093) or even "splinter skills" (p. 1095). However, a relationship between such knowledge and skill cannot always be assumed: "although such unique skills do exist in individuals with ASD, this occurs less than 10 percent of the time and is hypothesized to be related to the cognitive style of ASD (e.g., restricted interests, focus on detail)" (Vital et al., 2009). In any case, incorporating these into everyday routines can support motivation, learning, and development, and "embedding these interests into the curriculum can make previously difficult and 'boring' tasks more interesting for the student with ASD" (Mancil & Pearl, 2008, p. 3). Kluth and Schwarz (2008) suggest 20 ways to use such strengths to encourage characteristics such as risk-taking and cooperation, and skills such as literacy and numeracy. Special interests, according to the authors, can be incorporated into classroom expectations, for example, through project-based learning. Even if a student has already explored an area of special interest, adaptations are possible, such as:

- Focusing on supported, related, curricular-linked skills (e.g., note-taking);
- Examining new content (e.g., moving from writing to drawing);
- Exploring a connected topic, such as a subspecialty (Kluth & Schwarz, 2008).

Simply embedding these special interests into lessons can increase engagement, such as by adding related visuals to resources (see Figure 6.1) using a planning process such as the one described in Table 6.1.

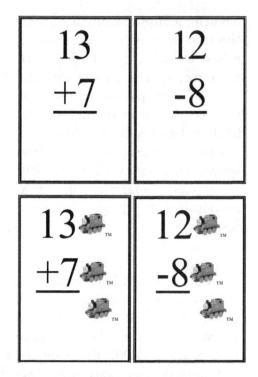

Figure 6.1: Classic Flash Cards versus Thomas the Tank Engine Flash Cards
Source: Mancil & Pearl, 2008, p. 5.

Read about it. Think about it. Write about it.

Describe how you would use an antecedent-based strategy to increase academic engagement in a student who has a particularly strong area of special interest.

Differential Reinforcement

Differential reinforcement utilizes differentiated responses for positively reinforcing—or not positively reinforcing—target behaviours. It was shown to be evidence-based for preschool-aged children up to adulthood, and "can be used effectively to address social, communication, behavior, joint attention, play, school-readiness, academic, motor, and adaptive skills" (Kucharczyk, 2013, p. 4). For example, a child may eat only food that is white, causing dietary concerns from his medical team. To help encourage a wider range of food preferences, that child may be offered a range of food items on his or her dinner plate, providing

Table 6.1: Planning Strategies that Incorporate Strengths and Interests

---

To plan a motivating strategy, consider following this structure:

1. *List* the strengths, interests, and talents of the student. Challenge yourself to write as many as possible!

2. *Identify* the student's specific area of need. Is the student's need behavioural, academic, social, or emotional?

3. *Consider* which research-supported strategies could be used to address the need. Consult recent literature or strategies found in journals like Intervention in School and Clinic.

4. *Pair* the strategy with a strength, interest, or talent creatively. Ensure that the interest is an inherent part of the strategy itself to increase the student's motivation.

Here are some of the strengths and interests our students have shared with us. It was our goal to teach with, through, and about these areas.

Strengths	Interests	Talents
• Reading stamina • Hyperlexia • Attention to detail • Computation • Ability to focus on areas of interest • Using the computer Creativity	• Titanic • Sharks • Transportation • Godzilla • Riddles • Waste management • Elevators • Anime	• Conceiving of imaginary worlds • Map making • Creating silly poems • Vocabulary • Creating collections • 3-D design • Creating comics

Source: Lanou, Hough, & Powell, 2012, p. 180.

opportunities for eating non-white food. While eating, that child may be given verbal praise, a high five, or a tickle for eating a food that is green (e.g., broccoli), but not given that positive reinforcement for eating white food that is already part of his or her food repertoire (e.g., french fries). This differential reinforcement will help to increase how often broccoli and other

Differential Reinforcement: "Reinforcing a child when he or she performs the target behavior in the presence of the target stimulus and not reinforcing the child if he or she does not perform the desired behaviour" (Barton & Harn, 2012, p. 134).

non-white foods are eaten and decrease how often white foods are eaten. See Table 6.2 for the more commonly known types of differential reinforcement.

Table 6.2: Common Types and Examples of Differential Reinforcement

Type	Definition
Differential reinforcement of alternative behaviour (DRA)	• Reinforcing a desired alternative behaviour (e.g., talking to peers about a popular television show) • Withholding reinforcement for a problem behaviour (e.g., talking to peers only about race cars)
Differential reinforcement of incompatible behaviour (DRI)	• Reinforcing a desired behaviour that cannot happen simultaneously with the problem behaviour (e.g., talking to peers about a popular television show that does not include race cars) • Withholding reinforcement for a problem behaviour (e.g., talking to peers only about race cars)
Differential reinforcement of other behaviour (DRO)	• Reinforcing the absence of a problem behaviour (e.g., not talking to peers only about race cars)

Source: Cooper, Heron, & Heward, 2007.

The three types of differentiated reinforcement outlined in Table 6.2 (DRA, DRI, and DRO) combined meet the criteria of being an evidence-based intervention, based on 26 single-case design studies in the *EBI Report* (Kucharczyk, 2013; Wong et al., 2014). One example of a related study is Nuernberger, Vargo, and Ringdahl's (2013) demonstration of the effectiveness of DRO as one element in a successful intervention designed to reduce repetitive hair, eyebrow, and eyelash pulling in a 19-year-old woman with ASD.

In the classroom environment, for example, a grade 3 student's difficulty with repetitive hand-flapping causes him to not engage in gym class activities (e.g., gymnastics) because he would rather hand-flap than tumble, use the rings, or swing on the parallel bars. Hand-flapping might then be prioritized as a problem behaviour as it is affecting his ability to be engaged in the activities of both the Ontario curriculum and the socialization opportunities that come along with participation in the inclusive classroom environment. This student's team might decide, then, that it is important to reduce hand-flapping in the gym using differential reinforcement; specifically, differential reinforcement of incompatible behaviours (DRI). Since the student's team already knows that attention—both teacher attention and peer attention—is a very powerful positive reinforcer for this student, they might plan to positively reinforce any gym class activities, such as a swinging on the rings, swinging from the parallel bars, and standing on his head or hands, by giving the student attention (e.g., smiling, praise, high fives, etc.) but not positively reinforcing (e.g., ignoring) him when he is hand-flapping. Since he cannot hand-flap and engage in these gym activities at the same time, this student will quickly learn that swinging on the rings, swinging from the parallel bars, and standing on his head or hands is an easy way to obtain attention, which he loves!

Read about it. Think about it. Write about it.

Explain how you might use differential reinforcement in a curricular area beyond physical education class.

Exercise

Exercise is one example of how to decrease disruptive behaviours, in general, and assist those who need support with interfering repetitive and restrictive behaviours (Wong et al., 2014). According to Cox (2013), exercise, as defined, is a new evidence-based intervention, with three single-subject designs and three group studies showing its effectiveness with preschoolers to early adolescents.

> **Exercise:** Exercise, in the context of evidence-based interventions and the field of ASD, is defined as "increase in physical exertion as a means of reducing problem behaviors or increasing appropriate behavior" (Cox, 2013, p. 60).

Exercise-based interventions have been used to:

- Decrease problem behaviours;
- Increase acceptable behaviours (e.g., school readiness-related skills);
- Increase motor skills; and,
- Increase physical fitness.

Characteristics of exercise-based interventions include that they:

- Occur regularly;
- Are pre-planned;
- Typically include both warm-up and cool-down phases;
- Often include stretching, aerobic, and strength training;
- May take place outside, inside, or in a swimming pool; and
- Are often used with other, concurrent strategies (e.g., visuals).

Nicholson, Kehle, Bray, and Van Heest (2010), for example, studied the effects of antecedent physical activity on the academic engagement of four nine-year-old boys with ASD, and found that an exercise-based jogging intervention of about 20 minutes, three times per week, resulted in increased academic engagement. Specific to the characteristic area of repetitive and restricted patterns of behaviour, Celiberti, Bobo, Kelly, Harris, and Handleman (1997) examined the relationship between such exercise and self-stimulatory behaviour. Using walking and jogging as an intervention for a five-year-old individual with ASD, they found that approximately 10 minutes of jogging was a successful intervention in decreasing stereotypical self-stimulation, in addition to other problem behaviour. Visual and physical stereotypy was targeted due to its interference with the development of functional skills and academic learning. For other individuals with ASD, then, exercise-based interventions (e.g., jogging) may help to decrease repetitive behaviours (e.g., twirling) and allow students to focus on other important areas of skill building that promote future independence.

Read about it. Think about it. Write about it.

Imagine how you might use an exercise-based intervention to support behaviour change in a family member, friend, or colleague.

Extinction

Extinction is a foundational strategy in the practice of ABA utilized in the field of ASD treatment, particularly in interventions related to restricted areas of interest and problematic, repetitive behaviours. It is an evidence-based intervention, based on one group design and four single-subject research studies, with evidence emerging from early childhood to early adolescence (Sullivan & Bogin, 2010a). A downfall of extinction, however, is that its side effects can include aggression. Often the behaviour may get worse before it gets better.

Extinction: Extinction is "weakening an undesirable behavior by withholding the reinforcer previously associated with it" (Dunn Buron & Wolfberg, 2008, p. 369).

Extinction is further described as a strategy that is "used to reduce or eliminate unwanted behaviour. Extinction involves withdrawing or terminating the positive reinforcer that maintains an inappropriate interfering behaviour. This withdrawal results in the stopping or extinction of behavior" (Sullivan & Bogin, 2010a, p. 1). Extinction is synonymous with decrease, and is especially relevant for targeting behaviours that are interfering with everyday functioning and opportunities for learning and causing distress. When ritualized and repetitive behaviours occur related to autism, Wolff, Hupp, and Symons (2012) emphasize that options for intervention are limited. In one example, the authors successfully intervened in two of three adults with both a cognitive delay and ASD who demonstrated "ritual and compulsive behaviours" (p. 1741) (e.g., hyper-vigilance around common household items), using an intervention package of response blocking and extinction. Aiken and Salzberg (1984) also used extinction with white noise in two children with ASD to successfully decrease vocal stereotypic behaviours (e.g., snorting), which were being maintained by sensory consequences. In general, the steps to implementing extinction are: 1) identification of the target interfering behaviour; 2) identification of data collection methods along with baseline data collection itself; 3) identification of the function or cause of the behaviour; 4) creation of an intervention plan to ensure that the target behaviour does not receive reinforcement; 5) implementation of the planned intervention; 6) collection of intervention data; and 7) review of the implemented intervention (Sullivan & Bogin, 2010b).

Extinction is inappropriate in some situations, such as dealing with extremely harmful behaviours or those that might be imitated to an intolerable level. There are two important additional considerations in the use of extinction. First is the typical occurrence of an extinction burst, where the target behaviour not only persists following the initial use of extinction but might temporarily increase in either force or amplitude. Second is the possibility of spontaneous recovery, when an extinguished behaviour returns without reinforcement. Both of these are temporary if intervention is applied with appropriate procedures (Cooper, Heron, & Heron, 2007). The use of extinction "requires sound, mature, humane, and ethical professional judgment," and should only be considered after more positive strategies have been attempted without success (Sullivan & Bogin, 2010a, p. 467).

Read about it. Think about it. Write about it.

In detail, explain some of the concerns around using extinction for interfering behaviours.

Functional Behaviour Assessment

Functional behaviour assessment (FBA) is a foundational component in planning successful interventions for a range of problematic behaviours, including those with repetitive and restricted patterns. It meets the standards for evidence-based interventions (with one group design and five single-subject designs); its effectiveness was demonstrated with preschool-aged children to adolescents; and it is typically focused on interventions in the communication and behaviour domains (Collet-Klingenberg, 2008).

Functional Behaviour Assessment: Functional behaviour assessment is defined as "a process for gathering information that can be used to maximize the effectiveness and efficiency of behavioral support" to understand why a behaviour is occurring so that appropriate interventions can be designed to change the reinforcers maintaining the behaviour (O'Neill et al., 1997, p. 3).

FBAs can be compiled indirectly (e.g., interviews, questionnaires), directly (e.g., systematic observation), and experimentally. The latter is termed a functional behaviour analysis, where conditions are set up by the clinician to understand which situations elicit target problem behaviours and the functions of the behaviours themselves (O'Neill et al., 1997). All approaches can provide information about "when, where, and why problem behaviors occur" (p. 6) through data-based evidence. An FBA determines if a problem behaviour is maintained by direct or socially mediated consequences (Cipani & Schock, 2011), as well as its underlying purpose, typically understood as either attention, avoidance, tangible, automatic, or a complex combination (Collet-Klingenberg, 2008; Neitzel & Bogin, 2008). Neitzel and Bogin (2008) describe a seven-step process for FBA (see Table 6.3).

Read about it. Think about it. Write about it.

Have you ever utilized an FBA or elements of an FBA, either formally or informally, to help develop an intervention approach? Explain. If not, explain how you might use this in a future situation.

Table 6.3: Steps of Functional Behaviour Assessment

Step	Description
1	Gather a multidisciplinary team (e.g., educators, clinicians)
2	Identify and operationalize the problem behaviour
3	Collect baseline data (i.e., questionnaires, interviews, observations)
4	Develop a functions-based hypothesis
5	Test the hypothesis
6	Develop intervention strategies (i.e., accommodations, resources, strategies, data collection)
7	Monitor effectiveness

Source: Neitzel & Bogin, 2008.

Response Interruption/Redirection

Response interruption/redirection, or RIR, is an evidence-based intervention that is especially advantageous for certain types of behaviours, such as repetitive behaviours, stereotypies, behaviours that have a defined sensory function, and behaviours that are persistent or resistant. In detail:

> **Response Interruption/Redirection:** Response interruption/redirection is defined by Neitzel (2009a) as interrupting an interfering behaviour and redirecting such behaviour to one that is more socially acceptable.

> RIR is particularly useful with persistent interfering behaviors that occur in the absence of other people, in a number of different settings, and during a variety of tasks. These behaviors are not often maintained by attention or escape. Instead, they are more likely maintained by sensory reinforcement and are often resistant to intervention attempts. RIR is particularly effective with sensory-maintained behaviors because teachers/practitioners interrupt learners from engaging in interfering behaviors and redirect them to more appropriate, alternative behaviors. (Neitzel, 2009a, p. 1)

RIR has met the standards for an evidence-based intervention in ASD with five successful single-subject studies, including preschool-aged children to high-school aged adolescents. For example, Ahearn, Clark, and MacDonald (2007) decreased significant levels of vocal stereotypy or "any instance of noncontextual or non-functional speech and included singing, babbling, repetitive grunts, squeals, and

---

Box 6.1: Functions of Behaviour

Escaping situations, tasks, or people
Sometimes children may engage in challenging behaviour to escape from situations, tasks, or people. For example, if your child throws food on the floor and is told "dinner is over," then your child may learn that throwing food on the floor means that he doesn't have to eat it.

Attention (adult or peer)
Sometimes children may engage in challenging behaviour to get attention from others (e.g., parent, sibling, teacher, peer, etc.). Attention can take many forms (e.g., looking at your child, talking with your child, giving help, laughing at the child, and even using a firm voice with the child). Sometimes your child may be looking for attention in any way possible. This could mean praise or even getting angry with them. For example, a child cries whenever you are on the phone, and then the parent yells, "Stop crying, I'm on the phone!" The child may learn that crying when parents are on the phone will result in attention.

Tangible items
Sometimes children may engage in challenging behaviour to receive a tangible item or a desired activity. Tangible items can include: food, toys, computer time, a turn at a game, etc. For example, a child goes up to his sibling at home and pushes her, and as a result gets the toy car; the child may by consequence learn that pushing others will result in gaining access to the toy car.

Automatic
Sometimes children may engage in challenging behaviours because it is internally reinforcing. It is important to note that a behaviour's appearance does not give an indication of its function. For example, if your child flaps his hands, he may not be doing so to meet an automatic need; it depends on what happens after the behaviour and where the behaviour occurs. Behaviours that serve as automatic function will occur across all environments, with a variety of different people and even when others are not there.

Source: ErinoakKids, 2012a.

---

phrases unrelated to the present situation. Examples include 'ee, ee, ee, ee'" (p. 266) using RIR-based language prompts (e.g., social questions). Neitzel (2009a) provides examples of alternative behaviours to replace such vocal stereotypies, as well as motor stereotypies, self-injury, pica, and echolalia (Table 6.4) and suggests four steps to RIR implementation (Table 6.5).

Table 6.4: Alternative Behaviours in RIR Use

Interfering behaviour	Description	Possible alternative behaviours
Motor stereotypy	Movement of body parts that has no apparent function and movement that is not directed toward another individual (e.g., hand-flapping, hand mouthing, putting fingers in ears, fanning/spreading fingers, positioning hands in front of face)	• Redirecting to put body parts somewhere other than mouth (e.g., on table, on lap) • Handing preferred toys/objects to learners one at a time • Providing an object to hold and/ or play with (e.g., squishy ball, play dough) • Teaching learner to put hands together
Vocal stereotypy	Vocalizations that have no apparent function and are not directed toward another individual (e.g., echolalia, non-contextual laughing/giggling, non-contextual words/phrases, non-recognizable words)	• Teaching learner to say, "I don't know" in response to a question • Teaching learners to use more appropriate language when they engage in vocal stereotypy (e.g., rather than giggling/laughing during social interventions, teach the learner to say, "Hello" to peers)
Self-injury	Any aggressive behaviour that is directed towards oneself (e.g., hitting, scratching, biting)	• Providing preferred toys and/or objects • Having learner engage in heavy work (e.g., pulling wagons, heavy lifting)
Pica	Ingesting non-food items such as pencils, paint chips, dirt	• Providing a food item to eat (e.g., popcorn, raisins) • Having learner chew gum, on a rubber tube, etc.
Echolalia	Repeating words, phrases, or vocalizations	• Teaching learner to say, "I don't know" in response to a question • Teaching learners to use more appropriate language when they engage in vocal stereotypy (e.g., rather than giggling/laughing during social interventions, teach the learner to say, "Hello" to peers)

Source: Neitzel, 2009b, p. 3.

Table 6.5: Implementation Steps to RIR

Step	Description	Essential activities
1	Identify the target interfering behaviour	• Use direct assessment (e.g., ABC—antecedent, behaviour, consequence) • Create a hypothesis • Choose alternate behaviour
2	Collect baseline data	• Choose type and format • Utilize multiple data collectors
3	Implement RIR intervention	• Use prompting, blocking, and reinforcement (see Neitzel, 2009b, for additional detail)
4	Monitor implementation	• Collect additional data • Adapt interventions as necessary

Source: Neitzel, 2009b.

Read about it. Think about it. Write about it.

Explain how you might use a verbal "block" for verbal stereotypy.

Self-Management

Self-management is a well-researched, important, and often-utilized evidence-based intervention to help individuals manage and reinforce their own behaviours. When self-management happens, children, adolescents, and adults with ASD learn to discriminate, monitor, and record their own target behaviours (Heflin & Alaimo, 2007; Neitzel & Busick, 2009). This may include conversational skills, self-help skills, and academic task completion. Overall, these techniques can "help a person be more effective and efficient in his daily life, replace bad habits with good ones, accomplish difficult tasks, and achieve personal goals" (Cooper, Heron, & Heward, 2007, p. 579).

Self-Management: Self-management can be defined as the ability to personally monitor one's own behaviours to reach a specific goal (Heflin & Alaimo, 2007).

Heflin and Alaimo (2007) emphasize that this is an especially important skill during academic learning. The evidence for self-management ranges from early childhood studies to interventions with high-school students in the areas of "play, social, adaptive, behavior, and language/communication skills" (Neitzel & Busick, 2009, p. 1) as well as the reduction of problem behaviours, such as stereotypies. Koegel and Koegel (1990) summarize the literature around this strategy specifically in the area of repetitive behaviours as follows: "Self-management treatment packages have two potential strengths for the reduction or elimination of stereotypic behavior: (a) self-management may be used for extended periods of time in the absence of a treatment provider, and (b) self-management techniques are easily adapted and used in a wide variety of settings" (p. 119).

They successfully utilized such a self-management package for four children with ASD considered severely disabled, quickly reducing sensory-based rituals (e.g., flapping, jumping, humming, etc.) to near-zero levels using check boxes and individualized reinforcers. Mancina, Tankersley, Kamps, Kravits, and Parrett (2000) also successfully reduced interfering vocalizations (e.g., repetitive words and phrases) in multiple settings for a 12-year-old girl with both ASD and a cognitive delay. Developing a self-management system can be summarized in four steps (Busick & Neitzel, 2009), using easy-to-use strategies for self-managed data collection, such as tally marks on paper, blocks in egg cartons, digital counters, poker chips placed in a jar (Scheuermann & Webber, 2002), or specialized software (Cooper, Heron, & Heward, 2007).

Table 6.6: Steps to Self-Management

Step	Description	Essential activities
1	Preparation	• Defining target behaviour • Identifying reinforcers • Planning data collection
2	Instruction	• Demonstrating target behaviour • Recording data • Managing reinforcement system
3	Implementation	• Providing materials or teaching gathering of materials
4	Independence	• Checking in • Changing criterion, session, and interval length

Source: Busick & Neitzel, 2009.

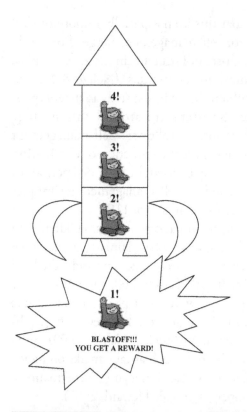

Figure 6.2: Sample Self-Management Data Collection Sheet

Instructions: Each time the student raises her hand to ask a question, she circles the picture of the girl raising her hand. She starts at four and counts down to one (for a total of four hand raises). When she gets to one, she earns a reinforcer.

Source: Busick & Neitzel, 2009, p. 13.

Read about it. Think about it. Write about it.

Explain how you have used any elements of self-management to change your own behaviour.

Task Analysis

Task analysis is breaking down complex behaviours into smaller, discrete steps that can be taught using multiple steps (Barton & Harn, 2012). Ontario's ErinoakKids Centre for Treatment and Development defines task analysis as synonymous with terms like "skills break down" and "sequencing" (ErinoakKids, 2012b, p. 1), and explains that demonstrating how to make a sandwich, following a recipe for making soup, and teaching a child how to brush their teeth are all examples of routines where one follows a task analysis. As of 2014, task analysis had

> **Task Analysis:** Breaking down complicated tasks into steps or parts that are teachable (Boutot & Smith Myles, 2011).

eight single-subject studies and is considered an evidence-based intervention (Fleury, 2013). For example, Luscre and Center (1996) taught three children with autism to cooperate with a dental exam using a step-by-step process as part of a treatment package, and Alcantara (1994) trained three children with a task analysis and other strategies to purchase items in a grocery store. Task analyses can help to teach functional routines to a child, youth, or adult, or help her or him adhere to a non-functional routine. For example, a task analysis may be useful in the case of an adolescent with a part-time job within walking distance from home who takes a route to work that is particularly lengthy—making him exhausted before he even starts—and is resistant to learning an efficient way to get there.

Scheuermann and Webber (2002) suggest that task analysis is part of individual curriculum development, and that the number of steps in any task analysis is dependent on an individual's ability. Those who are functioning at a lower level may require more steps in order to break down the task and learn the components of the entire skill. Cooper, Heron, and Heward (2007) add that the subject's age and experience also affect development of a task analysis, because this will influence the number of steps. Ontario's Grand Erie District School Board (2003) has developed a Life Skills Program Planner that consists of task analyses for life skills (e.g., making a bed), and functional academics (e.g., printing first name). Another Ontario resource is "A4: Assessing Achievement in Alternate Areas: A Place for Ideas, Resources and Sharing" (A4 Idea People, n.d.), which breaks down skills and alternatives to the Ontario curriculum, such as personal life management, social skills, and fine and gross motor skills, including downloadable planning, inventory, and assessment charts.

Task analyses can be developed in three ways:

- Watching a skilled person perform the task;
- Consulting with an expert on the task; or
- Personally completing the tasks (Cooper, Heron, & Heward, 2007).

Table 6.7: Types of Chaining

Type	Description
Forward chaining	Complex behaviours are taught from beginning to end
Backward chaining	Complex behaviours are taught from the last behaviour to the first behaviour in a chain

Source: Cooper, Heron, & Heward, 2007.

Table 6.8: Steps of Task Analysis

Step	Description
1	Identify the final target skill that needs to be taught
2	Identify all prerequisite skills and any materials needed to teach them
3	Break down the target skill into smaller components
4	Try out the task analysis to ensure that it is complete and accurate
5	Choose methods for teaching skills in the task analysis
6	Implement the intervention and monitor its success through data collection

Sources: Franzone, 2009a; Szidon & Franzone, 2009.

Read about it. Think about it. Write about it.

Create a task analysis for a complex skill you would like to teach or learn, such as making a drink in a blender or taking out the trash.

After the development of a task analysis, they are often taught through two well-known types of chaining: forward chaining and backward chaining (Table 6.7), utilizing "prompting, instructing, and reinforcing procedures" (Cooper et al., p. 437) to build new skills, though other options exist. Szidon and Franzone (2009) suggest six steps for implementation of a task analysis (Table 6.8).

Time Delay

Time delay is an evidence-based intervention in the ASD field, with such evidence emerging from five peer-reviewed, effective single-subject designs (Wong et al., 2014). Successes have been demonstrated in clinical interventions for 6- to 11-year-olds related to social, play, and language and communication skills, as well as academic areas of need (Neitzel, 2009). In time delay interventions, an item being learned, such as a new word (i.e., the

Time Delay: Time delay is "fading the use of prompts during instructional activities. This practice is always used in conjunction with prompting procedures ... a brief delay is provided between the initial instruction and any additional instructions or prompts" (Neitzel, 2009).

stimulus or instruction), is immediately paired with a picture (i.e., the prompt), but over time, space (the time delay) is added to allow a learner to respond before the prompt is shown (Akçin, 2013). It is important to emphasize that "there is no delay between the instruction and prompt when a learner is first learning a skill" (Neitzel, 2009, p. 1). Canadians Ingenmey and Van Houten (1991) used time delay successfully to increase the spontaneous speech of a 10-year-old boy with ASD who used hand gazing as a self-stimulatory behaviour, specifically targeting "spontaneous and task-appropriate speech during play" (p. 591).

According to Neitzel (2009), there are two evidence-based types of time delay (see Table 6.9).

Table 6.9: Types of Time Delay

Type	Description
Constant	Inserting a fixed amount of time after the instruction but before a prompt
Progressive	Inserting a gradually increasing amount of time after the instruction but before a prompt

Source: Neitzel, 2009.

For children with ASD who have restricted areas of interest or repetitive behaviours, time delay can be an effective intervention. For example, a child with ASD may be preoccupied with attending to a specific area of interest, and may not demonstrate an interest in other elements of the environment around him or her, which may be characterized by a lack of questions. One of the purposes of Taylor and Harris's (1995) intervention was the use of time delay to teach three children with ASD to ask, "What's that?" in order to gain additional information about objects and their surroundings. This intervention was successful with all three children. Neitzel and Wolery (2009) suggest a seven-step procedure for planning to teach a skill or behaviour using a time delay procedure (Table 6.10) and four steps for implementing it (Table 6.11), using essential features of ABA such as data collection and reinforcement (see Neitzel & Wolfrey, 2009, for details).

Read about it. Think about it. Write about it.
In your own words, explain the purpose of time delay.

Table 6.10: Seven Steps of Time Delay

Step	Name	Explanation
1	Target skill identification	What needs to be learned (i.e., behavioural goal)
2	Assessment of current skill level	Observing prerequisite skills (e.g., imitation, waiting)
3	Selection of stimulus and cue	Choosing a clear and consistent, "event, thing, or situation to which the learner with ASD should respond" (Neitzel & Wolery, 2009, p. 5) and a cue to use (e.g., phrase, picture, sound)
4	Choice of controlling prompt	Select a controlling prompt very successful in evoking behaviour
5	Identification of reinforcers	Choose reinforcers appropriate to the learner and as natural as possible in the particular context
6	Selection of response interval	Choose constant or progressive types according to characteristic task and learner
7	Choice of teaching times and activities	Identify regular times and the number of trials when skills/ behaviour can be taught

Source: Neitzel & Wolery, 2009.

Visual Strategies

Visual strategies have a strong evidence base for supporting students with ASD, and have been well utilized in both research and practice in home and school settings for all ages, meeting evidence-based criteria from preschool to pre-adolescence (Hume, 2008). For example, Dettmer, Simpson, Myles, and Ganz (2000) successfully decreased the latency in transition times for two boys with ASD in multiple settings using a visual schedule, and Pierce and Schreibman (1994) used pictorial self-management to train three children with ASD in daily living skills (e.g., getting dressed).

Visual supports are "part of everyone's communication system" (Rao & Gagie, 2006, p. 26). When teaching complex concepts, for example, "students with ASD benefit from having [a graphic or visual organizer] already developed for them.

Table 6.11: Four Steps of Implementing Time Delay

Step	Description
1	Teachers/practitioners: a. Provide learners with materials needed to use the self-management system at the appropriate time, or b. Teach learners to independently gather the necessary materials.
2	Teachers/practitioners provide learners with cues (e.g., verbal instruction, visual aid) that signal them to begin using self-management systems.
3	Teachers/practitioners teach learners how to self-record their behaviour in the target setting by: a. Prompting them (as needed) to self-record accurately at the appropriate time, b. Reinforcing all accurate self-recordings at the appropriate time (prompted and unprompted), and c. Fading prompts until learners self-record (without prompts) with accuracy 80% of the time.
4	Teachers/practitioners teach learners to gain access to reinforcement when the criterion is reached by: a. Prompting learners (as needed) to acquire reinforcement when the criterion is reached, and b. Fading prompts until learners consistently and independently acquire reinforcement when the criterion is reached.

Source: Neitzel & Wolery, 2009.

By visually representing the information, these students can call on their strong abilities to visualize information" (Marks et al., 2003, p. 51). Visuals are concrete, structured resources (e.g., maps, labels, scripts, etc.) (Hume, 2008) that can also support information processing, attention, focus, organization, and anxiety reduction in students with ASD—even "help[ing] the student express his or her thoughts" (Rao & Gagie, 2006, p. 26)—and provide instructional supports such as rules, models, instructions, scripts, schedules, and reminders, as well as depicting areas of interest (e.g., trains). Their use can support both academic and social learning in clinical and school environments, and help to increase independence, decrease the need for teacher prompting, and support behavioural learning, such as on-task behaviour (Goodman & Williams, 2007; Marks et al., 2003).

Careful consideration must be given to individual needs and the context when using a visual support, such as sociocultural considerations, required effort, clarity, size, age-appropriateness, and so on. It is essential to remember that, to be effective, the use of any visual supports should be taught, and the use assessed and adjusted as needed, using data-based decision making (Meadan, Ostrosky, Triplett, Michna, & Fettig, 2011). Many organizations provide easily accessible information, resources, and interactive tools for visual supports, such as the Visual Supports and ASD

Visual Schedule: According to Banda, Grimmett, and Hart (2009), a visual schedule is "a visual support system that combines photographs, images, or drawings in a sequential format to represent a targeted sequence" (p. 17).

Tool Kit (Autism Speaks, n.d.), PictureSET (Special Education Technology British Columbia, n.d.), and Ontario's Visuals Engine (ConnectABILITY, n.d.) and e-Learning Visuals (Geneva Centre, 2008) (the latter is available in both English and French).

Visual schedules are one example of a visual support used to assist students with ASD, typically in the classroom environment, and are also used in inclusive settings by all students, from class-wide schedules on the blackboard or white board to individualized electronic or paper schedules in a student's binder. Visual schedules remain as students develop in skills, functioning, age, and grade, though the format may change (e.g., moving from real items, photos, line drawings, to words). Schedules are helpful, as they provide information beforehand to individuals with ASD, who often struggle with change and thrive on routine and preparedness. Schedules can be used to depict the schedule of an entire day, the schedule of activities in a context (e.g., the school day), or how to complete a particular task (i.e., mini-schedules) using task analysis. They visually depict what is happening, what is next, when it's done, and if any plans have been changed (Meadan et al., 2011); they are particularly useful in allowing a student with restricted interests to see when a preferred activity will occur next. Visual schedules are useful for supporting both everyday, minor transitions as well as major transitions. For example, a visual schedule may help a student move from a highly preferred activity (e.g. stacking blocks) to a less preferred activity (e.g., completing a math worksheet), which might otherwise lead to them trying to escape the situation (escape-based disruptive behaviours), decreasing potential opportunities for learning. Visual schedules also help with communication (e.g., conversational skills), daily living skills (e.g., preparing meals), and challenging behaviours (e.g., compliance issues) (Banda, Grimmett, & Hart, 2009). Banda, Grimmett, and Hart (2009) suggest 12 steps for using visual schedules in inclusive classrooms (Table 6.12).

Table 6.12: Steps of Using Visual Schedules

Step	Description	Example
1	Identify target transition	Changing classroom activities
2	Collect baseline data	Frequency of target problem behaviour
3	Choose the type	Steps of the whole day versus steps of one activity
4	Choose a mode	Strip with hook-and-loop tape
5	Choose a medium	Colour photos versus black-and-white line drawings
6	Choose a location	On a wall with a "done" envelope
7	Teach the student	Modelling, prompting, and praise
8	Collect intervention data	Decrease in problem behaviour
9	Add new items	Lengthen the period of time
10	Fade prompts	Move to gestural prompts
11	Fade its prominence	Move to a binder
12	Encourage generalization	Apply to other settings

Source: adapted from Banda, Grimmett, & Hart, 2009.

Read about it. Think about it. Write about it.

Visit an online site for creating visual supports and explain how its use can help make the creation of visuals more effective or efficient.

Reinforcement

Reinforcement has a lengthy, effective history in research and applied practice, in clinical, educational, home, and community settings, as one of the foundational elements of applied behaviour analysis (Cooper, Heron, & Heward, 2007). Its use meets evidence-based standards from preschool until early adulthood, with 10 successful single-subject studies (Neitzel, 2009). For example, Pelios, MacDuff, and Axelrod (2003) used reinforcement as part of a treatment package to increase on-schedule and on-task independent work in three children with autism, and Todd and Reid (2006) also used an intervention package for three adolescents with autism to increase physical activity. In the latter study, verbal encouragement, preferred edibles, and tokens were used with success. Simply stated, reinforcement happens when the future likelihood of a behaviour increases; for example, when a child is verbally praised for putting dishes in the dishwasher, he or she is more likely to do that in the future (if parental praise is meaningful to him or her). For individuals who have special or restricted areas of interest, access to that interest often acts as a strong preference, and likely a reinforcer.

Reinforcement: "A relationship between learner behavior and a consequence that follows the behavior. This relationship is only considered reinforcement if the consequence increases the probability that a behavior will occur in the future, or at least be maintained" (Neitzel, 2009, p. 1), and will help children with ASD—and all learners—learn and use new skills (Neitzel, 2009).

Two types of reinforcement exist; both increase the likelihood of a given target behaviour, like putting the dishes in the dishwasher after a meal, happening again in the future.

Table 6.13: Types of Reinforcement

Type	Description	Future behaviour change
Positive reinforcement	The delivery of a reinforcer immediately following a target behaviour	Target behaviour increases
Negative reinforcement	The removal or lessening of an aversive immediately following a target behaviour	Target behaviour increases

Source: Cooper, Heron, & Heward, 2007.

A first-then arrangement is an example of positive reinforcement, and is based on the Premack principle. This means that, first, an individual completes a less preferred activity— for example, reading an assigned novel for 15 minutes. Then, that person is given an opportunity to participate in a highly preferred activity, such as scrolling through images of inukshuks on the computer for 15 minutes, or bouncing on a large exercise ball for 15 minutes.

Premack Principle: The Premack principle is defined as "contingent access to the opportunity to engage in a behavior that occurs as a high rate (i.e. eating preferred foods) upon engaging in a low frequency behavior (i.e. eating non-preferred or novel foods)" (Seiverling, Kokitus, & Williams, 2012, p.12).

First   **Then**

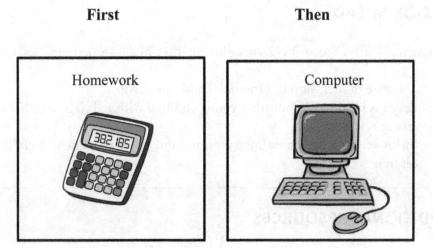

Figure 6.3: Example of a First-Then Board

Read about it. Think about it. Write about it.

Explain how you have, perhaps unknowingly, used a first-then strategy on yourself, or explain how you might in the future.

A LOOK BACK

Chapter 6, "Behaviour-Based Interventions," focused on:

- The repetitive and restricted patterns of behaviour that individuals with ASD exhibit;
- How these patterns of behaviour differ from other diagnoses, such as obsessive compulsive disorder (OCD); and
- Evidence-based interventions to work with repetitive and restricted behaviours, including antecedent-based interventions, differential reinforcement, exercise, extinction, functional behaviour assessment, response interruption/redirection, self-management, task analysis, time delay, visual supports, and reinforcement.

A LOOK AHEAD

Chapter 7, "Autism Spectrum Disorder in Ontario Child Care Settings," focuses on:

- The state of inclusion in Ontario's child care field;
- Responsibilities of supporting young children with red flags for ASD (e.g., service referrals); and
- Inclusive, evidence-based interventions and related research in child care centres.

ADDITIONAL RESOURCES

- A4: Assessing Achievement in Alternate Areas (A4 Idea People, n.d.): www.thea4ideaplace.com/
- Implementation checklist for task analysis (Franzone, 2009): autismpdc.fpg.unc.edu/sites/autismpdc.fpg.unc.edu/files/imce/documents/Task-analysis-Complete-10-2010.pdf
- Life Skills Planner (Grand Erie District School Board, 2003): autismbeacon.com/images/uploads/Life_Skills_Program_Planner.pdf
- Visual Supports & ASD Tool Kit (Autism Speaks, n.d.): www.autismspeaks.org/science/resources-programs/autism-treatment-network/tools-you-can-use/visual-supports
- PictureSET (Special Education Technology British Columbia, n.d.):
- www.setbc.org/pictureset/
- Time Delay Module (Neitzel & Busick, 2009): autismpdc.fpg.unc.edu/sites/autismpdc.fpg.unc.edu/files/imce/documents/TimeDelay_Complete.pdf
- Visuals Engine (ConnectABILITY, n.d.): connectability.ca/visuals-engine/
- E-Learning Visuals (Geneva Centre, 2008): visuals.autism.net/main.php?g2_itemId=25

REFERENCES

A4 Idea People. (n.d.) A4: Assessing achievement in alternate areas: A place for ideas, resources, and sharing. Retrieved from www.thea4ideaplace.com/

Adcock, J., & Cuvo, A. J. (2009). Enhancing learning for children with autism spectrum disorder in regular education by instructional modifications. *Research in Autism Spectrum Disorder, 3*(2), 319–328. doi: 10.1016/j.rasd.2008.07.004

Ahearn, W. H., Clark, K. M., & MacDonald, R. P. F. (2007). Assessing and treating vocal stereotypy in children with autism. *Journal of Applied Behavior Analysis, 40,* 263–275.

Aiken, J. M., & Salzberg, C. L. (1984). The effects of a sensory extinction procedure on stereotypic sounds of two autistic children. *Journal of Autism & Developmental Disorders, 14*(3), 291–299.

Akçin, N. (2013). Comparison of two instructional strategies for students with autism to read sight words. *Eurasian Journal of Educational Research*, (51), 85–106.

Alcantara, P. R. (1994). Effects of videotape instructional package on purchasing skills of children with autism. *Exceptional Children, 61*(1), 40–55.

American Psychiatric Association. (2013). *Diagnostic and statistical manual: DSM-5* (5th ed.). Washington, DC: Author.

Attwood, T. (1998). *Asperger syndrome: A guide for parents and professionals.* Philadelphia: Jessica Kingsley.

Attwood, T. (2003). Understanding and managing circumscribed interests. In M. Prior (Ed.), *Learning and behavior problems in Asperger syndrome* (pp. 126–147). New York: Guilford Press.

Autism Speaks. (n.d.). Visual supports and autism spectrum disorder tool kit. Retrieved from www.autismspeaks.org/science/resources-programs/autism-treatment-network/tools-you-can-use/visual-supports

Banda, D. R., Grimmett, E., & Hart, S. L. (2009). Activity schedules: Helping students with autism spectrum disorders in general education classrooms manage transition issues. *TEACHING Exceptional Children, 41*(4), 16–21.

Barton, E. E., & Harn, B. (2012). *Educating young children with autism spectrum disorder.* Thousand Oaks, CA: Corwin.

Belcher, C., & Maich, K. (2014). Autism spectrum disorder in popular media: Storied reflections of societal views. *Brock Education: A Journal of Educational Research and Practice, 23*(2), 1–19. doi: 10.1177/1088357609356094

Bejerot, S., Nylander, L., & Lindström, E. (2001). Autistic traits in obsessive-compulsive disorder. *Nordic Journal of Psychiatry, 55*(3), 169–176.

Bejerot, S. (2007). An autistic dimension: A proposed subtype of obsessive-compulsive disorder. *Autism, 11*(2), 101–110.

Boutot, E. A., & Smith Myles, B. (2011). Autism spectrum disorder: Foundations, characteristics, and effective strategies. Upper Saddle River, NJ: Pearson.

Busick, M., & Neitzel, J. (2009). Self-management: Steps for implementation. Chapel Hill, NC: National Professional Development Center on Autism Spectrum Disorder, Frank Porter Graham Child Development Institute, The University of North Carolina. Retrieved from http://csesa.fpg.unc.edu/sites/csesa.fpg.unc.edu/files/ebpbriefs/SelfManagement_Steps.pdf

Celiberti, D. A., Bobo, H. E., Kelly, K. S., Harris, S. L., & Handleman, J. S. (1997). The differential and temporal effects of antecedent exercise on the self-stimulatory behavior of a child with autism. *Research in Developmental Disabilities, 18*(2), 139–150.

Cipani, E., & Schock, K. M. (2011). *Functional behavior assessment, diagnosis, and treatment: A complete system for education and mental health settings.* New York, NY: Springer Publishing Company.

Collet-Klingenberg, L. (2008). Overview of functional behavior assessment. Madison, WI: The National Professional Development Center on Autism Spectrum Disorder, Waisman Center, The University of Wisconsin.

ConnectABILITY. (n.d.). Visuals Engine. Retrieved from http://connectability.ca/visuals-engine/

Cooper, J. O., Heron, T. E., & Heward, W. L. (2007). *Applied behaviour analysis* (2nd ed.). Upper Saddle River, NJ: Pearson.

Cox, A. W. (2013). Exercise (ECE) fact sheet. Chapel Hill: The University of North Carolina, Frank Porter Graham Child Development Institute, The National Professional Development Center on Autism Spectrum Disorder.

Dettmer, S., Simpson, R. L., Myles, B. S., & Ganz, J. B. (2000). The use of visual supports to facilitate transitions of students with autism. *Focus on Autism & Other Developmental Disabilities*, *15*(3), 163.

Dunn Buron, K., & Wolfberg, P. (2008). Learners on the autism spectrum: Preparing highly qualified educators. Shawnee Mission, KS: Autism Asperger Publishing Co.

ErinoakKids. (2012a). Functions of behaviour. Retrieved from http://www.erinoakkids.ca/getattachment/Resources/Growing-Up/Autism/Applied-Behaviour-Analysis/ABA-for-Families-Functions-of-Behaviour.pdf.aspx

ErinoakKids. (2012b). Task Analysis. Retrieved from http://www.erinoakkids.ca/getattachment/Resources/Growing-Up/Autism/Applied-Behaviour-Analysis/ABA-for-Families-Task-Analysis.pdf.aspx

Fleury, V. P. (2013). Task analysis fact sheet. Chapel Hill, NC: University of North Carolina, Frank Porter Graham Child Development Institute, The National Professional Development Center on Autism Spectrum Disorders

Franzone, E. (2009a). Implementation checklist for task analysis. Madison, WI: The National Professional Development Center on Autism Spectrum Disorder, Waisman Center, University of Wisconsin.

Franzone, E. (2009b). Overview of task analysis. Madison, WI: National Professional Development Center on Autism Spectrum Disorder, Waisman Center, University of Wisconsin.

Geneva Centre for Autism. (2008). Visuals. Retrieved from http://visuals.autism.net/main.php

Gillberg, C. (1991). Clinical and neurobiological aspects of Asperger syndrome in six family studies. In U. Frith (Ed.), *Autism and Asperger syndrome* (pp. 142–146). New York: Cambridge University Press.

Goodman, G., & Williams, C. M. (2007). Interventions for increasing the academic engagement of students with autism spectrum disorder in inclusive classrooms. *TEACHING Exceptional Children*, *39*(6), 53–61.

Grand Erie District School Board. (2003). Life skills planner: A framework for the development of programs for pupils who experience developmental delays. Retrieved from autismbeacon.com/images/uploads/Life_Skills_Program_Planner.pdf

Helfin, J., & Alaimo, D. F. (2007). *Students with autism spectrum disorder: Effective instructional practices.* Upper Saddle River, NJ: Pearson.

Hume, K. (2008). Overview of visual supports. Chapel Hill, NC: National Professional Development Center on Autism Spectrum Disorder, Frank Porter Graham Child Development Institute, The University of North Carolina. Retrieved from autismpdc.fpg.unc.edu/sites/autismpdc.fpg.unc.edu/files/imce/documents/VisualSupports_Complete.pdf

Hume, K. (2013). Antecedent-based intervention (ABI) fact sheet. Chapel Hill: The University of North Carolina, Frank Porter Graham Child Development Institute, The National Professional Development Center on Autism Spectrum Disorder. autismpdc.fpg.unc.edu/sites/autismpdc.fpg.unc.edu/files/imce/documents/ABI-complete-2010.pdf

Ingenmey, R., & Van Houten, R. (1991). Using time delay to promote spontaneous speech in an autistic child. *Journal of Applied Behavior Analysis*, *24*(3), 591–596.

Kanner, L. (1973). *Childhood psychosis: Initial studies and new insights.* Washington, DC: Winston.

Kern, L., & Clemens, N. H. (2007). Antecedent strategies to promote appropriate classroom behavior. *Psychology in the Schools*, *44*(1), 65–75. doi:10.1002/pits.20206

Klin, A., Volkmar, F. R., & Sparrow, S. (2000). *Asperger syndrome*. New York: Guilford Press.

Kluth, P. (2015). Paula Kluth: Toward inclusive classrooms and communities. Retrieved from www.paulakluth.com/books-and-products/

Kluth, P., & Schwarz, P. (2008). *"Just give him the whale!": 20 ways to use fascinations, areas of expertise, and strengths to support students with autism*. Baltimore, MD: Paul H. Brookes Pub. Co.

Koegel, R. L., & Koegel, L. K. (1990). Extended reductions of stereotypic behavior of students with autism through a self-management treatment package. *Journal of Applied Behavior Analysis, 23*(1), 119–127.

Kucharczyk, S. (2013). Differential reinforcement of alternative, incompatible, or other behavior (DRA/I/O) fact sheet. Chapel Hill: The University of North Carolina, Frank Porter Graham Child Development Institute, The National Professional Development Center on Autism Spectrum Disorder.

Lanou, A., Hough, L., & Powell, E. (2012). Case studies on using strengths and interests to address the needs of students with autism spectrum disorder. *Intervention in School and Clinic, 47*(3), 175–182.

Leekam, S. R., Prior, M. R., & Uljarevic, M. (2011). Restricted and repetitive behaviors in autism spectrum disorder: A review of research in the last decade. *Psychological Bulletin, 137*(4), 562–593. doi:10.1037/a0023341

Luscre, D. M., & Center, D. B. (1996). Procedures for reducing dental fear in children with autism. *Journal of Autism & Developmental Disorders, 26*(5), 547–556.

Mancil, G. R., & Pearl, C. E. (2008). Restricted interests as motivators: Improving academic engagement and outcomes of children on the autism spectrum. *TEACHING Exceptional Children Plus, 4*(6). Retrieved from escholarship.bc.edu/education/tecplus/vol4/iss6/art7

Mancina, C., Tankersley, M., Kamps, D., Kravits, T., & Parrett, J. (2000). Brief report: Reduction of inappropriate vocalizations for a child with autism using a self-management treatment program. *Journal of Autism & Developmental Disorders, 30*(6), 599.

Marks, S. U., Shaw-Hegwer, J., Schrader, C., Longaker, T., Peters, I., Powers, F., & Levine, M. (2003). Instructional management tips for teachers of students with autism spectrum disorder (ASD). *TEACHING Exceptional Children, 35*(4), 50–54.

Meadan, H., Ostrosky, M. M., Triplett, B., Michna, A., & Fettig, A. (2011). Using visual supports with young children with autism spectrum disorder. *TEACHING Exceptional Children, 43*(6), 28–35.

Miltenberger, R. (2012). *Behaviour modification: Principles and procedures*. Belmont, CA: Wadsworth.

Moyes, R. (2002). Addressing the challenging behaviour of children with high-functioning autism/Asperger syndrome in the classroom: A guide for parents and teachers. London, UK: Jessica Kingsley Publishers.

Myles, B. S., & Adreon, D. (2001). *Asperger syndrome and adolescence: Practical solutions for school success*. Shawnee Mission, KS: Autism Asperger.

Myles, B. S., & Simpson, R. L. (2003). *Asperger syndrome: A guide for educators and parents*. Austin, TX: PRO-ED.

National Autism Center. (2015). Findings and conclusions, national standards project, phase 2. Retrieved from http://www.nationalautismcenter.org/national-standards-project/

Neitzel, J. & Bogin, J. (2008). Steps for implementation: Functional behavior assessment. Chapel Hill, NC: The National Professional Development Center on Autism Spectrum Disorders, Frank Porter Graham Child Development Institute, The University of North Carolina. Retrieved from http://csesa.fpg.unc.edu/sites/csesa.fpg.unc.edu/files/ebpbriefs/FBA_Steps_0.pdf

Neitzel, J. (2009a). Overview of response interruption/redirection. Chapel Hill, NC: The National Professional Development Center on Autism Spectrum Disorders, Frank Porter Graham Child Development Institute, The University of North Carolina. Retrieved from http://csesa.fpg.unc.edu/sites/csesa.fpg.unc.edu/files/ebpbriefs/ResponseInterruption_Overview.pdf

Neitzel, J. (2009b). Steps for implementation: Response interruption/redirection. Chapel Hill, NC: The National Professional Development Center on Autism Spectrum Disorders, Frank Porter Graham Child Development Institute, The University of North Carolina. Retrieved from http://csesa.fpg.unc.edu/sites/csesa.fpg.unc.edu/files/ebpbriefs/ResponseInterruption_Steps.pdf

Neitzel, J. (2009c). Overview of reinforcement. Chapel Hill, NC: The National Professional Development Center on Autism Spectrum Disorder, Frank Porter Graham Child Development Institute, The University of North Carolina.

Neitzel, J. (2009d). Overview of time delay. Chapel Hill, NC: National Professional Development Center on Autism Spectrum Disorder, Frank Porter Graham Child Development Institute, The University of North Carolina.

Neitzel, J. & Busick, M. (2009). Overview of self-management. Chapel Hill, NC: National Professional Development Center on Autism Spectrum Disorder, Frank Porter Graham Child Development Institute, The University of North Carolina

Neitzel, J., & Wolery, M. (2009). Steps for implementation: Time delay. Chapel Hill, NC: The National Professional Development Center on Autism Spectrum Disorder, Frank Porter Graham Child Development Institute, The University of North Carolina.

Nicholson, H., Kehle, T. J., Bray, M. A., & Van Heest, J. (2010). The effects of antecedent physical activity on the academic engagement of children with autism spectrum disorder. *Psychology in the Schools*, *48*(2), 198–213. doi: 10.1002/pits

Nuernberger, J., Vargo, K., & Ringdahl, J. (2013). An application of differential reinforcement of other behavior and self-monitoring to address repetitive behavior. *Journal of Developmental & Physical Disabilities*, *25*(1), 105–117. doi:10.1007/s10882-012-9309-x

O'Neill, R. E., Horner, R. H., Albin, R. W., Sprague, J. R., Storey, K., & Newton, J. S. (1997). *Functional assessment and program development for problem behaviour: A practical handbook* (2nd ed). Belmont, CA: Wadsworth Cengage Learning.

Pelios, L. V., MacDuff, G. S., & Axelrod, S. (2003). The effects of a treatment package in establishing independent academic work skills in children with autism. *Education and Treatment of Children*, *26*(1), 1–21.

Pierce, K. L., & Schreibman, L. (1994). Teaching daily living skills to children with autism in unsupervised settings through pictorial self-management. *Journal of Applied Behavior Analysis*, *27*(3), 471.

Rao, S. M., & Gagie, B. (2006). Learning through seeing and doing: Visual supports for children with autism. *Teaching Exceptional Children*, *38*(6), 26–33.

Reichow, B., & Reichow, T. (2012). Evidence-based strategies for teaching children with autism spectrum disorder: Skill acquisition and fluency. In E. E. Barton & B. Harn (Eds.), *Educating young children with autism spectrum disorder* (pp. 127–150). Thousand Oaks, CA: Corwin.

Richler, J., Huerta, M., Bishop, S. L., & Lord, C. (2010). Developmental trajectories of restricted and repetitive behaviors and interests in children with autism spectrum disorder. *Development and Psychopathology, 22*(01), 55–69.

Ruta, L., Mugno, D., D'Arrigo, V. G., Vitiello, B., & Mazzone, L. (2010). Obsessive–compulsive traits in children and adolescents with Asperger syndrome. *European Child & Adolescent Psychiatry, 19*(1), 17–24.

Scheuermann, B. & Webber, J. (2002). *Autism: Teaching does make a difference.* Belmont, CA: Wadsworth Cengage Learning.

Seiverling, L., Kokitus, A., & Williams, K. (2012). A clinical demonstration of a treatment package for food selectivity. *Behavior Analyst Today, 13*(2), 11–16.

Special Education Technology British Columbia. (n.d.). PictureSET. Retrieved from https://www.setbc.org/pictureset/

Sullivan, L., & Bogin, J. (2010a). Overview of extinction. Sacramento: CA. National Professional Development Center on Autism Spectrum Disorder, M.I.N.D. Institute. University of California at Davis Medical School.

Sullivan, L. & Bogin, J. (2010b). Steps for implementation: Extinction.

Sacramento, CA: The National Professional Development Center on Autism Spectrum Disorder, M.I.N.D Institute, University of Californiaat Davis School of Medicine.

Szidon, K., & Franzone, E. (2009). Task Analysis. Madison, WI: National Professional Development Center on Autism Spectrum Disorder, Waisman Center, University of Wisconsin.

Tanidir, C., & Mukaddes, N. M. (2014). Referral pattern and special interests in children and adolescents with Asperger Syndrome: A Turkish referred sample. *Autism: The International Journal of Research and Practice, 18*(2), 178–184.

Tantam, D. (1991). Asperger syndrome in adulthood. In U. Frith (Ed.), *Autism and Asperger syndrome* (pp. 147–183). New York: Cambridge University Press.

Taylor, B. A., & Harris, S. L. (1995). Teaching children with autism to seek information: Acquisition of novel information and generalization of responding. *Journal of Applied Behavior Analysis, 28*, 3–14.

Todd, T., & Reid, G. (2006). Increasing physical activity in individuals with autism. *Focus on Autism and Other Developmental Disabilities, 21*(3), 167–176.

Vital, P. M., Ronald, A., Wallace, G. L., & Happé, F. (2009). Relationship between special abilities and autistic-like traits in a large population-based sample of 8-year-olds. *Journal of Child Psychology & Psychiatry, 50*(9), 1093-1101. doi:10.1111/j.1469-7610.2009.02076.x

Winter-Messiers, M. A. (2007). From tarantulas to toilet brushes: understanding the special interest areas of children and youth with Asperger syndrome. *Remedial & Special Education*, (3), 140.

Wolff, J. J., Hupp, S. C., & Symons, F. J. (2012). Brief report: Avoidance extinction of treatment for compulsive and ritual behaviour in autism. *Journal of Autism & Developmental Disorders, 43*, 1741–746.

Wong, C., Odom, S. L., Hume, K. Cox, A. W., Fettig, A., Kucharczyk, S.,…Schultz, T. R. (2014). *Evidence-based practices for children, youth, and young adults with autism spectrum disorder.* Chapel Hill: The University of North Carolina, Frank Porter Graham Child Development Institute, Autism Evidence-Based Practice Review Group.

Zandt, F., Prior, M., & Kyrios, M. (2007). Repetitive behaviour in children with high functioning autism and obsessive compulsive disorder. *Journal of Autism and Developmental Disorders, 37*(2), 251–259.

SECTION III

A LOOK
ACROSS THE LIFESPAN

SECTION 3, A LOOK ACROSS THE LIFESPAN, TAKES A SPECIFIC look at autism spectrum disorder (ASD) services across Ontario. This starts in chapter 7 with the child care context, describing inclusive principles and practices as well as red flags and referrals to agencies should child care educators suspect a diagnosis. Services for ASD in the school setting are explored in chapter 8, where the spectrum of placement options are examined from inclusive to alternate settings, while exploring the details of the Individual Education Plan (IEP). Chapter 9 looks at current history and supports for treating adults with ASD, examining the transition to adulthood in addition to recreation, housing, schooling, and employment options and supports in Ontario. Chapter 10 describes the changing view of ASD in the family, from negative historical views to current views, including a survey of supports for families across the province. The section is designed to aid understanding of how policies, services, and supports are laid out and made available in Ontario for individuals with ASD.

CHAPTER 7

AUTISM SPECTRUM DISORDER IN ONTARIO CHILD CARE SETTINGS

In chapter 7, the significant changes in Ontario's child care field are briefly reviewed, including the state of inclusion both in a general context and in the specific context of inclusion for students with autism spectrum disorder (ASD). Responsibilities of the child care field in the case of young children with ASD are outlined, including recognition of red flags for ASD, referral for additional service provision, individual program plans, and the need to provide inclusive, evidence-based interventions onsite at child care centres. An example is given of utilizing visual supports to support students with ASD and all young children in a child care centre. Provincial research on young children with ASD in child care settings is presented, interwoven throughout these principles and practices. Three feature stories are included in chapter 7: one reflection of a front-line early childhood educator teaching a child with ASD, and two stories of exemplary, inclusive local programs which include support and care for children with ASD in their child care settings.

INTRODUCTION

Ontario's field of licensed early childhood education and care—an area of provincial responsibility with little federal direction—is in a state of change (Ferns & Friendly, 2014). In 2008, the Ontario College of Early Childhood

Educators (CECE) accepted its first member, a registered early childhood educator (RECE) (Ontario College of Early Childhood Educators, 2014), following the 2007 Early Childhood Educators Act (Service Ontario e-laws, 2007). The Early Childhood Educators Act established the registered early childhood educator credential and serves to regulate and govern early childhood education to protect the public interests (Service Ontario e-laws, 2007). The regulatory body of the CECE provides foundational

Ontario's College of Early Childhood Educators: "The professional self-regulatory body for early childhood educators (ECEs) in Ontario. The College's mandate is to protect the public interest and ensure quality and standards in the practice of early childhood education" (Ontario College of Early Childhood Educators, n.d., para. 1).

services to its member RECEs, such as professional registration and governance, ethics and standards of practice, resource publications, and professional advisories.

Another significant change occurred when RECEs became employed in school-based settings: "In 2010, Ontario began to implement a new province-wide, government-sponsored initiative for all early learners—including children with special needs—which continues to be piloted in school boards until its full implementation, namely, full-day kindergarten" (Ontario Ministry of Education, 2010; Ontario Ministry of Education, 2013), now fully implemented in the province. In this model, full-day kindergarten for four- and five-year-olds was rolled out to every school in the province over multiple years, in which an Ontario Certified Teacher and an RECE worked together on a play-based curriculum. Subsequently, Ontario's Education Act (Service Ontario e-laws, 2014) was updated to include the roles and responsibilities of designated early childhood educators in the school system. One of these inevitable responsibilities in today's inclusive settings is supporting students with exceptionalities, including ASD, in child care settings. McLennan, Huculak, and Sheehan (2008) examined four centres of specialized service provision across Canada, including two located in Ontario, and found that 39 percent of surveyed parents reported receiving daycare services, though a picture of service receipt overall was difficult to clarify.

Read about it. Think about it. Write about it.

Choose one or more of these changes in Ontario's child care field and explain how you think services for children with ASD in child care settings could be affected.

INCLUSIVE PRACTICES IN ONTARIO CHILD CARE SETTINGS

The practice of inclusion varies across Ontario's licensed child care centres. Currently, "legislation and policy that make it illegal to exclude children with special needs are lacking" (Crowther, 2010, p. 44), and child care centres are permitted to refuse children with special needs. Even when special needs children can access such settings, multiple issues remain, including the absence of proper funding, resources, facilities, and training. Some individual centres and geographic regions struggle with inclusion, and others are firmly committed to inclusion as an essential practice. Provincially, it is recognized that "inclusive early education is not just about placement in a program, but also active participation in social interactions and the development of children's abilities and skills" (Underwood, 2013, p. 1). St. Matthew's House is an example of such an inclusive environment, aided by three elements that Underwood emphasizes: supportive policies, leadership, and staff.

Box 7.1: St. Matthew's House: Where Hope Lives

- St. Matthew's House (SMH) is a charitable, non-profit, multi-service agency local in the inner city of Hamilton. We have been providing services to the most vulnerable in our community since the mid-sixties.
- Our goal is to instill hope in people's lives, improve their quality of life and increase their capacity to participate in the community.
- Our Early Childhood Integration Support Services (ECISS) serves preschool children with special needs who are enrolled in child care centres in the city of Hamilton. (St. Matthew's House, n.d.)

Hamilton's child care centres are in a state of "new beginnings," according to Susan Lepore, Program Manager at the Early Childhood Integration Support Services, one of the many services at St. Matthew's House and one of five services that make up the Integration Resources Hub. The Integration Resources Hub is a group of agencies that receive special needs resourcing funding to support preschool children with special needs in licensed child care centres in the city of Hamilton.

"We utilize our funding," Susan explains, "to support preschool-aged children with identified special needs and support them in licensed child care settings."

"Our municipality has completed a special needs resourcing review and we are waiting for that report to become public, to formally find out what we are doing well and where the gaps are." But while they wait, many positive, inclusive practices and programs are happening every day in Hamilton, Ontario. "We do not turn children away," Susan emphasizes with passion. "We do not turn away children with ASD. But we do have parents of children with ASD who are surprised that their children are allowed to continue.... All of our centres are inclusive, but not all are yet accessible: the best fit between centre and child is extremely important. Child care is very accommodating, all-embracing, and we work very well with families."

Children come to the St. Matthew's-based child care centres in

Integration Resources Hub: The Integration Resources Hub is a group of five agencies in the city of Hamilton—Early Childhood Integration Support Services (St. Matthew's House), McMaster Children's Hospital (Chedoke), Red Hill Family Centre (City of Hamilton), Community Living (Hamilton), and Hamilton and District of Cooperative Preschools Corporation—which are provided with special needs resourcing to support a range of programs.

various ways. Hamilton also has a "Check It Out: Do you have questions about your child's development?" postcard for quick, face-to-face consultations with various professionals, such as an occupational therapist, a speech-language pathologist, and a public health nurse. "Parents simply check boxes and write their concerns, then have a chance to meet with various professionals every month," summarizes Susan. "This can be one of the ways we get referrals.... When we get a referral for any child with special needs—not just ASD—we have a process." Educators from St. Matthew's follow a strengths-based approach. They have an onsite play visit; meet the child and the family; find out about reinforcers, barriers, communication style, and clinical supports; and develop strengths, goals, and a profile. Then, they begin! "What is tricky," Susan cautions, "is if the child care centre thinks they need more than resource consultant support for students on Individual Program Plans, which is called a 'support facilitator,' extra staff placed in the centre as a means of supporting the centre, for three to four months before we reassess. This is not intended as one-to-one support, but as a means of improving the overall ratio and building capacity." If any child, including those with ASD, has complex medical needs, then staff is trained to meet those needs, and a medical plan is put in place. If a child with ASD is receiving intensive behaviour intervention (IBI), for example, IBI sometimes happens in the centre, but not in the classroom. If a child needs an Individualized Program Plan (IPP), that child has to have a one-year delay in two areas of development. But if a centre is not yet sure of a child's needs, and they encounter a not-yet-diagnosed child who might have ASD, staff members watch for and document any red flags of development. They wait a little for the parents to approach the RECE in the classrooms, while in the meantime supporting that student in joining in—even if it is just for a minute at a time. "Red flags usually start around speech and language development," Susan emphasizes. "We make sure the concerns are not scary, and have no stigma. We would introduce the family to a resource consultant; we might refer to a speech-language program, other clinical supports, or maybe suggest the parents talk to the family doctor. Or, one of us might refer a family directly to a clinical setting, and they will direct the process accordingly, beginning with a pediatric appointment." Centres that have students with ASD can be provided with multi-disciplinary training, individual staff members might attend training or conferences as part of their own continuous learning plan, or a range of community-based training is available to train staff at all of the centres. "Children with ASD are all unique and different," Susan recognizes. "They tend to have trouble with similar things—like a lack of social learning—but their personalities, barriers, reinforcers, and special interests are all different. There is no magic formula to support and teach a child with ASD. You have to be a good observer, and look at each child and that child's gifts, because communication can be very subtle." Transitioning successfully to school is an important time for a child with ASD. To support this significant transition, comprehensive planning is necessary. For example, parents complete a package of information about their child, the school boards come together for an information night, and transition meetings happen, along with on-site observations. "We don't really have them for very long: maybe from age one to age three," Susan reflects. St. Matthew's-based child care centres support all students in an inclusive environment—including children with ASD—leading the way to model effective inclusion for all children in child care settings in Ontario.

Tools do exist to help examine inclusive practices specific to child care centres. Many sites in Ontario make use of the SpeciaLink Early Childhood Inclusion Tool (Irwin, 2009). This tool is not ASD-specific, but does give a general sense of a centre's overall approach to inclusion, consisting of the SpeciaLink Child Care Inclusion Practice Profile and the SpeciaLink Child Care Principles Scale (Crowther, 2010).

The SpeciaLink Early Childhood Inclusion Quality Scale is a tool for assessing inclusion quality in early childhood centres and for helping centres move toward higher quality inclusion. The Scale provides a picture of sustainable and evolving inclusion quality — an emerging issue as more children with special needs attend community-based centres and as inclusion pioneers leave their centres and a new generation of directors and early childhood educators take on the inclusion challenges. (The National Centre for Child Care Inclusion, 2010)

Inclusive practices for young children with exceptionalities, including those with ASD, can be categorized in the following manner: inclusive programs (e.g., environmental adaptations), support services (e.g., clinical services), and specialized programs (e.g., IBI) (Crowther, 2010). In many instances, support services and specialized programs can be invited in or hosted by child care centres, whereby clinicians (e.g., a speech-language pathologist) who are working with an individual can come into the centre, or the IBI team may come into the centre for part of the day to implement the ASD support program with the child. However, inclusive programs also take individual initiative and responsibility to provide inclusive environments. An example of such an environmental arrangement is the use of visual strategies.

It is inevitable that many eager, innovative educators will continue to adopt novel, emerging practices that are not yet supported by a sustained research base, such as the use of iPads and children's picture books that include characters with ASD (e.g., King, Thonrieczek, Voreis, & Scott, 2014; Maich & Belcher, 2012; Murdock, Ganz, & Crittendon, 2013). Although most best practices for including and supporting students with ASD in child care settings are evidence-based interventions offered in other settings to diverse age groups (chapter 3), some are important to highlight in the specific context of the child care setting. Visual strategies are one such evidence-based intervention that fits well into typical child care practice from a universal design approach (Ontario Ministry of Education, 2005) (see chapter 8) and can be incorporated in everyday practice. The goal of visual strategies is to help a child develop a particular behavioural or social skill, or to attain independence, without prompts from others (Wong et al., 2014). Types of visual strategies that can be individualized for children with ASD, as well as used with all children in inclusive environments, are listed in Table 7.1.

Visual strategies can use objects, photos, line drawings, or words, depending on the needs of the students. Visual strategies can be organized through their structure (e.g., inherent prompts), their organization (e.g., consistent sequence), and their clarity (e.g., colour coding). Before utilizing a visual strategy individualized for the needs of a student with ASD, its purpose should be clarified, the appropriate type should be selected, the child should be specifically taught its use, and its implementation should be monitored and adapted, as needed (Meadan, Ostrosky, Triplett, Michna, & Fettig, 2011). Visual strategies can also be used to teach specific social and behavioural skills, such as play, with social scripts that indicate what to do or say, visual cards that remind students to play with one another, or visual indicators of whose turn it is (Mavropoulou, Papadopoulou, & Kakana, 2011).

Table 7.1: Visual Strategies for Young Children with ASD

Type of visuals	Purpose
Schedules	Support transitions
Environmental	Decrease prompting
Scripts	Increase social skills
Cards	Understand behavioural expectations
Task analysis	Build complex skills

Source: Meadan, Ostrosky, Triplett, Michna, & Fettig, 2011.

Hampshire and Hourcade (2014) emphasize that while inclusive settings are becoming more common for young children with ASD, environmental inclusion is not sufficient to establish high levels of social interaction—including play. Rather, play skills need to be taught systemically, utilizing visual strategies as a strengths-based instructional strategy. Five steps to teaching play skills are suggested by Hampshire and Hourcade (2014):

1. Identify reinforcing play resources
2. Develop a task analysis of a specific play sequence
3. Visually structure resources (i.e., allow resources to be instructions)
4. Teach using prompting strategies (e.g., least-to-most)
5. Expand and generalize new skills

Read about it. Think about it. Write about it.

Choose an evidence-based or innovative, promising strategy for children with ASD, and explain how you might use this effectively for all the children in a child care centre.

RED FLAGS AND EARLY DETECTION

Two of the keys to supporting young children with ASD are early detection and early intervention. In addition to being educated on potential interventions for young children, professionals supporting students with ASD in child care centres are responsible for identifying concerns or red flags in young children with ASD who might not yet be diagnosed, as well as documenting and communicating concerns related to foundational skills like imitation, joint attention, and peer interest (Barton & Harn, 2012). Being aware of easily accessible screening tools, such as the Modified Checklist for Autism in Toddlers (M-CHAT-R), can be beneficial (Robins, Fein, & Barton, 1999). However, the experience of staff members with red flags for ASD may vary widely. Autism Ontario has provided a poster for display in professional environments, which can be used to inform professionals, parents, and collaborative partners in child care centres about common red flags that might indicate that a child has ASD (Box 7.2). Some of these red flags are:

- Difficulty with language development;
- Little reciprocal social responding;
- Unusual, repetitive hand movements;
- Lack of functional play; and
- Unusual preoccupations (Autism Ontario, 2015).

In 2010, the Ontario Middlesex-London Health Unit completed the third revision of "Red Flags: For Infant, Toddler, and Preschool Children: A Quick Reference Guide for Early Years Professionals." "Red Flags" is intended as a helpful guiding tool for informed, educated professionals supporting young learners. As well as including helpful information about the difficult task of talking with parents or caregivers about potential developmental concerns (red flags), this resource includes a section specific to ASD, as well as other areas that may also be implicated (e.g., language, behaviour). Its explanation of red flags for ASD focuses on their unique outward presentation in each child, which "represents a pattern of behaviours. As there is no one specific behaviour which identifies autism, it is important to look at a child's overall developmental pattern and history" (p. 41). Three overall areas are presented as raising potential concerns: social, communication, and behavioural. Within each of these three areas are between six and nine red flags, which, when recognized, should lead to a specialized medical or psychological referral (e.g., pediatrician). Referrals may include services from the Ontario Early Years Centres across the province, Best Start–based initiatives, and many other support services, following regional-specific referral pathways, built upon generic pathways such as the visual overview of local information found in the the On Track Guide, as featured in Figure 7.1.

These red flags and their next steps in resources provided for the child care field underlie the importance of taking immediate action if there is the potential for a future ASD diagnosis (Middlesex-London Health Unit, 2014): "the earlier the intervention, the greater the likelihood of positive changes in the child's behaviour" (Allen, et al., 2015, p. 212). For staff members who are not yet comfortable referring to written guides, helpful video examples are also available through Autism Speaks' online Video Glossary (2009). The video glossary includes specific red flags videos, which "show a wide range of intensity, symptoms, and

Box 7.2: Signs of ASD in Early Childhood

If you observe items on the following list, it may mean that your child is developing differently. Parents should discuss this with their family doctor or pediatrician and ask about a referral for further assessment.

- Doesn't point to show others things he or she is interested in
- Inconsistent or reduced use of eye contact with people outside the family
- Rarely smiles when looking at others or does not exchange back and forth warm, joyful expressions
- Does not spontaneously use gestures such as waving, reaching or pointing with others
- Does not respond to gestures and facial expressions used by others
- More interested in looking at objects than at people's faces
- May be content to spend extended periods of time alone
- Doesn't make attempts to get parent's attention; doesn't follow/look when someone is pointing at something; doesn't bring a toy or other item to parent to show them
- Inconsistent in responding when his or her name is called
- Seems to be in his or her "own world"
- Doesn't respond to parent's attempts to play, even if relaxed
- Avoids or ignores other children when they approach or interact
- No words by 16 months or no two-word phrases by 24 months
- Any loss of previously acquired language or social skills
- Odd or repetitive ways of moving or holding fingers, hands or whole body (rocking, pacing). Walks on toes.
- Displays a strong reaction to certain textures, sounds or lights (e.g., may reject clothing or want to be completely covered, put hands over ears, stare at lights)
- May appear indifferent to pain or temperature
- Lacks interest in toys, or plays with them in an unusual way (e.g., lining up, spinning, smelling, opening/closing parts rather than using the toy as a whole)
- May engage in prolonged visual inspection of objects (e.g., may stare along edges, dangle string or move items closely in front of his/ her eyes)
- Insists on routines (has to perform activities in a special way or certain sequence; requires a particular route or food and is difficult to calm if even small changes occur)
- Preoccupation with unusual interests, such as light switches, doors, fans, wheels – difficult to distract from these activities
- Unusual fears but may not seek comfort from adults

Source: Autism Ontario, 2015, p. 2

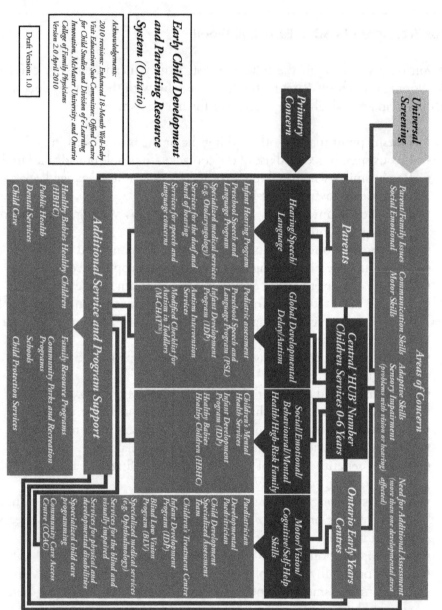

Figure 7.1: London's "On Track" Guide: Early Child Development and Parenting Resource System, Ontario

Source: Best Start, 2015, p. 144.

behaviours in children affected by ASD. The signs are as varied as the number of children affected. These signs can be subtle or, to the untrained eye, easy to miss" (Autism Speaks, 2009). Although RECEs do not diagnose ASD, it can be helpful to be educated on how to talk to parents about possible signs and characteristics of ASD, should the occasion arise where you suspect ASD or want a family to consider getting an outside opinion. Autism Speaks (2013) emphasizes that "if you suspect a developmental delay or autism, speak up! Your intervention can change a child's life" in its Early Childhood Milestone Map and Talking to Parents about Autism Training video resources; however, caution and care in documenting and describing concerning characteristics and appropriate next steps are always essential to appropriate, beneficial communications with parents (see chapter 10).

Read about it. Think about it. Write about it.

Have you ever been in the position of documenting and sharing red flags for ASD in a young child? Explain what happened throughout this process. If not, what are the first steps you would take if you noticed these early signs of what might be ASD?

INDIVIDUAL PROGRAM PLANS

A child who is already diagnosed with ASD can qualify for "Social/Learning Adaptation Disorder" (Allen et al., 2015), and is likely to have an Individualized Program Plan (IPP) in a child care setting.

IPPs and their development also include:

- A supportive team made up of parents and a number of professionals (Allen et al., 2015);
- Intentional planning for the child's time in child care and information sharing (Underwood, 2013);
- A process that includes problem identification, implementation of strategies, and adaptation of the program if changes are needed (Crowther, 2010);
- Staff and funding (Underwood, 2013);
- Direction and structure (Allen et al., 2015);
- A profile (Crowther, 2010);
- Access to multidisciplinary services (Underwood, 2013);
- An outline for implementation of the plan (Allen et al., 2015); and
- A method to evaluate the plans created and adapt (Allen et al., 2015).

Individualized Program Plan: An Individualized Program Plan is "an approach to providing services to individuals with special needs: the process involves developing a written plan based on the child's strengths, needs, and interests" in order to provide a plan for educating and supporting the child in an inclusive manner in the child care environment (Allen et al., 2015, p. 279).

The five components of an IPP are:

1. Observation and assessment
2. Identification of strengths, needs, and interests
3. Setting of goals and objectives
4. Creation of an implementation plan
5. Evaluation (adapted from Allen et al., 2015, p. 280).

PROFESSIONAL PREPARATION IN EXCEPTIONALITIES AND ASD

In Ontario, as well as across Canada, universal access to child care is an important objective (Killoran, Tymon, & Frempong, 2007). For children with exceptionalities, this includes "the dire need to focus on our preschool settings and the inclusion of young children with disabilities. Very few children are attending their community preschools. If we envision an inclusive community, young children must begin their school years with their peers" (Killoran, Tymon, & Frempong, 2007, p. 92).

In many areas of Canada—including Ontario—health care, social services, and education are responding to increasing numbers of children diagnosed with ASD (Ouellette-Kuntz et al., 2014). For example, one study of 354 Toronto-based preschool environments found that ASD was the most common diagnosis in enrolled children (Killoran, Tymon, & Frempong, 2007). Yet, parents report having difficulty finding child care supports, perhaps, for example, due to rejection from a centre or centres (Killoran, Tymon, & Frempong, 2007). This type of difficulty with service provision might contribute to the finding that "many parents never get a break from their child as it is often extremely difficult to obtain suitable child care arrangements" (Factor, Perry, & Freeman, 1990, p. 139). One reason for this finding, however, is that families may have access to formal means of support, such as respite care (Factor, Perry, & Freeman, 1990) or licensed child care for their children diagnosed with ASD. Issues of inclusion for students with special needs, including ASD, and issues of preparation for educators who will inevitably support students with ASD in either the child care system or the school system—or both—have perhaps not yet caught up to the breadth and depth of change in recognizing early childhood educators as credentialed professionals. For example, one study found that up to 79 percent of centres perceived barriers: "the four greatest barriers were identified as physical, training, funding, and ratios" (Killoran, Tymon, & Frempong, 2007, p. 91).

Although inclusion is a respected and desired element in child care settings across Canada, Crowther (2010) describes its implementation as inconsistent, haphazard, and "lack[ing] appropriate guidelines, policies and proactive legislation that address

Read about it. Think about it. Write about it.

How might parents react to the inability to find a space for their child with ASD in a child care setting? What is one way that we might work towards solving this issue?

Box 7.3: A Beautifully Orchestrated Symphony of Chaos
By Sheri Mallabar, RECE/OCT, Master of Education Student

At any given time you could walk into my preschool classroom and experience what can only be described as a beautifully orchestrated symphony of chaos. There was learning happening everywhere. Children were reading, role-playing, problem-solving, and working on beautiful, creative masterpieces. The classroom was filled with sounds of tiny voices and laughter. For the 11 students in my classroom, this was how they learned. From the outside looking in, it appeared that all of the children's needs were being met. They had the opportunity to interact with one another while they built on their rapidly growing knowledge repertoire. It looked like the perfect classroom.

If you took a closer look, you may have noticed one of my students acting differently than many of the others. He could be running around the room with his hands covering his ears, avoiding eye contact with anyone. He could be standing alone in the classroom fixated on a picture hanging on the wall. He could be sitting alone on the carpet gazing at his hands making gestures with his tiny fingers. He was identified as having autism spectrum disorder (ASD).

I knew it was my responsibility to develop a program for my class that supported his needs. I was educated, I had attended the training, but sometimes, there just wasn't enough *time* to be inclusive. With 11 other children in the group, it was often hard to give him as much attention as he needed. I knew that the lights were a little too bright, and that there was a lot going on with the other children, but I struggled with having to adapt the environment and behaviours of all of the other children in the class just for one boy. How could I expect a group of three- and four-year-olds to understand that they must play quietly or that it is upsetting for someone else if they giggle too loud? On certain days, it seemed there was a lot going on, or I had something that needed to be done; it was just easier to leave him not-quite-fully-engaged. As long as he wasn't hurting himself or someone else, I was happy. I knew it wasn't the right thing to do, but I felt, then, that when you were in classroom with so many different types of needs, sometimes you had to choose.

As these days began to happen more often I knew something had to change. I looked to colleagues, my supervisor, and a local child development organization for some help. Slowly, I began to transform my classroom environment. As it changed, I let go of the idea that I was asking the children in my class to make sacrifices for this boy. The changes that were happening were benefiting all of them. I could see it almost instantly. One of the most significant changes I made in my classroom was creating a sense of awareness and advocating for social justice. During our circle time we began talking about people, and how their needs are different. We shared stories about things that happen that make us sad, or afraid, as well as things that make us happy. It started as a way to encourage empathy among classmates and quickly turned in to a project that had immeasurable success. Preschoolers transformed before my eyes into empathetic members of our small classroom community. Suddenly, I didn't feel the same burden I often felt when I wasn't able to give the student with ASD my attention, because he was allowing peers to attend to some of his needs. The small boy who often played alone was slowly becoming comfortable with his peers, just as they were becoming more comfortable with him. The other children in the class who had often told me they were afraid to play with this boy were not only inviting him into their play, but oftentimes letting him take over. The children did not feel they were missing out on things because they couldn't yell in the classroom; they were understanding, and encouraged each other in order to support their friend. They were still part of our beautifully orchestrated symphony of chaos, except now everyone had a chance to take part. Together we took a step in the right direction toward inclusion.

... the inclusion of children with special needs" (p. 40). Some centres are physically inaccessible (in one study, over 35 percent of centres in the region), some provide onsite clinical services for children with special needs, but others are associated only with off-site services for children with complex needs (Killoran, Tymon, & Frempong, 2007).

Crowther also notes that across Canada, no additional training is required to support inclusive practices for the 1.6 percent of children with special needs in the birth to four age range; not even half of the nation's children, overall, can utilize inclusive child care settings. However, overall, "young students diagnosed with ASD increasingly are receiving their educational programs in inclusive settings, learning side by side with typical peers" (Hampshire & Hourcade, 2014, p. 26). In addition to the RECEs supporting inclusion, other human resource supports are available. For example, resource consultants work to build capacity in multiple child care centres for children with special needs; they work onsite and in the community to provide supports to educators and help to promote inclusion for children with disabilities in these environments (Underwood, 2013). The only centre- or agency-based staff, however, who currently require additional training in supporting children with ASD and other disabilities are resource consultants. Resource consultant roles do require additional post-secondary training—a one-year graduate certificate at an Ontario colleges. It is a specialized role to support students with exceptionalities and the RECEs who in turn support children, including those with ASD and their families, in the child care environment. The role of a resource consultant is explained by RECE Debbie Hanna-Jacklin:

> My main role as a resource consultant is to assess the needs of early learning and care programs and support them through training, modelling and coaching so that children with special needs are included in all aspects of their program. I also support the optimum development of the child with special needs. As I am not a centre-based resource consultant, I rely very much on educators' input as they are with the children more than I am. Another part of my job is creating a team service plan for a child with special needs. I coordinate a meeting with the parents, educators and therapists and the team gives an overview of what the child's doing in the program and at home. I ask parents and the program about their priority areas and help them create achievable short and long-term goals for the child. (Ontario College of Early Childhood Educators, 2013, para. 4–6)

Although there is no course of training specific to ASD for Ontario's child care centres, educators can take advantage of centre-based, community-based, local, provincial, national, and international opportunities for professional development. According to Crowther (2010), "one of the components of high-quality care is the amount of education and training early childhood educators receive" (p. 40). For Ontario RECEs, like their professional partners across the country, this can take many forms, initiated either by individuals looking for additional learning opportunities or agencies offering training. One opportunity is an optional, ongoing initiative called Raising the Bar, designed to ensure RECEs receive additional training to promote standards in best practice (e.g., Affiliated Services for Children and Youth, 2015). This may come in the form of arrangements made by a single child care centre to provide training to meet the needs of individual or small groups of RECEs; a series of workshops presented collaboratively onsite (i.e., clinical and educational collaboration);

Resource Consultants: A resource consultant is a registered early childhood educator with a diploma or degree in early childhood education and an additional post-secondary program that is focused on children with exceptionalities (Childcare Resource and Research Unit, 2014).

or taking advantage of either advertised courses (Geneva Centre training and certificate programs); conferences (e.g., Early Childhood Resource Teacher Network of Ontario); opportunities developed by professional agencies, including online webinars; or post-secondary programs (e.g., Autism and Behaviour Science Ontario Colleges graduate certificate). Allen and colleagues (2015) suggest that child care centres supporting children with ASD should seek out training in "successful early intervention programs" (p. 213), such as applied behaviour analysis (ABA), discrete trial training (DTT), pivotal response training (PRT), and incidental teaching. In addition, they should have the skills to build in structured routines, individualized programs, and validated instructional strategies.

Read about it. Think about it. Write about it.

Investigate one way for early childhood educators to learn more about young children with ASD. Fully describe this resource, course, program, certificate, diploma, or degree.

Box 7.4: The Child Care and Learning Centre at the University of Guelph: Putting Children First and Disabilities Second
By Dr. Tricia van Rhijn, PhD, RECE, Assistant Professor of Family Relations and Human Development, University of Guelph

The Child Care and Learning Centre (CCLC) at the University of Guelph provides a high-quality, inclusive program for children with ASD (as well as other special needs and disabilities) and their families. The CCLC provides integrated programming with full participation of children with special needs in all facets of the centre. Children are never turned away based on their unique needs. Staff put "children first and disabilities second," recognizing that all children are unique and learn in different ways. By doing so, they provide a safe and supportive emotional environment for the children, their parents, and even their siblings.

Establishing trust with families is a vital part of the CCLC's practice. Parental input is highly valued; parents are recognized as being the experts on their child whose input is necessary to best meet the children's needs and support their development. Communication between parents and staff, during times of both success and challenge, provides opportunities for shared learning over time. The knowledgeable and skilled program staff are prepared to create a community of support to help families adapt to and handle the challenges and successes that accompany their child's growth and development. This may happen as families move through various emotional stages, including grief, anger, disappointment, wonder, pride, and joy. Supporting resiliency in the children and their families and focusing on strengths rather than deficits alone helps to provide stability. The power of sharing reduces feelings of confusion, isolation, and stress often felt by families. As the central partner in their child's learning, parents are invited to be involved in other ways, such as serving on the Parental Advisory Council, volunteering in the playrooms, partnering with and supporting other parents with children with ASD, or taking part in extracurricular parent programs.

Staff members at the CCLC are highly trained and knowledgeable. Many are pursuing or have attained post-secondary education beyond their ECE training, including bachelor's and master's degrees, as well as Ontario College of Teachers and Resource Teacher qualifications. The staff are creative, caring, and skilled; they participate in ongoing training and professional development opportunities. The child care cook and kitchen staff work with the families and registered dieticians, using varying approaches to accommodate food and preparation requirements to meet each child's nutritional needs. All staff use and develop their observation skills to better support all children in their care, trying to understand the children's unique perspectives in order to open themselves to "see the world in different ways."

The CCLC employs a collaborative, team-based approach to support children with ASD. This approach is supported by Growing Great Kids, a partnership of organizations that facilitates access to community-based inclusion support services for children with developmental or behavioural needs from before birth to age six in Guelph and Wellington County. Families make the final decisions for their children and are supported in making educated choices by an inclusion team made up of program staff (e.g., playroom ECEs, centre supervisor, centre director, inclusion facilitators) and external support service providers (e.g., early childhood resource consultant, occupational therapist, physiotherapist, speech-language pathologist, social development consultant). Individual Program Plans are created for the child through consultation and collaboration. Applications are made for required support services or funding on an as-needed basis in partnership with parents.

Individualized strategies are practiced for each child by building on the child's strengths as well as "outside the box" thinking on behalf of the program staff. Playroom iPads are utilized to provide daily contact with parents (e.g., sending text or photos via email), create pedagogical documentation, and to offer assistive technology options for the children (e.g., augmentative language applications). Alternative approaches, such as Intensive Behaviour Intervention

(IBI), are integrated within the playrooms, with staff not only accommodating but also supporting these approaches by learning about and practicing them in their playrooms. Peer play is facilitated with other children in the classrooms; all children are supported in being respectful and inclusive peers, resulting in high levels of social inclusion and their being very warm and welcoming toward their peers with ASD and other special needs.

The CCLC staff also looks to the future and works to support children's transitions to the school system. They fully support the children and their families throughout the transition by utilizing unique collaborative solutions to better prepare them for the school environment. One example of an approach is a child's lunch being prepared and packed into a lunchbox by the kitchen to prepare for school lunch routines. All milestones, big and small, are celebrated. The staff "walk and talk" their values, advocate for the children, and focus on the children's perspectives; they remind themselves to be light-hearted, joyful, and full of wonder, like the children with whom they have the privilege to work. When asked about children with ASD, the staff are quick to point out that even though children with ASD can be very challenging at times, they are the most rewarding!

A LOOK BACK

In Chapter 7, "Autism Spectrum Disorder in Ontario Child Care Settings," significant practices and processes in supporting young children with ASD were reviewed. This included:
- The state of inclusion in Ontario's child care field;
- Responsibilities of supporting young children with red flags for ASD (e.g., service referrals); and
- Inclusive, evidence-based intervention and related research in child care centres.

A LOOK AHEAD

Chapter 8, "Autism Spectrum Disorder in Ontario Schools," includes options, practices, and services for students in Ontario. It reviews:
- Fully inclusive settings in Ontario schools;
- Specialized or alternate provincial settings for students with ASD;
- Ontario-based resources for educators teaching students with ASD; and
- Legislated supports for Ontario students identified as exceptional (e.g., Individual Education Plans).

ADDITIONAL RESOURCES

- Affiliated Services for Children and Youth: Raising the Bar:
  ascy.ca/raising-the-bar/
- Autism in Education: An Atlantic Partnership:
  www.apsea.ca/aie/
- Behavioural Science Programs at Ontario Colleges:
  www.ontariocolleges.ca/SearchResults/EDUCATION-COMMUNITY-
  SOCIAL-SERVICES-BEHAVIOURAL-SCIENCE/_/N-ll0t
- Best Start "On Track" Guide (Best Start, 2015):
  www.beststart.org/OnTrack_English/1-introduction.html
- Early Childhood Resource Teacher Network:
  www.ecrtno.ca/
- Early Childhood Milestone Map (Autism Speaks, 2013):
  www.autismspeaks.org/sites/default/files/docs/talking_to_parents/autism_
  brochure_2013_v2.pdf
- Signs of Autism Spectrum Disorder in Early Childhood (Autism Ontario, 2015):
  www.autismontario.com/Client/ASO/AO.nsf/object/DR2013/$file/2013+A
  O+Pediatrician+tearoffs+EN+web+%282%29.pdf
- Geneva Centre Training:
  www.autism.net/training.html
- M-CHAT-R (Robins, Fein, & Barton, 1999):
  www.autismspeaks.org/what-autism/diagnosis/mchat
- Ontario College of Early Childhood Educators:
  www.college-ece.ca/en/AboutUs/Pages/History-.aspx
- "Quick and Easy Adaptations and Accommodations for Early Childhood
  Students":
  journals.cec.sped.org/cgi/viewcontent.cgi?article=1151&context=tecplus
- Red Flags (Middlesex-London Health Unit, 2010):
  www.beststart.org/OnTrack_English/local_resources/18_Month/Middlesex
  LondonRedFlags_2010.pdf
- St. Matthew's House (Hamilton):
  www.stmatthewshouse.ca
- Talking to Parents about Autism Action Kit (2015):
  www.autismspeaks.org/what-autism/learn-signs/talking-parents-about-autism-
  action-kit
- Talking to Parents about Autism Training Video (2015):
  www.autismspeaks.org/what-autism/learn-signs/talking-parents-about-autism-
  action-kit
- The State of Early Childhood Education and Care in Canada 2012 (2014):
  childcarecanada.org/sites/default/files/StateofECEC2012.pdf

- The SpeciaLink Early Childhood Inclusion Tool (The National Centre for Child Care Inclusion, 2009): www.specialinkcanada.org/about/rating%20scales.html

REFERENCES

Allen, K. E., Cowdery, G. E., Paasche, C. L., Langford, R., Nolan, K., & Cipparrone, B. (2015). *Inclusion in early childhood programs: Children with exceptionalities* (6th ed.). Toronto, ON: Nelson.

Autism Ontario. (2015). Signs of autism spectrum disorder in early childhood. Retrieved from www.autismontario.com/Client/ASO/AO.nsf/object/DR2013/$file/2013+AO+Pediatrician+tearoffs+EN+web+%282%29.pdf

Autism Speaks. (2009). Autism speaks video glossary. Retrieved from www.autismspeaks.ca/community-services/resources/video-glossary/

Autism Speaks. (2013). Early childhood milestone map. Retrieved from www.autismspeaks.org/sites/default/files/docs/talking_to_parents/autism_brochure_2013_v2.pdf

Autism Speaks. (2015). Talking to parents about autism action kit. Retrieved from www.autismspeaks.org/what-autism/learn-signs/talking-parents-about-autism-action-kit

Barton, E. E. & Harn, B. (2012). *Educating young children with autism spectrum disorder*. Thousand Oaks, CA: Corwin.

Best Start. (2015). On track: Local information. Retrieved from www.beststart.org/OnTrack_English/7-howtouse.html

Breitfelder, L. M. (2008). Quick and easy adaptations and accommodations for early childhood students. *TEACHING Exceptional Children Plus, 4*(5), 1–15.

Childcare Resource and Research Unit. (2014). Ontario provincial context. Retrieved from www.childcarecanada.org/sites/default/files/ON.pdf

Crowther, I. (2010). *Inclusion in early childhood settings: Children with special needs in Canada* (2nd ed.). Toronto, ON: Pearson.

Factor, D. C., Perry, A., Freeman, N. (1990). Brief report: Stress, social support, and respite care use in families with autistic children. *Journal of Autism & Developmental Disorders, 20*(1), 139–146.

Ferns, C., & Friendly, M. (2014). The state of early childhood education in Canada 2012. Retrieved from childcarecanada.org/sites/default/files/StateofECEC2012.pdf

Fletcher, P. C., Markoulakis, R., & Bryden, P. J. (2012). The costs of caring for a child with an autism spectrum disorder. *Issues in Comprehensive Pediatric Nursing, 35*(1), 45–69. doi:10.3109/01460862.2012.645407

Hampshire, P. K., & Hourcade, J. J. (2014). Teaching play skills to children with autism using visually structured tasks. *Teaching Exceptional Children, 46*(3), 26–31.

Irwin, S. H. (2009). The specialink early childhood inclusion quality scale. Retrieved from www.specialinkcanada.org/about/rating%20scales.html

Killoran, I., Tymon, D., & Frempong, G. (2007). Disabilities and inclusive practices within Toronto preschools. *International Journal of Inclusive Education, 11*(1), 81. doi:10.1080/13603110500375473

King, A. M., Thonrieczek, M., Voreis, G., & Scott, V. (2014). iPad use in children and young adults with autism spectrum disorder: An observational study. *Child Language Teaching & Therapy, 30*(2), 159–173. doi:10.1177/0265659013510922

Maich, K., & Belcher, E. C., (2012). Using picture books to create peer awareness about autism spectrum disorder in the inclusive classroom. *Intervention in School and Clinic, 47*(4), 206–213. doi: 10.1177/1053451211424600

Maich, K., & Hall, C. (2014). Are we ready? Examining the level of preparedness of early childhood education students for school-based special education. *Canadian Children, 39*(3), 42-52. Retrieved from cayc.ca/content/canadian-children-vol-39-no-3

Mavropoulou, S., Papadopoulou, E., & Kakana, D. (2011). Effects of task organization on the independent play of students with autism spectrum disorder. *Journal of Autism & Developmental Disorders, 41*(7), 913–925.

Meadan, H., Ostrosky, M. M., Triplett, B., Michna, A., & Fettig, A. (2011). Using Visual Supports with Young Children with Autism Spectrum Disorder. *TEACHING Exceptional Children, 43*(6), 28–35.

McLennan, J. D., Huculak, S., & Sheehan, D. (2008). Brief report: pilot investigation of service receipt by young children with autistic spectrum disorders. *Journal of Autism and Developmental Disorders, 38*(6), 1192–1196. doi:10.1007/s10803-007-0535-5

Middlesex-London Health Unit. (2014). Red flags: A Quick Reference Guide for Early Years Professionals in Middlesex-London. Retrieved from https://www.healthunit.com/.../red-flags-early-id-quick-reference.pdf

Murdock, L., Ganz, J., & Crittendon, J. (2013). Use of an iPad play story to increase play dialogue of preschoolers with autism spectrum disorder. *Journal of Autism & Developmental Disorders, 43*(9), 2174–2189. doi:10.1007/s10803-013-1770-6

Ontario College of Early Childhood Educators. (2013). Conversation with an RECE. Retrieved from www.college-ece.ca/en/Public/News/Pages/Conversation-with-an-RECE.aspx

Ontario College of Early Childhood Educators. (2014). History of the college. Retrieved from www.college-ece.ca/en/AboutUs/Pages/History-.aspx

Ontario College of Early Childhood Educators. (n.d.). Becoming an RECE in Ontario. Retrieved from www.college-ece.ca/en/Documents/Become_an_RECE.pdf

Ontario Ministry of Education. (2005). Education for all: The report of the expert panel on literacy and numeracy instruction for students with special education needs, kindergarten to grade six. Retrieved from www.edu.gov.on.ca/eng/document/reports/speced/panel/speced.pdf, 137–138

Ontario Ministry of Education. (2010). Full day kindergarten schools. Retrieved from www.edu.gov.on.ca/kindergarten/fulldaykindergartenschools2.asp

Ontario Ministry of Education. (2013). Full day kindergarten: A question and answer guide for parents. Retrieved from www.edu.gov.on.ca/eng/multi/english/FDKFactSheetEN.pdf

Ouellette-Kuntz, H., Coo, H., Lam, M., Breitenbach, M. M., Hennessey, P. E., Jackman, P. D., & ... Chung, A. M. (2014). The changing prevalence of autism in three regions of Canada. *Journal of Autism And Developmental Disorders*, (1), 120.

Robins, D., Fein, D., & Barton, M. (1999). The modified checklist for autism in toddlers, revised. Retrieved from www.autismspeaks.org/what-autism/diagnosis/mchat

Service Ontario e-laws. (2007). Early childhood educators act. Retrieved from www.e-laws.gov.on.ca/html/statutes/english/elaws_statutes_07e07_e.htm

Service Ontario e-laws. (2014). Education act. Retrieved from www.e-laws.gov.on.ca/html/statutes/english/elaws_statutes_90e02_e.htm#BK418

St. Matthew's House. (n.d.) St. Matthew's house: Where hope lives.

Szatmari, P., Bryson, S. E., Streiner, D. L., Wilson, F., Archer, L., & Ryerse, C. (2000). Two-year outcome of preschool children with autism or Asperger's syndrome. *The American Journal of Psychiatry, 157*(12), 1980–1987.

The National Centre for Child Care Inclusion. (2010). The specialink early childhood inclusion tool. Retrieved from www.specialinkcanada.org/about/rating%20scales.html

Underwood, K. (2013). Everyone is welcome: Inclusive early childhood education and care. Retrieved from www.edu.gov.on.ca/childcare/Underwood.pdf

Wong, C., Odom, S. L., Hume, K. Cox, A. W., Fettig, A., Kucharczyk, S.,...Schultz, T. R. (2014). *Evidence-based practices for children, youth, and young adults with autism spectrum disorder.* Chapel Hill: The University of North Carolina, Frank Porter Graham Child Development Institute, Autism Evidence-Based Practice Review Group.

CHAPTER 8

AUTISM SPECTRUM DISORDER IN ONTARIO SCHOOLS

IN THIS CHAPTER:

- Inclusive Practices in Ontario Schools
- Alternate Settings in Ontario Schools
- The Identification, Placement, and Review Committee
- Individual Education Plans
  - Accommodations
  - Modifications
  - Alternative Courses
- Continuing Education for Ontario Certified Teachers

Students with autism spectrum disorder (ASD) and their educators have a range of options, practices, and services available in Ontario schools, from fully inclusive settings to specialized, alternate settings; supports include the development of individual education plans with their processes and intricacies. In chapter 8, these topics—and more—are introduced, and feature boxes highlight unique contexts in meeting the needs of students with ASD.

INCLUSIVE PRACTICES IN ONTARIO SCHOOLS

Since the release of Bill 82 in 1980, Ontario schools have emphasized movement toward inclusion—rather than segregation—in neighbourhood communities with same-aged peers for all students, including those with ASD (Ryan, 2009). Using proactive, flexible approaches such as universal design and differentiated instruction, inclusion means that "the regular classroom teacher [is] taking ownership of all students in his or her class" (Bennett, 2009, p. 2), a model funded by a complex, multi-part Special Education Grant of close to three billion dollars. Of the 186,545 students identified as students with exceptionalities in

Ontario's 72 publicly funded boards, 9.4 percent (17,600) are identified as "Communication: Autism" in the 2012/13 school year—an increase from a previous 8.6 percent (Finlay, 2015).

However, it can be argued that inclusion is not yet wholly a smoothly running, fully supported method of instruction in Ontario schools. Killoren et al. (2013) emphasize a not-yet-accomplished reality of one fully inclusive system:

> The reality is we have two clearly delineated streams, general and special education. In Ontario, teachers are often constrained by legislation, terminology and board practices that do not fully embrace the shift towards a reconceptualization of schooling that supports inclusive learning environments for all children. Until legislation changes we must work within a system that has enough room for adaptations, yet few explicit requirements for accountability regarding inclusion. (p. 242)

Alternatives to inclusive settings remain in most Ontario jurisdictions, though major initiatives are also underway to emphasize fully inclusive environments for all students—including those with ASD.

Bill 82: Bill 82, or the Education Amendment Act (1980), changed the provision of services to students with special needs from optional to a legislated requirement for Ontario boards of education (Bennett, 2009).

Universal Design for Learning (UDL): "A set of principles for curriculum development that give all individuals equal opportunities to learn. UDL provides a blueprint for creating instructional goals, methods, materials, and assessments that work for everyone—not a single, one-size-fits-all solution but rather flexible approaches that can be customized and adjusted for individual needs" (Center for Applied Special Technology, 2013, para.1). UDL is inspired by the commitment to architectural accessibility (Ontario Ministry of Education, 2005).

Differentiated Instruction: Carol Ann Tomlinson describes differentiated instruction as a common-sense, flexible way of teaching diverse groups of students by meeting students at their individualized levels in order to support their "essential understandings and skills" (Tomlinson, 1999; Tomlinson, 2000, p. 27).

Box 8.1: Inclusion for Students with ASD.
By Dr. Sheila Bennett, Teacher Education, Brock University

Inclusion for students with ASD is an ever-changing and somewhat idiosyncratic landscape. Advances have been made on educational approaches to working with students with ASD, and advocacy across many fronts is clearly evident. While not an absolute, in general, service delivery approaches that rely on a more clinically based model, associated with what would have been considered a "medical model" approach focused on fixing, tend to choose a more segregationist route. In contrast, those educational settings that blend clinical and educational approaches within a "social model" of service delivery, focused on examining the environment and collaboratively adjusting all the participants to create a space in which students with ASD can engage successfully, choose a more inclusive model of service delivery. Currently in Ontario, service delivery is often dependent on the philosophical orientation of a specific school board. It is worth aspiring to a rights-based model of schooling that assumes that each student has a place in a classroom, in a school, and in a community, and demands that environments are created with accessible curriculum for everyone. We have believed for too long that special services require special places. Denying access for students with ASD to the larger school community as an equal and denying access for students in the regular class to develop meaningful relationships with a more diverse population is equally devastating on both sides. A well-developed curriculum, best practices in clinical approaches, supports where necessary, and a robust educational experience is the right of every student. This can only be accomplished when we insist on excellence for all students, including those with ASD, in an inclusive setting. Access to friendships, the larger community, and the building of social capital does not need to be the price paid for services supposedly rendered.

Inclusion: School-based inclusion can be defined as children with disabilities "being educated alongside their typically developing peers" (Boer, Pijl, Minnaert, & Post, 2014, p. 72), but can and should be extended to all students in the whole school community (Bennett, 2009).

Read about it. Think about it. Write about it.

How has school inclusion changed over your lifetime?

ALTERNATE SETTINGS IN ONTARIO SCHOOLS

Although inclusion is the standard model for students with ASD—and 83 to 86 percent of all students with exceptionalities in the 2012/13 school year (Finlay, 2015)—in Ontario's public school system, some self-contained or alternative settings persist, which focus on the needs of students with ASD in environments with low teacher to student ratios. One example of such a setting within the publicly funded school system is at Streetsville Secondary School, in Peel District School Board, part of the Greater Toronto Area. Streetsville describes this specialized program as "one of the sites for the Secondary Regional Communications Program—Autism Spectrum Disorder (ASD). This program provides students identified with ASD with specialized learning and technological support" (Peel District School Board, 2013, para. 2). This program, well-known in the province and also recognized by the moniker "Room 150," is touted as a potential model by the Toronto Star (Rushowy, 2012), which described it as a transition program that "focuses on a child's unique skills, while creating a low-stress, high-interest atmosphere" (para. 7) through which students earn credits in a carefully arranged physical—and emotional—high school environment.

Section 23 school settings, so named for their legislative roots under Funding for Educational Programs in Care and/or Treatment, Custodial and Correctional Facilities in Ontario's Education Act, may serve as collaborative facilities to congregate students with ASD, when students struggle with maintaining placement in inclusive school environments and need a more goal-oriented treatment approach. When students are admitted to such programs, they are no longer formally considered "pupils of the board" (Ontario Ministry of Education, 2014a, p. 6), but are referred to as clients of an approved facility, which delivers collaborative, multidisciplinary, school-board-associated education programs with the support of qualified teachers and through a Memorandum of Understanding.

A range of privately funded schools also exist across Ontario, which may combine a private funding model with ministry approval for Applied Behaviour Analysis (ABA) therapy (see Autism Ontario's Spirale website to find provincial professional services). This type of model offers greater flexibility in combining academic teaching with onsite, clinical supports. Such schools may combine academic instruction with a more clinical or intense approach to ABA, and have multidisciplinary educators and clinicians on staff in instructor therapist and senior therapist roles. The Joy of Learning Centre in Burlington, for example, has a registered social worker and a board-certified behaviour analyst onsite, and its program is supervised by a clinical psychologist (The Joy of Learning Centre, n.d.). Similarly, the Gregory School for Exceptional Learning

Box 8.2: The Gregory School

Angeline Savard, principal of The Gregory School for Exceptional Learning, had long aspired to start her own school. She attained her Bachelor of Science Degree, her Bachelor of Education Degree, and became certified as an Ontario Certified Teacher with the Ontario College of Teachers, then began working at Toronto's Hospital for Sick Children in a learning disabilities research unit. It was there that she was introduced to direct instruction, a teaching and learning methodology embedded in an ABA framework.

Direct Instruction: Direct Instruction is an ABA-based teaching and learning methodology, defined by Carter, Stephenson, and Strnadová (2011) as "academically focused, teacher-directed learning with sequenced, structured materials and high levels of student responding" (p. 50).

With her strong background in tutoring, teaching, and research, and now herself a mother to a seven-year-old son with exceptionalities, she began to consider how she could further implement direct instruction in an environment that would support students in a full day of learning, and also provide services for her own son. Though the affordability of such a venture had always been a concern, greater concern closer to home was a strong motivator in moving forward. In 2002, the Gregory School and its intertwined clinical service provider, Kalyana Systems, began in a church hall in Ancaster, supporting the individual educational and clinical needs of six students. This was Savard's introduction to ASD; yet,

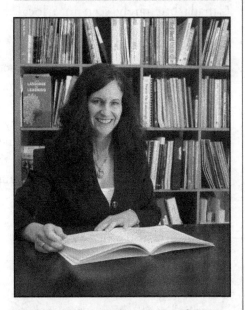

Figure 8.1: Angeline Savard, OCT

the complex needs of children with ASD have dominated the program since then. By the end of the first year, the school grew to 8 students, and since then they have further expanded to a steady 15 to 20 school-aged students each year, typically between the ages of 4 and 15. Two years later, the school's clinical service provision began, and officially formed its parent company in

2010, Kalyana Support Systems. In 2012 the school moved to Brant County, purchasing the former Brant County municipal building.

Due to its private status, the school is not regulated by provincial legislation, but chooses to follow innovations, such as new directions from the Ministry of Education. It is primarily funded by Ontario's direct funding option and individual tuition, with some subsidy for personal care needs (e.g., feeding, dressing) through the Community Care Access Centre.

The Gregory School, formally considered a private school in a unique blend of school and clinic—common outside of Ontario and Canada but rarely seen in a local context—is now housed in a calm two-floor building with impressive

Direct Funding Option (DFO): Ontario's direct funding option for the Autism Intervention Program permits parents to "receive funding directly. The family then arranges for services from a private service provider" (para. 2). Alternatively, service provision can come directly from regional service providers in the direct service option (Ontario Ministry of Children and Youth Services, 2011b).

noise control, in a peaceful, pastoral setting with multiple classrooms, offices, meeting spaces, a huge yard, and a fenced outdoor play area. Students live mostly in Brantford and Ancaster, but many come from as far away as Burlington or Dorchester, each about 45 minutes by car or taxi, for a partial or full day of instruction that is similar to the framework of most schools. They begin at nine a.m., start with homeroom, and then move on to academics. Academics at the Gregory School, however, are taught through individualized instruction

Discrete Trial Teaching: Discrete trial teaching (DTT) is an evidence-based, data-driven teaching strategy built on the foundations of ABA. It is described as efficient, structured, and individualized, focused on teaching, maintaining, and generalizing specific skills (Gongola & Sweeney, 2012).

in a one-to-one ratio of instructors to students using strategies like direct instruction or discrete trial teaching. Like the enrolled students, instructors have diverse backgrounds, including university graduates from the fields of education, psychology, disability studies, and ABA with undergraduate, professional, or master's degrees as well as college graduates in child-youth work or autism and behaviour science.

DTT Example

Teacher Instruction:	What color? [presenting a *red* card]
Student Response:	Red.
Teacher Consequence:	Great job saying red!
Teacher Instruction:	What color? [presenting a *green* card]
Student Response:	Red. [incorrect response]
Teacher Consequence:	No. Try again.
Teacher Instruction:	What color? Green. [presenting a *green* card paired with a full verbal prompt as an error correction procedure]
Student Response:	Green.
Teacher Consequence:	Good! [and a high five]
Teacher Instruction:	What color? [presenting a *green* card]
Student Response:	Green.
Teacher Consequence:	Yes! Green! Nice work! [paired with providing the student access to a preferred toy]

Source: Gongola & Sweeney, 2012, p. 184.

Group sessions include music, art, science, gym, and drama, which continue a focus on individual goals and skill development. For example, physiotherapy recommendations may be integrated into gym class, communication goals into music, fine motor skills into art, and instruction goals—such as attending to the instructor—into all subject areas.

Other unique practices that make the Gregory School a distinctive experience for students with ASD and other exceptionalities include its "combination of intervention (ABA) that works, but also a real school atmosphere, [and] the ability to interact with children who have around the same comprehension level. Students can learn specific skills from peers at the same level where they might otherwise be overwhelmed: it's ABA intervention plus positive social interactions," describes Savard. All such goals, strategies, and assessments are described either within a unique, regularly updated Individual Education Plan (IEP), typically a lengthy 16 pages, or within a required individual service plan; both approaches utilize goals in every developmental or academic domain, dependent on each child's needs.

Beyond these innovations, the Gregory School works with a range of placement students in multiple disciplines, and is considering supplementing their program with high school credit options. The school is committed to research, and enthusiastic about the future development of a laboratory classroom.

is located outside of Brantford, offering a spacious school on rural grounds, with both individualized educational programs and specialized therapeutic interventions, such as behaviour therapy, social skills training, music therapy, art therapy, and tutoring in individual and small group settings (Kaylana Support Systems, 2013).

For teachers in specialized settings and educators supporting inclusive classrooms, ongoing professional development about students with ASD is a necessary requirement for meeting professional standards. Opportunities for professional learning can be employer-initiated, through mandatory or optional workshops for example, but are often teacher-driven in the search for excellence. Regardless of its origins, professional development is widely available from school boards, ministry initiatives, and union-funded workshops as well as community-based, course-based, and degree-based learning. The most widely recognized system of professional development is Additional Qualifications courses (discussed later in this chapter).

Box 8.3: W. Ross Macdonald School for the Blind and Visually Impaired

Jennifer McMillan, Ontario Certified Teacher at W. Ross Macdonald School in Brantford, first began her teaching career supporting students who were both deaf and blind, moving on to teaching students who were blind and visually impaired. Along the way, she noticed a great quantity of students with multiple and complex needs in her school environment, including students with autism spectrum disorder in addition to their sensory impairments. To support her own professional learning, and with

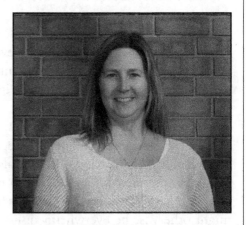

Figure 8.2: Jennifer McMillan, OCT

encouragement from her school leadership, she signed up for what was—at the time—a brand-new Additional Qualifications course focused on supporting students with ASD. Here is an excerpt from one of the papers she wrote:

> The majority of programs that are intended for children who fall within the diagnosis of Autism Spectrum depend heavily on visual support mechanisms. This presents several major challenges when teaching a student who is diagnosed with both Autism Spectrum Disorder,

(ASD), as well as a Visual Impairment, (VI). A number of strategies need to be implemented in order to effectively teach students with Autism Spectrum Disorder. When another diagnosis besides Autism is present, such as a Visual Impairment, it is imperative to adapt using strategies suggested within both fields. It is also very important to recognize that each student is unique and there is no standard method that is guaranteed to yield success with every child ... although development in children with Autism Spectrum Disorder and Visual Impairment presents many obstacles, hope exists that by implementing adapted strategies and effective education practices, students will be enabled to achieve to their highest potential. It is important to have an understanding of both disabilities and their implications on the student and ability to learn.

With this professional learning in hand, she was assigned to a small classroom of students diagnosed with both ASD and serious vision issues and taught this class for five years. As far as Jennifer knows, although it was not officially labelled as such, it was the only one of its kind in the province. Perhaps not surprisingly, she found very little research on the topic.

To prepare for her students, she read books, and consulted with resource and board-level specialists through the ministry's Provincial Schools Branch, and the Autism Spectrum Disorder School Support Program consultants from McMaster Children's Hospital—all of whom were a "huge support"—and found that her background areas of specialization were a significant help. For example, she found that concrete, tactile materials like a calendar, a first-then board, and a daily schedule, all made with small objects that students could touch, were very helpful.

ASD and VI: Li (2009) explains that students with both ASD and visual impairment (VI) also include those with "low vision (i.e., visual acuity of 20/70 to 20/200 in the better eye with correction) and those who are legally blind (i.e., acuity below 20/200 or visual field is restricted to no more than 20 degrees in the better eye with correction)" (p. 22).

Day to day, Jennifer reported that "I tried to stay as close to routine as I could." Her class took advantage of in-school educational and multidisciplinary services like the indoor sensory-based swimming pool, music class, rhythm band, music therapy, and physiotherapy. Jennifer also utilized the physio room every morning, both to meet the proprioceptive needs of students (e.g., riding bike, treadmill, swings, large balls) and to provide a large indoor activity that

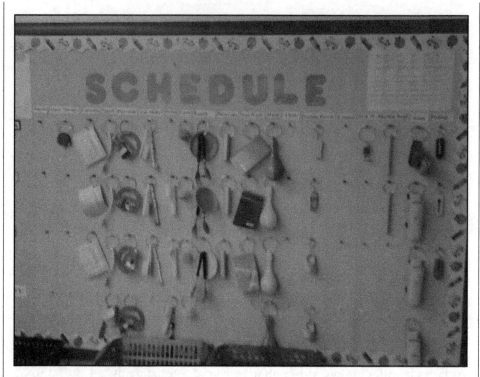

Figure 8.3: Tactile Calendar

allowed for whole-body movement and exploration. "This kept the rest of the day in focus and allowed them to concentrate on academic tasks," she noted. For academic tasks and skills building, she used a structured teaching classroom approach and task boxes created using resources like *Tasks Galore* (Fennell, Hearsey, & Eckenrode, 2013) and *How Do I Teach This Kid? Visual Work Tasks for Beginning Learners on the Autism Spectrum* (Henry, 2005) in addition to support of an educational assistant, working individually with students in 5 to 15-minute intervals.

Jennifer describes one of the challenges of teaching such a unique group of individuals as the lack of research and programs available, which encouraged her to "be very creative in my teaching and think outside the box a lot," making dollar stores one of her go-to resources. One of the innovations Jennifer used was a unique program that links together music keys on the piano with letters of the alphabet for teaching written language to musically strong students. One of the many benefits that Jennifer emphasized is that "my students taught me patience, how to be creative, and reinforced the concept that every student can learn. It might take a full year to reach a particular goal, but when they reach that—no matter how big or how small—they can do it. One small thing is still worth doing."

> **Read about it. Think about it. Write about it.**
>
> Would you send your own child or student to one of these alternate settings? Why or why not?

THE IDENTIFICATION, PLACEMENT, AND REVIEW COMMITTEE

The Identification, Placement, and Review Committee (IPRC) is a legislated team that undertakes the task of formally identifying whether or not a student in the Ontario school system is considered exceptional, including students diagnosed with ASD. It is important to know that while clinicians diagnose, the IPRC team identifies. The two roles differ in process, purpose, and outcome.

In the clinical setting, a child, adolescent, or adult would typically encounter a lengthy, multidisciplinary, team-based process consisting of observation and formal assessment leading, potentially, to a diagnosis. In Ontario, a diagnosis of ASD in a child of student age is often provided by a medical practitioner, such as a developmental pediatrician or a child psychiatrist, who would provide a written outcome of this evaluation and any resulting diagnoses. The parent of that student could then request in writing to the principal that an IPRC must convene to decide on the identification and placement of their child, which are the committee's two main areas of responsibility (Ontario Ministry of Education, 2014b).

Students with ASD—like all students with exceptionalities if deemed exceptional under the provincial definitions by this team meeting, including an administrator or designate, parent, and advocate—would be identified with the category and subcategory of Ontario's categorical special education model. Similar to the clinical categorization, the school system would be likely to identify a student with ASD with the exceptionality "communication: autism." The purpose of identification would be to recognize that student as exceptional, and to label that student with one or more of Ontario's categories of exceptionality. All of this, then, helps the student access services and allows the system to prioritize access to services. The categorical model does not necessarily mirror clinical language, but retains similar features.

Reading on an Individual Education Plan, then, that a student's IPRC-assigned exceptionality is "communication: autism" does not mean she or he necessarily has an exact diagnosis of autism, but rather that this is the category in which that student fits. A student would not be identified as "communication: autism," however, without written evidence of a formal, clinical diagnosis of autism spectrum disorder. On the other hand, it may happen that the IPRC rules that although a student has a diagnosis of ASD, this diagnosis is not affecting school performance sufficiently to drive identification as an exceptional student. Clinicians and advocates in the area of ASD, for example, may be surprised to learn that not all students who are diagnosed are also identified, and may advocate against this practice. Certainly, parents might feel similarly and choose to formally appeal such decisions. If a decision is not appealed, and is documented on a letter of decision, the school setting then has 30 days in which to develop an Individual Education Plan for that newly identified student (Ontario Ministry of Education, 2014b).

INDIVIDUAL EDUCATION PLANS

To reiterate, an IEP is one of the services that is a legislated outcome of the IPRC process of school-based identification. However, if school personnel, the parent(s), or the involved student choose not to proceed to the formal process of the IPRC, that student can still be provided with an IEP. In alignment with key directions from the seminal *Special Education Transformation* (Bennett & Wynne, 2006), many students—including those with an ASD diagnosis—are provided with an IEP without the identification process. In 2012/13, this number reached 44 percent of students receiving special education services in Ontario classrooms (Finlay, 2015).

Some more universal principles for IEP development do exist, such as developing individualized skills-based programs in areas of need or deficit such as communication, social, behaviour, sensory, adaptive, and academic domains (Wilczynski, Menouek, Hunter, & Mudgal, 2007); these are not unique to the Ontario context. There are few elements specific to Ontario schools that must be included in IEPs for students with ASD, beyond a transition plan and the inclusion of ABA-based programming from PPM 140 (Ontario Ministry of Education, 2004). The emphasis on applied behaviour analysis in IEPs for students with ASD leads to accompanying emphasis on specific and measurable goals and a focus on data collection, especially with the consultative and training support of Ontario's clinically based School Support Program (McDougall et al., 2009) and its more recent role development for ABA specialists in all boards (Ontario Ministry of Children and Youth Services, 2011a).

Publicly accessible training specific to school-based practices in Ontario exists, but finding and using resource examples can be challenging. For example, few publicly accessible examples of Ontario-based IEPs exist, with the exception of those samples available on EduGains (2015). These sample IEPs include some that are specific to students with ASD, and are offered in French and English. Training specific to the design of Ontario IEPs is similarly difficult to find. The Learning Disabilities Association of Ontario, however, provides other resources for effective IEP development, specific to the Ontario context but not to ASD, entitled "IEP 101" (2011).

However, the set framework inherent in Ontario IEPs does offer opportunities for flexibility and individualization for students with ASD, through accommodations, modifications, and especially the development of alternate courses.

Accommodations

In the context of Ontario IEPs, accommodations are examples of differentiation in the areas of instruction, environment, and assessment, which may overlap with examples of strong pedagogy already in use by skilled teachers of inclusive classrooms. However, when documented in an IEP, it is typically assumed that students have a greater need for these accommodations, such as scribing for assessments, than most students in the classroom. For students with ASD—or other students supported by IEPs—who do

Accommodations: Accommodations can be defined as "supports or services that are not provided to the general student population but that are required by individual students with special needs to help them achieve learning expectations and demonstrate learning" (Ontario Ministry of Education, 2004, p. 6).

not need modifications or alternate courses, classroom accommodations are the most important component of such individualized programming. When accommodations are recorded in the IEP, they are assumed relevant across all subject areas unless otherwise indicated. It is important to keep in mind, however, that drop-down menus built into IEP software typically require choosing the "best" accommodations from a list, rather than developing individually suited wording. Another issue to consider is the quantity of accommodations. Is it better to inclusively list all the accommodations a student may need, or prioritize three to five accommodations in each area that the classroom teachers are more likely to retain, emphasize, and fulfill? Likely, it is the latter.

Modifications

If a student is unable to meet the standards of the provincial curriculum at grade level, courses can be modified or, in the case of a student with ASD or other exceptionalities, changed. This is a decision that should be taken seriously by the IEP team, as changes to the provincial curriculum have implications for high school streaming, diploma completion, and post-secondary options. Is it better to achieve a "low" evaluation with a grade-level curriculum, or to achieve a "high" evaluation on a modified curriculum? Curriculum can also be modified for students who are gifted and have ASD, allowing them to study subjects above grade level. If courses are modified, accommodations still apply, but an additional component of the IEP must be completed: the Special Education Program. If more than one modified or alternate course is developed, this component is repeated for each course. Typically, modified courses are also drawn from other areas of the provincial curriculum, but three to five learning expectations are prioritized per term. The important tools in developing a modified curriculum are the provincial curriculum, the classroom teacher's long-term plan, report cards, past IEP, and formal assessments. Alternatives to developing modified courses include modifying existing courses at grade level by, for example, decreasing the number or complexity of grade-level outcomes expected to be achieved. Each individual outcome from the curriculum can also be revised to meet needs.

Modification: In the context of Ontario IEPs, modifications are "changes made in the age-appropriate grade-level expectations for a subject or course in order to meet a student's learning needs. These changes may involve developing expectations that reflect knowledge and skills required in the curriculum for a different grade level and/or increasing or decreasing the number and/or complexity of the regular grade-level curriculum expectations" (Ontario Ministry of Education, 2004, p. 25–26).

Alternative Courses

Alternative courses are the third component of the IEP that can be individualized for any student, including those with ASD. This component stands out as the most creative way to individualize curriculum. Alternative courses can be utilized in addition to the courses of the provincial curriculum, or in place of the provincial curriculum (Ontario Ministry of Education, 2004). Provincially approved courses might be replaced if the student's skills are below those goal areas where a K-12 provincial curriculum exists, for example, if the student's math skills are below the goal areas in the kindergarten program, or if the goals are not suitable for that child's needs. This type of program—like modifying courses—is a serious step that should be carefully discussed on an individual basis by the IEP team. Alternative courses are typically built on more formal, either norms-referenced or criterion-referenced assessments that make each student's skills and next steps evident. An example of such assessments might be the Woodcock Johnson Test of Education Achievement or the Wechsler Individual Achievement Test, depending on the practices of the individual board or school, or the Assessment of Basic Language and Learning Skills (ABLLS) or Verbal Behavior Milestone Assessment and Placement Program (VB-MAPP) assessments from the clinical field. As with modified courses, three to five learning expectations are typically prioritized per term and written in a measurable manner, often referred to as "'SMART' goals: Specific, Measurable, Attainable, Routines-based, and Tied to a functional priority" (Jung, 2007, p. 54). Other commonly utilized tools for building alternative courses can be task analyses of basic life skills, such as the one developed by the Grand Erie District School Board (n.d.), which provides a task analysis of seven different areas in what is termed a "developmental program": functional academics, communication, interpersonal, independent living, leisure, pre-vocational, and vocational skills. The number of alternative courses used in place of the typical program of studies would depend on the individual skills profile, strengths, needs, and assessments of each student.

Alternative courses can also be used to supplement the provincial curriculum in an area of need that extends beyond the academic focus areas of the typical program of studies. For example, a student with ASD may need a course developed in communication, social, behavioural, and sensory skills (Wilczynski, Menouek, Hunter, & Mudgal, 2007), or in areas such as use of assistive technology, learning about ASD, and whatever topics are deemed needful by that student's team. Although these courses remain assessment driven and have a similar structure (i.e., three to five learning expectations are prioritized per term), few formalized resources are available for their development. In these cases, educators need to seek out professional and academic resources, such as books, articles, and manuals, to support these individualized courses; no collaborative database exists. One example of such a support is the online resource "A4: Assessing Achievement in Alternate Areas," which provides a fully accessible bank of alternative course examples (e.g., personal life management), lesson suggestions (e.g., task analyses), and ideas for assessment and evaluation (e.g., rubrics).

Alternate Courses Development Example: Social Skills
Part of the diagnostic criteria for students with ASD is significant difficulty with functional social communication skills (American Psychiatric Association, 2013); which is a problem because this area is a predictor of long-term life success (Division of Behavioural and Social Sciences and Education of the National Research Council, 2001). Many students with ASD may not pick up and absorb social skills from examples of adult or peer social skills via simple day-to-day modelling in everyday social settings. Even though such skills are foundational, they are rarely integrated into provincial, academic curricula (Maich, Hall, & Sider, 2013; Maich, 2010).

It is quite common, then, for students with ASD to need individual program development and direct instruction in social skills, and this instruction is best encapsulated in the writing of an alternate course, which provides goals, objectives, instructional strategies, and assessment methods.

Box 8.4: Reflections on Writing IEPs for Students with ASD
By Monique Somma, PhD Student, Brock University

IEPs for students with ASD can vary as much as the characteristics of ASD themselves. When developing an IEP for any student, I ask, "How can I modify the curriculum or provide accommodations to meet the learning needs of the student, while at the same time incorporating measurable goals into the overall goals of the class?" This is easier said than done and takes a lot of pre-planning, authentic attempts and trial and error to understand where the student is at and what level of support is needed. One of the biggest challenges is deciding what strategies will best benefit the student. For example, when implementing an expectation for a student to play a turn-taking card game with a peer, I did not realize that the organization of the cards would pose a challenge for this student. I had to reconsider the plan and adjust the strategies to best meet his learning needs by creating a card placeholder. This change in strategy allowed the student the appropriate level of support in order to be successful socially. Developing curriculum-derived or alternative program expectations for the IEP that include classmates allows the student with ASD to meet his expectations and develop relationships at the same time. By carefully selecting curriculum-derived expectations that align with the expectations of the class, we create a greater sense of belonging for the student—for example, having the class work on designing a board game where they are working through several curriculum expectations while at the same time incorporating IEP expectations for language, math, and social skills for the student with ASD. Another method is to parallel the IEP expectations in the lesson or activity; for example, using project-based learning tasks with various outcomes allows all students to work on a similar assignment with various options for the final product, providing necessary choice and alternatives for a student with ASD. Nonetheless, developing IEPs that have just the right amount of challenge and are appropriate for each student requires collaboration among those who know the student best—including the student himself! The IEP expectations are the most important things that I want the student to learn, but are by no means the only skills that the students will attain in a term. I need to select a few big expectations to focus on each term, for which I can monitor and track progress. As a working document, the IEP is designed to be tweaked and changed as the term goes on. If I make edits to an IEP 10 times over the course of the term, it doesn't mean that my IEP was poorly written; it means that I am taking the time to really get to know the student and adjust my teaching to better meet his needs.

Because children with ASD do have built-in difficulties in social skills, ignoring this area of instruction can leave them with a great disadvantage over time. Ideally, social skills teaching should be assessment-based, individualized, and intensive ... even better: social skills teaching should happen in the inclusive classroom for authentic practice with their peers. (Maich et al., 2013)

The first requirement in writing such a course is the presence of an assessment related to social skills. If the student does not have one already in place, there are some informal checklists that are widely accessible and can be administered by professionals with various training backgrounds. Some examples are found in *Building Social Relationships* (Bellini, Peters, & Hopf, 2007), and *Social Skills Solutions* (McKinnon & Krempa, 2002). Both resources have easy-to-use checklists or rating scales, which help to provide a baseline and next steps for building an alternate course in social skills.

Read about it. Think about it. Write about it.

What do you know about IEPs? Explain any involvement that you have had with IEPs or their related processes and practices.

CONTINUING EDUCATION FOR ONTARIO CERTIFIED TEACHERS

Continuing education for Ontario certified teachers is hosted, delivered, and regulated by the provincial professional regulatory body: the Ontario College of Teachers (OCT) (Ontario College of Teachers, 2014). The OCT is located in Toronto, and it can be found online at www.oct.ca. Currently, it is the only provincial or territorial college for professional certified teachers in Canada. Its graduates are Ontario Certified Teachers, and are both permitted and encouraged to utilize the regulated term OCT in professional nomenclature. The OCT also takes responsibility for hosting the public registry of its certified teachers, sharing information about each registrant's status and education, and listing any additional qualifications (AQ) course successfully undertaken.

One of the formal, documented means of obtaining additional knowledge, skills, and teaching credentials is through AQ courses, a province-wide initiative which is well-recognized provincially and an expected credential for many teaching positions in a range of roles. These courses can be taken onsite or through varied means of fully or hybrid distance education (e.g., part onsite and part online), by approved providers, which may be universities (e.g., Brock

Special Education Program

Subject or Course Code or Alternative Skill Area

Collaboration

Baseline Level of Achievement (usually from previous June report card):	Baseline Level of Achievement for Alternative Skill Areas:
Prerequisite secondary course (if applicable): Letter grade/mark: Curriculum grade level:	Student is able to describe the intent of a character from a book; however, in his own interactions he frequently misreads the intentions of others. Student verbally participates in conversations but needs to develop his listening skills in small groups of peers.

Annual Program Goal(s): A goal statement describing what the student can reasonably be expected to accomplish by the end of the school year (or semester) in a particular subject, course, or alternative skill area.

Will consistently respond positively to the ideas, opinions, values and traditions of others in his instructional small groups and during lunch/recess periods.

Learning Expectations	Teaching Strategies	Assessment Methods
Progress Report		
Demonstrate the difference between types of questions (social greeting questions, bridging questions, questions to sustain a topic) and ask 3 social greeting questions per day during classroom-based interactions using learned strategies.	Use comic strip conversations to teach the use of different types of social questions. Role play. Direct instruction on 2 strategies to ask a peer a question related to school work.	Conference with student to monitor self-reflection. Observation to monitor question technique used and result Antecedent, Behaviour, Consequence (ABC).
Demonstrate active listening skills daily during small group instruction.	Directly teach the student how to listen with one's whole body (using ears to hear, the mind to concentrate on what is being said, eyes to look for nonverbal information, the whole body to face the speaker).	Teacher observation noting active listening techniques used. Student self-reflection checklist. Conference with student to debrief small group participation.
Term 1		
Term 2		

Figure 8.4: Sample IEP for Collaboration

Source: EduGains, 2015.

University) or other professional bodies (e.g., Elementary Teachers' Federation of Ontario). For example, even early-career classroom teachers are expected to have successfully undertaken the Special Education Part One AQ course, the first in a series of three AQ courses leading to the designation "special education specialist," which can be taken immediately after graduation from an approved program of teacher education (e.g., bachelor of education). This type of AQ is called a schedule D. Indeed, "the most popular Additional Qualification courses in Ontario are those designed to support educators in meeting the needs of students with exceptionalities" (Killoran et al., 2013, p. 243).

Within the special education field, apart from this foundational three-part series, OCTs can choose specialty subject areas, which focus in depth on a single field within Ontario special education. One of these courses is the newly re-named "Teaching Students with Communication Needs (Autism Spectrum Disorder)," categorized as a schedule C course.

One of the more recent features of the OCT's website is the "Find an AQ" internal search engine, which assists OCTs searching for professional development opportunities. If an OCT wants to undertake the Teaching Students with Communication Needs (Autism Spectrum Disorder) AQ, the educator can simply search for the keyword "autism" within the OCT's dedicated search engine (www.oct.ca/members/additional-qualifications/findanaq) to find the full course name, and follow its pathway to view all institutional providers offering this subject area as well as their contact information.

This particular AQ course was first developed and taught in Ontario in 2009 through Redeemer University College, a private, faith-based undergraduate-focused post-secondary school (Maich, 2009). Following guidelines developed by the OCT, individual providers develop extensive course proposals, which undergo a careful approval process by the OCT prior to their being offered to teachers. The ASD AQ development followed a similar process; however, such subject areas have additional considerations given their politically weighty natures, and concerns for those who want to avoid being slotted into teaching students with ASD as a career focus as well as those who would prefer to take a more general course that leads to their special education specialist designation.

Further professional resources for educators range from academic and professional graduate degrees, certificate programs, workshops, and online learning, to written or electronic resources and school- or school-system–based human resources. For example, many community colleges (e.g., Fanshawe College, London) offer a post-graduate diploma in Autism and Behavioural Science in full-time, part-time, online, and weekend formats, and many universities (e.g., Brock University) offer graduate degrees with an ABA emphasis with similar flexibility. If OCTs choose to enhance their teaching credentials with approved course sequences, they can complete additional applied practice, supervision, and assessment to apply for their board certified behaviour analyst or board certified assistant behaviour analyst credentials through the Behavior Analyst Certification Board, based in Colorado, and can join the Ontario Association for Behaviour Analysis, Inc.

Many supplementary resources in the field of ASD are available to a wide geographical locale, some of which have emerged from the Ontario region. For example, one well-known resource is Toronto's Geneva Centre for Autism. For Ontario-based educators—and many others—the Geneva Centre offers a range of services related to professional development, such as both onsite and online learning, certificate courses, a biannual conference, and a lending library. The centre has also created and posted e-visuals in French and English, from templates, examples, and tip sheets, to implementation videos (Geneva Centre for Autism, 2008).

ConnectABILITY (n.d.), the website of Community Living (Toronto), though not specific to ASD, provides an easily navigated fully online Visuals Engine, with a set of templates and visuals that can be quickly created, printed, and saved.

Read about it. Think about it. Write about it.

What are your next steps for your own professional development in the field of ASD?

Many other additional resources exist provincially, nationally, and internationally to enhance knowledge, skills, and resources available for supporting students with ASD in school settings. Within schools, this includes resources in the school community, such as classroom teachers and school administrators with training and experience in ASD, onsite resource teachers with expertise in ASD, and educational assistants, who provide additional support staff to classroom teachers and school communities. Beyond the school walls, many provincial school boards have behaviour counsellors and every board has an ABA specialist.

A LOOK BACK

In Chapter 8, "Autism Spectrum Disorder in Ontario Schools," options, practices, and services for students in Ontario were reviewed. It included:
- Fully inclusive settings in Ontario schools;
- Specialized or alternate provincial settings for students with ASD;
- Ontario-based resources for educators teaching students with ASD; and
- Legislated supports for Ontario students identified as exceptional (e.g., Individual Education Plans).

A LOOK AHEAD

Chapter 9, "Supporting Ontario's Adults with Autism Spectrum Disorder," focuses on:
- The current status of services for adults with ASD in Ontario, including a historical perspective and current ministry investigations;
- A review of the most recent survey of adults with ASD in Ontario;
- An overview of post-secondary options for adults with ASD, including accommodations and advocating for one's education;
- A review of employment supports in Ontario and various support models that can be utilized; and
- A brief overview of recreation, financial, and housing supports in Ontario.

ADDITIONAL RESOURCES

- Community Care Access Centre:
  healthcareathome.ca/hnhb/en
- The Gregory School:
  www.gregoryschool.ca/The%20Gregory%20School/
- W. Ross Macdonald School:
  www.psbnet.ca/eng/schools/wross/index.html
- EduGains ASD Resources (2015):
  http://www.beta.edugains.ca/newsite/SpecialEducation/autism_spectrum_disorder.html
- EduGains IEP Samples (2015):
  http://www.beta.edugains.ca/newsite/SpecialEducation/transitions.html
- Geneva Centre for Autism:
  www.autism.net/
- ConnectABILITY Visuals Engine (Commmunity Living Toronto, n.d.)
  connectability.ca/visuals-engine/
- Spirale:
  www.autismontario.com/client/aso/spirale.nsf/ProvSearch?OpenForm
- Find a Teacher Ontario Certified Teacher Registry (Ontario College of Teachers, 2014)
  www.oct.ca/Home/FindATeacher
- Find an AQ (Ontario College of Teachers, 2014):
  www.oct.ca/members/services/findanaq?utm_source=homepage&utm_medium=web&utm_campaign=formembers&utm_content=FindAnAQ
- Behavior Analyst Certification Board:
  www.bacb.com/index.php?page=4

- "Ask Lindsay" Archives of Lindsay Moir (Ontario Association of Children's Rehabilitation Services, 2010):
  oacrs.com/en/AskLindsay
- Ontario Association for Behaviour Analysts, Inc.:
  www.ontaba.org/
- *Special Education Transformation* (Bennett & Wynne, 2006):
  www.edu.gov.on.ca/eng/document/reports/speced/transformation/transformation.pdf
- IEP 101 (Learning Disabilities Association of Ontario, 2011):
  www.ldao.ca/ldao-services/workshops-courses/iep-101-online-workshop-for-parents-and-students/
- Learning People Skills (Hall, Maich, & Sider, 2013):
  www.cea-ace.ca/education-canada/article/learning-people-skills
- A4: Assessing Achievement in Alternate Areas (The A4 Idea People, n.d.):
  www.thea4ideaplace.com

REFERENCES

American Psychiatric Association. (2013). DSM-5 Autism spectrum disorder fact sheet. Retrieved from www.dsm5.org/Documents/Autism%20Spectrum%20Disorder%20Fact%20Sheet.pdf

Bellini, S. (2006). *Building social relationships: A systematic approach to teaching social interaction skills to children and adolescents with autism spectrum disorder or other social difficulties.* Overland Park, KS: Autism Asperger Publishing Company.

Bellini, S., Peters, J. K., Benner, L., & Hopf, A. (2007). A meta-analysis of school-based social skills interventions for children with autism spectrum disorder. *Remedial and Special Education, 28*(3), 153–162.

Bennett, S. (2009). Including students with exceptionalities. *What works? Research into Practice Monograph Series #16.* Retrieved from www.edu.gov.on.ca/eng/literacynumeracy/inspire/research/Bennett.pdf

Bennett, S., & Wynne, K. (2006). *Special education transformation.* Toronto, ON: Queen's Printer. Retrieved from www.edu.gov.on.ca/eng/document/reports/speced/transformation/transformation.pdf

Boer, A., Pijl, S., Minnaert, A., & Post, W. (2014). Evaluating the effectiveness of an intervention program to influence attitudes of students towards peers with disabilities. *Journal of Autism and Developmental Disorders, 44*(3), 572–583. doi:10.1007/s10803-013-1908-6

Carter, M., Stephenson, J., & Strnadová, I. (2011). Reported prevalence by Australian special educators of evidence-based instructional practices. *Australasian Journal of Special Education, 35*(1), 47–60. doi:10.1375/ajse.35.1.47

Center for Applied Special Technology. (2013). What is universal design for learning? Retrieved from www.cast.org/udl/

ConnectABILITY. (n.d.). Visuals Engine. Retrieved from http://connectability.ca/visuals-engine/

Council of Ontario Directors of Education. (n.d.). IEP plans (samples): Resources to support the development and implementation of effective IEPs in Ontario. Retrieved from www.ontariodirectors.ca/IEP-PEI/en.html

Division of Behavioral and Social Sciences and Education of the National Research Council. (2001). *Educating children with autism.* Washington, DC: National Academy Press.

EduGains. (2015). Sample individual education plans. Retrieved from http://www.beta.edugains.ca/newsite/SpecialEducation/transitions.html

Fennell, L., Hearsey, P., & Eckenrode, K. (2013). *Tasks galore.* Raleigh, NC: Tasks Galore Publishing, Inc.

Finlay, B. (2015, January). An overview of special education. Presented to the Regional Special Education Committee.

Geneva Centre for Autism. (2008). E-learning visuals. Retrieved from visuals.autism.net/main.php

Gongola, L., & Sweeney, J. (2012). Discrete trial teaching: Getting started. *Intervention in School and Clinic, 47*(3), 183–190. doi:10.1177/1053451211423813

Grand Erie District School Board. (n.d.). Life skills program planner: A framework for the development of programs for pupils who experience developmental delays. Brantford, ON: Author.

Henry, K. A. (2005). *How do I teach this kid? Visual work tasks for beginning learners on the autism spectrum.* Arlington, TX: Future Horizons, Inc.

Jung, L. A. (2007). Writing SMART objectives and strategies that fit the ROUTINE. *Teaching Exceptional Children, 39*(4), 54–58.

Kaylan Support Systems. (2013). The Gregory school. Retrieved from www.gregoryschool.ca/The%20Gregory%20School/

Killoran, I., Zaretsky, H., Jordan, A., Smith, D., Allard, C., & Moloney, J. (2013). Supporting teachers to work with children with exceptionalities. *Canadian Journal of Education, 36*(1), 240–270.

Learning Disabilities Association of Ontario. (2011). IEP 101. Retrieved from www.ldao.ca/ldao-services/workshops-courses/iep-101-online-workshop-for-parents-and-students/

Li, A. (2009). Identification and intervention for students who are visually impaired and who have autism spectrum disorder. *Teaching Exceptional Children, 41*(4), 22–32.

Maich, K. (2009). ASD additional qualifications course. *Autism Matters, 6*(2), 24–25. Retrieved from www.autismontario.com/Client/ASO/AO.nsf/object/AM+Fall+2009/$file/AM+Fall+2009.pdf

Maich, K. (2010). *Opening a can of worms: Perceptions and practices of teachers in Newfoundland and Labrador incorporating the role of a therapist.* Saarbrücken, Germany: Lambert Academic Publishing.

Maich, K., Hall, C., & Sider, S. (2013). Learning people skills: Social literacy for students with autism spectrum disorder. *Education Canada, 53*(2). Retrieved from www.cea-ace.ca/education-canada/article/learning-people-skills

McDougall, J., Servais, M., Meyer, K., Case, S., Dannenhold, K., Johnson, S., & Riggin, C. (2009). A preliminary evaluation of a school support program for children with autism spectrum disorder: Educator and school level outcomes and program processes. *Exceptionality Education International, 19*(1), 32–50. Retrieved from http://ir.lib.uwo.ca/eei/vol19/iss1/4

McKinnon, K., & Krempa, J. L. (2002). *Social skills solutions: A hands-on manual for teaching social skills to children with autism.* New York, NY: DRL Books.

Ontario College of Teachers. (2014). Find an AQ. Retrieved from www.oct.ca/members/services/findanaq

Ontario Ministry of Children and Youth Services. (2011a). Applied behaviour analysis-based services and supports for children and youth with ASD. Retrieved from www.children.gov.on.ca/htdocs/English/topics/specialneeds/autism/guidelines/guidelines-2011.aspx

Ontario Ministry of Children and Youth Services. (2011b). Programs and services for children with autism. Retrieved from www.children.gov.on.ca/htdocs/English/topics/specialneeds/autism/programs.aspx

Ontario Ministry of Education. (2004). The individual education plan (IEP): A resource guide. Toronto, ON: Queen's Printer. Retrieved from www.edu.gov.on.ca/eng/general/elemsec/speced/guide/resource/iepresguid.pdf

Ontario Ministry of Education. (2005). *Education for all: The report of the expert panel on literacy and numeracy instruction for students with special education needs, kindergarten to grade six.* Toronto, ON: Queen's Printer. Retrieved from www.edu.gov.on.ca/eng/document/reports/speced/panel/speced.pdf

Ontario Ministry of Education. (2007). *Program/policy memorandum no. 140: Incorporating methods of applied behaviour analysis (ABA), into programs for students with autism spectrum disorder (ASD).* Retrieved from www.edu.gov.on.ca/extra/eng/ppm/140.html

Ontario Ministry of Education. (2014a). Guidelines for educational programs for students in government approved care and/or treatment, custody, and correctional (CTCC) facilities. Retrieved from faab.edu.gov.on.ca/Section_23/14-15/Guidelines_For_Educational_Programs_for_Students_In_Government_Approved.pdf

Ontario Ministry of Education. (2014b). Highlights of regulation 181/98. Retrieved from www.edu.gov.on.ca/eng/general/elemsec/speced/hilites.html

Peel District School Board. (2013). Streetsville secondary school. Retrieved from www.peelschools.org/schools/Pages/profile.aspx?sid=2552

Rushowy, K. (2012, November 12). The autism project: Streetsville school offers "home base" for autistic teens. The Toronto Star. Retrieved from www.thestar.com/news/investigations/2012/11/12/the_autism_project_streetsville_school_offers_home_base_for_autistic_teens.html

Ryan, T. G. (2009). Inclusive attitudes: a pre-service analysis. *Journal of Research in Special Educational Needs, 9*(3), 180–187. doi:10.1111/j.1471-3802.2009.01134.x\\

The Joy of Learning Centre. (n.d.). Programs. Retrieved from www.jolc.ca

Tomlinson, C. A. (1999). Mapping a route toward differentiated instruction. *Educational Leadership, 57*(1), 12–16.

Tomlinson, C. A. (2000). Differentiated instruction: can it work? *Education Digest,* (5), 25.

Wilczynski, S. M., Menouek, K., Hunter, M., & Mudgal, D. (2007). Individualized education programs for youth with autism spectrum disorder. *Psychology in the Schools, 44*(7), 653–666. doi: 10.1002/pits

CHAPTER 9

SUPPORTING ONTARIO'S ADULTS WITH AUTISM SPECTRUM DISORDER

IN THIS CHAPTER:

- The Ontario Movement for Adults with ASD
  - 2013 Ontario Survey of Adults with ASD
- Transitioning from Adolescence
- Post-Secondary Options
  - Accommodations
  - Taking Charge of One's Education
- Employment Opportunities
- Recreation and Leisure
- Financial Support
- Housing

Chapter 9 highlights the history of adult supports in Ontario, focusing on Developmental Services Ontario (DSO), and the frequent difficulty for those diagnosed with Asperger's disorder to get access to services. The chapter highlights the 2013 feedback and statistics on the status of adults living with autism spectrum disorder (ASD) in Ontario. Services and models for areas of adult life are highlighted for: 1) post-secondary, 2) employment, 3) recreation, 4) financial support, and 5) housing. Creative ideas for housing, and other stories from adults with ASD, demonstrate positive progress yet the need for further evolution of supports for adults with ASD in Ontario.

THE ONTARIO MOVEMENT FOR ADULTS WITH ASD

In Ontario, services for adults with autism spectrum disorder (ASD) are inconsistent and less available than those provided for the under-18 sector. Unlike services for children, there are no systematic, provincially funded services designed specifically for adults with ASD; rather, funding is focused on the developmental disabilities diagnostic category, according to law. Though many adults with ASD fall within this category, others do not. Individuals described as higher functioning were diagnosed with Asperger's disorder in the *Diagnostic and Statistical Manual of Mental Disorders, 4th Edition, Revised (DSM-IV-TR)* (American Psychiatric Association [APA], 2000) until 2013: "Up to 50% of individuals with ASDs do not have an intellectual disability (ID), yet their needs for support are as great as those with ASD and ID" (Autism Ontario, 2008, p. 13). In the current *DSM-5*, the sole diagnosis is autism spectrum disorder (ASD), rated on three levels of severity (APA, 2013). Funding to support daily living skills for those with ASD who do not have an intellectual disability is difficult to obtain (Autism Ontario, 2008).

In 2008, *Forgotten: Ontario Adults with Autism and Adults with Asperger's* (Autism Ontario) estimated that there are 70,000 individuals with ASD in

Developmental Disabilities: A developmental disability, according to the Services and Supports to Promote the Social Inclusion of Persons with Developmental Disabilities Act (Ontario Statutes, 2008), is defined as follows: "if the person has the prescribed significant limitations in cognitive functioning and adaptive functioning and those limitations,

(a) originated before the person reached 18 years of age;

(b) are likely to be life-long in nature; and

(c) affect areas of major life activity, such as personal care, language skills, learning abilities, the capacity to live independently as an adult or any other prescribed activity." (Ontario Statutes, 2008, s. 3 [1])

Ontario, including 50,000 adults. The National Epidemiologic Database for the Study of Autism in Canada has estimated that one in 94 children has ASD in Canada (2013). In 2013, it was estimated that there were 9,341,200 Ontarians between ages 16 and 64, so with a prevalence of one percent of the population, Stoddart and colleagues (2013) estimated that up to 93,412 adults with ASD are living in Ontario. It is estimated that, although the range of skill levels varies widely in children, this range is even greater in adulthood (Stoddart et al., 2013).

Many adults with ASD transition from childhood and adolescence with a diagnosis of ASD already in place, but some receive their first diagnosis in adulthood (Autism Ontario, 2008; Burke, 2005). For this latter group, such a diagnosis can be a relief after many years of concerns about fitting in, layered with many failed or awkward attempts at interacting with others (Burke, 2005).

Before Asperger's disorder was added to the *DSM-IV* in 1994, many such individuals were referred to as quirky or strange (APA, 1994; Stoddart, 2005). Although they may have functioned at average or above average levels for academics and other tasks of daily living, they struggled to feel like they were fitting in with a social group. Some suggest that celebrated intellectuals such as Albert Einstein and Bill Gates may have traits of ASD. Bill Gates, the founder of Microsoft and highly successful billionaire, for example, is often referenced as an adult with Asperger's: "He has often been seen rocking and tends to speak in monotones—both habits acknowledged to be symptoms" (CBC News, 2013, para. 14).

In Ontario, advocacy for adults with ASD continues to be an ongoing concern (Allen, 2014; Autism Ontario, 2008; Stoddart et al., 2013). Difficulties stem from a lack of funding, especially to those who are so-called "higher functioning", and include a lack of specialized services that meet the needs of those with ASD, all entangled with many potential comorbid mental health needs (Allen, 2014; Autism Ontario, 2008). The government continues to develop working groups in order to meet the different and unique services that both adults with ASD and mental health practitioners are calling necessary for this population (Allen, 2014).

The first major report highlighting the difficulties faced by adults with

Asperger's Disorder: In the *DSM-IV* (APA, 2000) Asperger's disorder was diagnosed via a qualitative impairment in social interaction and repetitive and restricted patterns of behaviour, having significant impact on everyday functioning, without a language delay before two years old, and no cognitive delays. It has since been removed from the *DSM-5* and grouped under the term *autism spectrum disorder*. (APA, 2000)

Intellectual Disability: An intellectual disability "(also commonly referred to as a developmental disability among other terms) is, simply stated, a disability that significantly affects one's ability to learn and use information. It is a disability that is present during childhood and continues throughout one's life. A person who has an intellectual disability is capable of participating effectively in all aspects of daily life, but sometimes requires more assistance than others in learning a task, adapting to changes in tasks and routines, and addressing the many barriers to participation that result from the complexity of our society." (Community Living Ontario, 2015, para. 1)

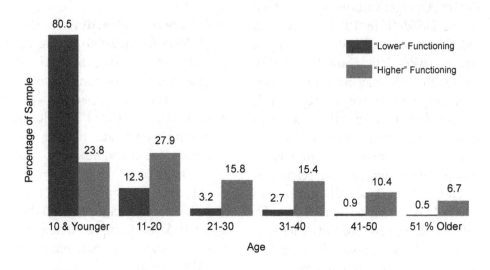

Figure 9.1: Age of Diagnosis in Ontario for Adults with ASD
Source: Stoddart et al., 2013, p. 18.

Read about it. Think about it. Write about it.

Reflect on the impact of social skill difficulties in adulthood. How would this influence a person's life? How would others in their environment respond?

ASD in Ontario and advocating for additional services was the *Forgotten* report (Autism Ontario, 2008), which provided three major recommendations: 1) regulated and sufficient services across sectors province-wide; 2) standard eligibility for services based on functional need rather than intellectual ability; and 3) the implementation of best practices for adults with ASD within the above services. See Box 9.2 for a more detailed description of these recommendations.

Since this report, the Services and Supports to Promote the Social Inclusion of Persons with Developmental Disabilities Act (Ontario Statutes, 2008), in order to support the individuality and equal treatment of all people with developmental disabilities, replaced the previous act, which was over 35 years old (Ontario Ministry of Community and Social Services [MCSS], 2012). This current act is for adults 18 years and older and focuses on activities of daily living, residential supports, caregiver respite supports, and person-directed planning supports (MCSS, 2012). It directly influenced the transformation of Developmental Services Ontario (DSO), which reviews each individual case

Box 9.1: ASD Diagnosis in Adulthood

For Pam, there was always something that felt different. She always did well in school, but struggled socially. In elementary and high school she remembered that although she was included in the popular groups, she always felt like she had to "fake it" in order to be accepted. There were never any concerns raised by family or teachers, as she was always polite, pleasant, well-behaved, and had good academic skills. She continued on to university, obtaining a degree in philosophy. She struggled a little more socially, but there were never any red flags, apart from major anxiety and depression. She was able to go to classes independently, work on her papers, demonstrate her giftedness in writing, and graduate successfully, after reducing to a part-time course load and even taking some time off of her studies. Afterwards, after having difficulties getting a job, she went on to attend community college in Ontario.

At this point, Pam enrolled in a hands-on program that focused on counselling. She began experiencing difficulties soon after entering the class. The class relied quite a bit on group work, field placements, and social interactions. In many classes, for example, she was expected to engage in role-play counselling sessions for the majority of the class time. She found this extremely challenging and was not attaining the same level of success as she did in previous academic experiences. The group dynamics were problematic; she recalls well the horrifying group dynamics, social exclusion, and difficulties of working with others. After a trip to counselling services herself, she was connected with the disabilities office. At that time, she requested a psychological assessment in the community, as she had long suspected Asperger's.

With opposing feelings of eagerness and apprehension, Pam undertook the psychological assessment provided by a community-based psychologist who specialized in ASD. Pam was 31 years old. The day that the psychologist told her that she had Asperger's disorder, Pam remembers feeling a tremendous sense of relief, as so many questions were finally answered. After the initial shock, and after doing some more reading, Pam felt that the diagnosis explained the situations where she struggled socially, and it definitely explained the difficulties she was having currently in school, and so much more. Although having a diagnosis sooner might have helped, the journey from diagnosis to where she is now was insightful and eye opening. She wonders, for example, if being labelled in childhood would have further contributed to her sense of otherness and possibly lowered her expectations of herself. She is now a successful member of her ASD community and is involved in advocacy events and talks, promoting ASD awareness. Obtaining a diagnosis in adulthood has overall been a positive experience for Pam, as it has provided opportunities for growth, self-acceptance, and helping others.

Box 9.2: Recommendations from *Forgotten*

Recommendation One
Ensure sufficient and regulated services for adults with ASD in the adult/child mental health, social service, colleges/universities and developmental sectors through an Ontario-wide cross-sector policy framework and devoted funding based on a provincial needs assessment. Specifically, this policy framework would ensure:

a) Financial supports which are not tied to "claw-backs" through the Ontario Disability Support Program (ODSP), Registered Disability Savings, and welfare programs;
b) Day supports including vocational and employment, educational, social and recreational services/opportunities;
c) Programs devoted to monitoring the well-being and safety of adults with ASDs;
d) A range of supported living options; and
e) Professional supports including psychological, medical, and psychiatric assistance, dental care, person-centered planning, case coordination, respite care, crisis supports and legal assistance.

Recommendation Two
Implement standard eligibility criteria to services for adults with ASD based on their functional needs rather than intellectual functioning through an Ontario-wide cross-sector policy framework.

Recommendation Three
Facilitate access to best practices education and research specific to adults with ASD across adult/child mental health, social service, colleges/universities and developmental sectors through a provincial knowledge exchange centre. This centre would:

a) Lead a provincial needs assessment.
b) Guide or seed, translate and disseminate best practice research;
c) Provide information to specialized and generic or developmental service providers;
d) Provide information to families and individuals with ASDs; and
e) Track adult services available throughout the province.

Source: Autism Ontario, 2008, p. 20.

for cognitive functioning, adaptive skills, and for a diagnosis before age 18 (Developmental Services Ontario [DSO], 2014).

In 2012, following the exposure of extreme cases where adults with developmental disabilities were in homeless shelters or jails in reaction to a dearth of placements (Ombudsmen Ontario, 2012), an emergency response to the adult service sector for those with developmental disabilities was undertaken by the Ontario Ombudsman to investigate adult services for those with developmental disabilities. This investigation was the result of many complaints that services were difficult to obtain and required long waiting lists after the individuals turned 18. By 2014, the Ombudsman received over 1,250 complaints about the services, and a report of recommendations was released in spring 2015 (Gordon, 2015; Ombudsman Ontario, 2015). The Ontario Ombudsman reports that he is dealing with the complaints on two levels, with broader systemic complaints and with the need for individual assistance to families in crisis: "housing these people in hospitals and nursing homes doesn't make sense. Many report that there is too much bureaucracy and not enough service. They feel like they are facing endless waiting lists" (Ombudsman Ontario, 2014, para. 6).

Activities of Daily Living: Activities of daily living "constitute a critical domain of adaptive behavior, which are defined as behaviors necessary for age-appropriate, independent functioning in social, communication, daily living, or motor areas" (Smith, Maenner, & Seltzer, 2012, p. 2).

Respite: Respite is defined as external social support that is available to families who are facing stressors and to provide support for the person with ASD who is requiring care, where the focus is on caregivers' needs, giving them a small break in order to regroup and refocus with the ongoing stresses of the continuous care for a child with varying needs (Harper, Dyches, Harper, Roper, & South, 2013).

Person-Directed Planning: Person-directed planning is an individualized approach to service planning where the individual's support circle is utilized, strengths rather than weaknesses are a focus, and the services that the individual needs are highlighted, rather than only what services are available (Mansell & Beadle-Brown, 2004).

2013 Ontario Survey of Adults with ASD

In 2013, Stoddart and colleagues finished a survey of adults with ASD in Ontario. A survey was administered online to 480 individuals with ASD, their parents, and service providers, dependent on the functioning level of the individual and his or her ability to self-report or have others report on his or her behalf (Stoddart et al., 2013). Of those involved, 72.5 percent were male, 27.5 percent female, 86.5 percent single, 9 percent married, and 2.3 percent separated or divorced (Stoddart et al., 2013, p. 15). Sadly, the wage of adults with ASD over 20 was low, with 32 percent earning below $10,000 and 73.2 percent earning less than $30,000. This puts many adults with ASD below the poverty level in Ontario, which is $19,930 (see Figure 9.2) (Poverty Free Ontario, 2015; Stoddart et al., 2013).

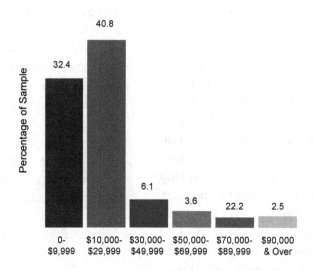

Figure 9.2: Annual Income for Adults with ASD 20 and Older
Source: Stoddart et al., 2013, p. 16.

Independence in Daily Life Skills
In the same report, when asked about the amount of help needed with services, over 64 percent required assistance with finding and using services, 59 percent required help with finances, 58 percent required assistance with household repairs, 54 percent required assistance in arranging appointments (52 percent with attending appointments) and 50 percent with shopping, groceries, and doing mail (see Figure 9.3) (Stoddart et al., 2013). These results demonstrate the consistent need for help with services, which is even more so considering that the largest group of respondents for the study had Asperger's disorder or high-functioning

autism (50 percent) (Stoddart et al., 2013). In addition, few resided on their own with no supports (13.6 percent), whereas the majority lived with their parents (59.8 percent) (see Figure 9.3) (Stoddart et al., 2013).

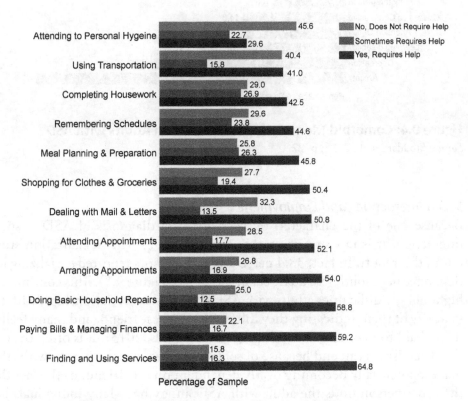

Figure 9.3: Amount of Help Required with Daily Life Skills
Source: Stoddart et al., 2013, p. 20.

Mental Health Concerns

Consistent with other literature, a diagnosis of ASD was found to be comorbid with other mental health concerns in Ontario's adults. Buck and colleagues (2014) found that 52.7 percent of adults with ASD were likely to have an anxiety disorder in their lifetime. Similarly, in Ontario, anxiety was the highest comorbid psychiatric disorder, followed by depression (Stoddart et al., 2013). See Figure 9.4 for a full breakdown of comorbid psychiatric conditions. In addition, 31 percent of adults with ASD who took the survey felt they had an undiagnosed psychiatric condition. Some of these individuals even needed emergency room services for behavioural, psychiatric, or psychological services (Stoddart et al., 2013).

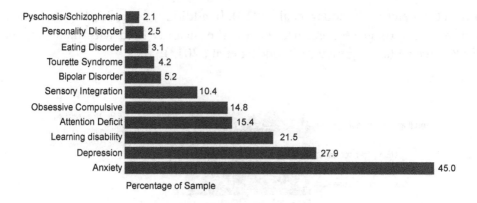

Figure 9.4: Comorbid Mental Health Concerns in Adults with ASD
Source: Stoddart et al., 2013, p. 22.

Social Interactions and Employment

Because one of the characteristic elements of a diagnosis of ASD is social interaction, it is not surprising that the difficulties with socialization stood out in this report. In fact, 38.4 percent of participants reported socializing less than once per month (Stoddart et al., 2013) (see Figure 9.5). This continues to highlight the difficulties adults with ASD have in social relationships, with the majority of them indicating they did not have a best friend, and many feeling it was hard to maintain friendships (Stoddart et al., 2013). It is often the case that friendships can end because of social mistakes that the person with ASD makes, potentially becoming overly dependent on one friend, or the fact that the other person finds the adult with ASD annoying. Many individuals had their family as the primary means of socialization, turned to online avenues for socialization, and felt that there were few social activities and programs available (Stoddart et al., 2013). Very few of the respondents were employed, and a high number of participants engaged in recreation in the community for their daily activities; yet, many indicated that their primary daily activities included watching TV, playing on the computer, or staying home with their caregivers (Stoddart et al., 2013).

Services in Ontario

A wide variety of various service options were discussed in the survey, including issues and concerns. Sixty percent of individuals utilized the Ontario Disability Support Program (ODSP) (Stoddart et al., 2013). Others stated that frequent advocacy was necessary; for example, "[we] had to fight for every single penny our

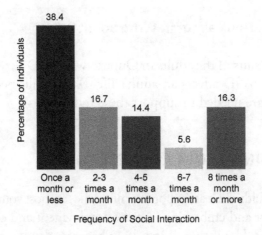

Figure 9.5: Frequency of Social Activities
Source: Stoddart et al., 2013, p. 28.

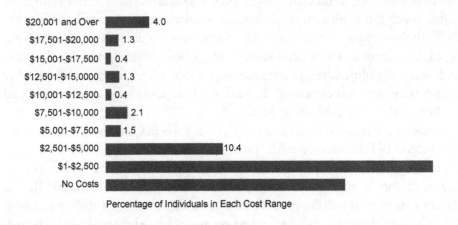

Figure 9.6: Costs Incurred for Services in the Previous 12 months
Source: Stoddart et al., 2013, p. 38.

son receives in support of his dignity, independence, integration, and equality of opportunity" (Stoddart et al., 2013, p. 35). Some indicated that although they met the criteria for their adaptive functioning being within the guidelines of the DSO, their cognitive ability was not, disqualifying them from additional funding and services (Stoddart et al., 2013). This left many individuals paying for their own services (see Figure 9.6).

Read about it. Think about it. Write about it.

Based on the results of the adults in Ontario with ASD survey, summarize the main ways that ASD affects an adult's life. What skills need to be targeted? What services are needed to support these individuals?

TRANSITIONING FROM ADOLESCENCE

Transition into adulthood is an important milestone for most youth, who are becoming more independent and embarking into the employment and educational world for their future careers. However, this transition becomes daunting when one has ASD. First, funding sources change from the programs under the Ministry of Children and Youth Services and Ministry of Education, to the Ministry of Community and Social Services (MCSS) and the Ministry of Training, Colleges, and Universities (MCTU). Within these ministries are different programs, different methods for accessing funding, and often much more onus on the individual to advocate for the services he or she needs. With these changes come new worlds to navigate. As difficult as this is for most young adults, it becomes that much more complex when navigating additional services for and with a disability. Given that transitions are difficult for individuals with ASD in general, transitions to new settings in adulthood can cause substantial anxiety and stress (APA, 2013; Alcorn MacKay, 2010).

For those attending publicly funded secondary schools in Ontario, all students who have an Individual Education Plan (IEP) are required to have a transition plan for each year, including (where appropriate) their exit from high school to the community, to further education, or to employment (Ontario Ministry of Education, 2013). It is important that these transition processes start as soon as the individual enters high school, to ensure that goals can be worked on and achieved throughout their high school career, to make the transition as successful as possible. In the last years of high school, this may involve experiencing work placements, undergoing educational preparation programs, and meeting with funding and accommodation services in the adult sector to prepare the adolescent and their family as much as possible.

CanChild (Centre for Childhood Disability Research) has also developed a youth kit, designed to help organize and prepare youth for their transition to adulthood (2010). The kit is designed to help the individual decide their goals and priorities for this transition, organize needed documents, and provide information in order to access the appropriate supports to attain goals (CanChild, 2010). It involves understanding social, work, school, health, life skills, and budget information. The kit is available to download for free from the CanChild website at: www.canchild.ca

The remainder of this chapter focuses on the five major transition avenues for adults with ASD to achieve success and integration into the community: 1) post-secondary options; 2) employment opportunities; 3) recreation and leisure; 4) financial support; and 5) housing. Within each of these areas, resources and information for adults with ASD in Ontario will be provided.

POST-SECONDARY OPTIONS

Just like any other student in the province, students with ASD can access numerous post-secondary options, including college, university, apprenticeship programs, and private career colleges (MCTU, 2015). At each college and university, there is an accessibility office, where supports to help students with disabilities access their programs and individual classes are provided (MCSS, 2015). Supports for adult students with ASD in post-secondary environments can include accommodations such as extra time for test writing, assistance with coaching on field placements, the hiring of note-takers for classes, or educational assistants to assist with tasks in the classroom for those with more substantial needs. Very little research is completed in this area, and the inclusion of those with ASD in post-secondary classrooms is somewhat new for disability offices (Alcorn MacKay, 2010).

Attending post-secondary school can be challenging for those with ASD because of a multitude of factors. First, navigating the large number of buildings amongst noise, crowded hallways, and little direction from educators can be overwhelming (Alcorn MacKay, 2010). Another difficulty is that individuals often have difficulty sustaining their interest in a course beyond their specific area of interest, making elective courses difficult to complete (Alcorn MacKay, 2010). In addition, with the rigidity that comes with the disorder, when in their specific area of interest, students have been known to challenge the professor, add additional information in the classroom (often uncalled for or without a raised hand), and get frustrated when the content does not match what or how it was envisioned. It was estimated that approximately 1,100 students with ASD would attend post-secondary institutions in Ontario from 2009 to 2011 (Alcorn MacKay, 2010).

Sometimes, community colleges can be a helpful place to start for individuals with ASD because of the smaller class sizes, smaller campuses, and ability for accessibility services to provide a more customized support system and accommodations (Adreon & Durocher, 2007). However, the difficulty is that smaller class sizes and hands-on approaches make the person with ASD more visible, making it then more difficult for the person to blend into the crowds (Adreon & Durocher, 2007). With the social challenges that these individuals face as part of the diagnosis, another potential area of struggle is group work, required more often in college classrooms (Alcorn MacKay, 2010; APA, 2013).

The Inclusive Education Program in Ontario Colleges, also called Community Integration through Cooperative Education, is another type of program available for adults with ASD. Such programs are offered in many Ontario colleges and are designed for those with intellectual disabilities, developmental disabilities, or other learning challenges (OntarioColleges.ca, 2015), and are individually tailored for each individual student based on his or her interests and skills. In this type of program, students attend multiple classes in different areas with a learning facilitator who also helps them with tutoring outside of class (OntarioColleges. ca, 2015). To enrol, students are required to have an Ontario Secondary School Diploma or equivalent or be a mature student (OntarioColleges.ca, 2015). Many of the programs also provide hands-on experiences through field placement programs and can lead to entry-level jobs depending on the course of study for the individual student (Ontariocolleges.ca, 2015)

Accommodations

Traditionally, accommodations for those with learning disabilities can also be accessed for individuals with ASD, such as test-taking in a quiet space, extra time for tests, special seating arrangements, and recorded lecture notes (Adreon & Durocher, 2007). For individuals in Ontario, such accommodations are accessed as part of the Ontario Human Rights Code (Alcorn MacKay, 2010). Individuals are still required to meet the course expectations, and program modifications cannot be made; however, accommodations are provided in order to level the playing field with peers (Alcorn MacKay, 2010). In order to receive accommodations, an assessment must be completed or documentation must be provided identifying a disability (Alcorn MacKay, 2010). Accommodations that may provide additional assistance for an individual with ASD may include the option to do group work individually, having assistance in selecting courses, permission to attend additional sections of the same course, and scheduling flexibility (Adreon & Durocher, 2007). A negative aspect is that because some individuals are required to take fewer classes, their financial obligations can be higher due to increased tuition over multiple terms (Alcorn MacKay, 2010).

Read about it. Think about it. Write about it.

List ways that accommodations may not be enough for individuals with ASD to succeed in their coursework. Come up with two creative solutions where the individual can still achieve the same outcome of the course, but use an accommodation that supports their ASD characteristics.

Taking Charge of One's Education

One significant difference between high school and post-secondary school is that the student is required to take the lead in requesting assistance and leading his or her educational journey (Alcorn MacKay, 2010; Manett & Stoddart, 2012; MCTU, 2015). This is done, in part, to recognize and acknowledge rights to independence and freedom as an adult, allowing the adult to make choices and have autonomy. In addition, because they are adults, the post-secondary institution requires written permission in order to talk to involved parents, sometimes preventing necessary additional communication from occurring that once occurred in high school (Manett & Stoddart, 2012). In ideal practice, accommodations must be arranged ahead of time in order to schedule classes and test-taking and provide professors with advance notice (Manett & Stoddart, 2012).

The difficulty with these practices, however well-intentioned they may be, is that taking charge, managing, organizing, and recognizing the need for assistance is sometimes difficult for those with ASD (Alcorn MacKay, 2010; Manett & Stoddart, 2012). Many individuals struggle with executive functioning and the ability to plan and organize appointments and strategies that are needed for success (Stoddart et al., 2013). In addition, the struggle with change, social skills, and communication can make this process increasingly difficult (Manett & Stoddart, 2012). Lastly, the individual with ASD may have difficulty with the introspection that would help him or her to realize that they are struggling, are behind, or to even recognize the hidden curriculum of what they should be doing in the post-secondary classroom environment (Lombardo & Baron-Cohen, 2011; Manett & Stoddart, 2012).

In a review of services provided to students with ASD in Ontario, Alcorn MacKay (2010) provided a summary of secondary and post-secondary school services, noting gaps in accommodations for students with ASD in the post-secondary education system. A summary of the findings is found in Table 9.1. It was recommended that post-secondary staff should: 1) be trained as ASD coaches; 2) obtain professional development in ASD; 3) provide safe spaces; 4) create transition plans whenever possible; 5) create partnerships with parents for planning and executing the post-secondary journey; 6) provide supports to those completing psychological assessments for adults with ASD, to provide helpful learner-specific recommendations for the institution; and 7) continue research in this area. See Box 9.3 for a story of misunderstandings in a postsecondary setting.

Box 9.3: A Therapist's Story of an Adult with ASD in Post Secondary
By Jocelyn Prosser, BSc, BCBA, Senior Therapist, Thames Valley Children's Centre

Late one afternoon, I received an email from a frantic support staff member from the university. She was concerned, asking me if I knew of an individual's whereabouts. I was puzzled, because I knew the student followed a detailed schedule and someone always knew where he was—he was always great at communicating what his plans were for the day. I tried my best to reach the student by phone and email, but there was no response. Ultimately, it turned out that he was okay, but I still questioned where he had been. At first he was not willing to share any information with me, seemingly embarrassed for what he had done. But when we entered a more private setting, he divulged all of the details.

He had been frustrated that day he went "missing," angry with himself, angry at the parts of his mind that hold him back from doing the things he wants to do. In that moment of anger, he began punching the walls in the hallway and talking to himself. He often used self-talk as a coping or calming mechanism for the times he found most difficult. When he was in the hallway, he was noticed by other students and was reported to security. Security was quick to approach him, giving him no opportunity to share how he was feeling. Security quickly called for a support vehicle and sent him to the hospital because they had suspected he was a threat to himself and was experiencing a psychotic break. At the hospital, his phone was removed, which was why no one could contact him that day.

In reality, the student was trying to cope with what had happened in his prior class. Upset with how he acted in class, and unsure on how to communicate this, he waited to get his frustration out until he was in the hall. It was apparent that the student did not understand why the situation ended the way it did. He did not know why people did not understand him, and why they proceeded in such an aggressive way. In that moment, I realized that the entire university community needed education about ASD, and not just the professors. Leaving the individual at the university, in an area we thought was safe, the team realized that not everyone knew the way to react to someone with ASD. This was my lesson in remembering to try and educate as many as possible that may come in contact with our university students with ASD.

Table 9.1: Services for Students with ASD in Ontario

Categories of services and supports: Human resources	
Helpful services and supports at secondary school	• resource teacher support • educational assistants assigned to student • designated mentor that they can go to in times of stress—"Safe Haven" • school board ASD teams or specialists • consultation with community-based agencies • interdisciplinary team consultations: speech-language pathologists, occupational therapists, physiotherapists, child and youth workers, social workers, psychologists, etc. • guidance teachers • regular contact with parents • peer tutors or mentors • job coaches
Current services and supports at postsecondary level	• disability counsellor/advisor (time limited) • general tutoring (peer and staff) • brief counselling support (not ASD specific) • referrals for more intensive community counselling support (if available) • referral for psychological assessments (if available)
Service gaps in postsecondary education	• autism specialists not generally available • designated staff with flexibility and availability to provide "Safe Haven" in times of stress not provided • no access to community-based agency supports with a mandate for adult support in most areas • no regular contact with parents generally arranged • ASD-specific tutoring and peer mentoring not available • no classroom assistants with ASD experience • no job coaches for placements • few psychological service providers current on adult recommendation for postsecondary environment

Categories of services and supports: Accommodations (Individualized Education Plan)	
Helpful services and supports at secondary school	• assistive technology and/or access to computer laptops • transition supports • reduced course load • extended time for tests and assignments • scribing or oral testing • distraction-reduced environment for tests • clarification or paraphrasing of test questions • note taker • recording of lectures
Current services and supports at postsecondary level	• assistive technology and/or access to computer laptops on a scheduled or limited basis • general orientation programs not specific to ASD needs • reduced course load • testing accommodations (scribing/oral, distraction reduced, extra time) • copies of instructor's and/or classmates' notes when available • recording of lectures when appropriate
Service gaps in PSE	• no ASD-specific orientation programs currently available • tutors are peers or generalists, not trained in the specific needs of students with ASD • class sizes may make recording of lectures problematic in some situations
Categories of services and supports: Professional development	
Helpful services and supports at secondary school	• staff training to develop awareness of ASD • training in behavioural strategies (e.g., ABA) • training instructional strategies (e.g., Differentiated Instruction)
Current services and supports at postsecondary level	• awareness training for disability service providers on an individual basis

Service gaps in PSE	• faculty PD on ASD for awareness and specific instructional strategies such as Universal Design for Instruction is done only on a voluntary basis • awareness training for residence and security staff specific to ASD potential issues not provided in general
Categories of services and supports: Learning Environment	
Helpful services and supports at secondary school	• sensory friendly, calming or "time-off" room • access to resource room • alternative lunch space • preferential seating arrangement—away from distractions • clearly structured day, with predictable routines • flexible timetables, with periodic breaks, late starts and/or early ends • opportunity to leave the class when needed to reduce stress • online courses • locally developed courses (developed at the school board level to accomplish specific goals for students with exceptionalities who can't access regular programs) • cooperative education and work experiences
Current services and supports at postsecondary level	• reduced course loads to adjust start/end of days and allow for periodic breaks if possible (however, this may have implications for program requirements and length of time in program) • opportunity to leave the class when needed to reduce stress • online courses for some courses • program placements (where part of a program)
Service gaps in PSE	• sensory-friendly, calming or "time-off" room not available in most campus locations due to restrictions on space availability and lack of staff to monitor • alternative lunch space not available

	<ul><li>preferential seating arrangement – away from distractions (currently self-managed and not always possible in some classroom settings)</li><li>insufficient institutional community understanding of the need for withdrawing from some situations due to stress</li><li>limited number of online courses available and little student support for these</li><li>ASD specialists not available to prepare and monitor placements (in addition to program staff)</li><li>no specialized orientation, course or program developed for students with ASD who require specialized transition experiences</li><li>insufficient support to promote adjustment in the residence environment</li></ul>
Categories of services and supports: Instructional Considerations	
Helpful services and supports at secondary school	<ul><li>monitoring of social-emotional needs</li><li>providing visual supports to facilitate comprehension</li><li>providing graphic organizers</li><li>breaking tasks down to make them more manageable</li><li>providing models of finished products</li><li>building on strengths and interests with differentiated instruction</li><li>repetition or clarification of concepts</li><li>clear expectations</li><li>reduced number of assignments</li><li>clarification of roles for group work</li></ul>
Current services and supports at postsecondary level	<ul><li>self-managed, limited access to general tutors for repetition or clarification of concepts when available</li><li>program selection in order to build on learning strengths and interests</li></ul>
Service gaps in PSE	<ul><li>insufficient monitoring of social-emotional needs</li><li>no ASD-specific tutors/coaches for graphic organizers, breaking tasks down, etc.</li></ul>

Categories of services and supports: Learning strategies training	
Helpful services and supports at secondary school	• social skills • managing sensory issues • organization and time management skills • structuring written assignments • self-advocacy skills • problem-solving skills
Current services and supports at postsecondary level	• disability advisors/counsellors available to guide development of problem-solving and self-advocacy skills on a very limited basis • LD-specific learning strategies training for students with coexisting learning disabilities on a limited basis
Service gaps in PSE	• no ASD-specific learning strategies or training/coaching in social skills, management of sensory issues, organization, time management, structuring written assignments, etc.

Source: Alcorn MacKay, 2010, pp. 30–34.

Manett and Stoddart (2012) have provided a range of suggestions for Ontario students with ASD to make their transition to post-secondary life easier. They suggest registering for any transitional or mentorship programs for the transition into college or university, as well as any social skills groups that may be offered at the institution. Many of these programs are available for any student entering college or university, with an ASD diagnosis, no diagnosis, or any diagnosis. Second, it is recommended that the student or parents connect with the disability office early, the year before enrolling, and again in the summer before the individual starts school. Bursaries are available for those with disabilities, and more information can be found in the funding section of this chapter. It is also important to plan out a course load that is specific and manageable for the student to set the stage for success. Beginning with fewer classes while learning the ins and outs of post-secondary education can be helpful. Lastly, strategically plan a method of assistance for communicating with the disability office, peers, professors, and others involved in the student's education. Because it is more difficult for the student to understand social norms, having a mentor, coach, or someone to help read and run things through before sending email, handing in assignments, or attending a meeting with a professor is helpful.

EMPLOYMENT OPPORTUNITIES

Employment is a significant area of concern for many adults with ASD. For example, only 13.9 percent of adults with ASD have full-time employment, and 6.9 percent have part-time employment in Ontario (Stoddart et al., 2013). In addition, many of these individuals are underemployed based on their skill set and education (Accardi & Duhaime, 2013). The fact remains that many individuals struggle to obtain and maintain employment due to difficulties in social skills, which emerge in the interview process and continue on in the navigation, understanding, and implementation of social rules in the workplace. Although individuals may have the skills required to do a given job, a lack of social skills may hinder those individuals from cooperating with others to successfully perform the job duties. See Box 9.4 for challenges individuals with ASD may face in the workforce.

Employment-related supports in Ontario are offered through the Ontario Disability Support Program (ODSP). These supports help individuals attain job skills and find employment, as well as implement self-employment strategies and plans (MCSS, 2013). Individuals are eligible for the supports if they are older than 16 years old, are able to work, and have a disability that makes it difficult for them to obtain and maintain employment (MCSS, 2013). These supports are provided on an individual basis with an employment support counsellor, depending on the individual's employment goal and readiness, and are available through various agencies in each city in Ontario (MCSS, 2013). Box 9.5 lists examples of job skill training that can be offered through ODSP. Individuals start the process by completing a form on the ODSP website and bringing it to the local ODSP office (MCSS, 2013). Effective in 2015, individuals with disabilities can apply for ODSP Employment Supports even if they are already receiving other types of employment supports (e.g., insurance policies, etc.) (MCSS, 2014).

There are many strategies to assist adults with ASD in learning job skills and their application to the workforce. Many of these focus on person-centred planning in order to understand the individual's interests, what types of potential jobs may fit with their skills, and strategies and adaptations that could be made in order for the individual to acquire the job. This also involves working with employers to understand the

Job Coach: A job coach is a hired person who assists the individual in preparing for the job site and attending the job site, as needed. This person helps the employee learn the skills required in the job, provides feedback, and provides additional training that may be needed to learn the job.

Box 9.4: Challenges in Employment for Adults with ASD

Challenges to Accessing Employment Faced by Youth and Adults with ASD:

- Preparing for and attending an interview—difficulties managing anxiety, reading social cues, communicating appropriate information
- Social interactions with colleagues, organizational skills and sensory challenges
- The work activities required might not be perceived as challenging, rewarding or meaningful
- Colleagues and bosses' misunderstanding of the individual's behaviours and challenges
- Lack of general awareness of the strengths that an individual with ASD can bring to the workplace
- Training which does not support the individual's specific needs related to ASD and other features
- Difficulty with self-advocacy: sharing information about personal needs and accommodations

Recommendations for the Community:

- Increase employment support programs geared to individuals with ASD
- Increase training for frontline workers in generic employment agencies to better understand the strengths and needs of the ASD population
- Customize existing employment programs to better support the ASD population
- Educate employers to understand how to cultivate talents and preferences of those with ASD
- Improve transitional services at the high school and post-secondary levels to ensure individuals are prepared to enter the workplace
- Increase research on vocational interventions specific to those with ASD to better understand and advocate for appropriate services
- Create opportunities for individuals with ASD who would like to pursue entrepreneurial activities—support with start-up costs, financial and management training, mentorship, etc.
- Increase employment coaching and support for individuals with ASD who have successfully entered the workforce, but may be struggling in their current position

Recommendations for the Individual and Family:

- Enroll in co-operative education opportunities in high school, volunteer in the community, and seek out summer employment to get experience in a variety of settings
- Enroll in programs that focus on employment, life skills, and social skills to prepare the individual for adult independence
- Connect the individual living with ASD to family and friends for informational interviews about specific jobs or careers
- Engage the individual in job-shadowing opportunities
- Develop strong self-advocacy skills so that personal strengths and needs can be communicated to the employer in an effective manner
- Begin career planning discussions as early as possible in adolescence to ensure a successful transition to the world of work
- Identify the individual's strengths, skills, interests, talents, and cognitive style
- Make use of psycho-vocational testing and assessment
- Don't just look for a job, but for a job that is "the right fit" for the individual
- When self-employment is viable, evaluate the individual's talents, whether he or she has a product or service that has the potential to be sold, strengthen the individual's entrepreneurial skills, and look for small business training and mentoring

Source: Accardi & Duhaime, 2013, p. 2.

benefits and supports when hiring an individual with a disability (MCSS, 2014). For instance, often the employment supports through ODSP can help provide a job coach, who can assist with job training and eventually reduce involvement to foster the transition to independence. See Box 9.6 for a list of various employment assistance strategies for adults with ASD.

Read about it. Think about it. Write about it.

Research creative jobs that individuals with ASD have worked in that highlight their strengths.

Box 9.5: Types of Employment Supports through ODSP

Everyone's path to employment is different. That's why there are many kinds of Ontario Disability Support Program Employment Supports. Here are some examples:

- help preparing for work
- help finding a job that is right for you
- help keeping a job
- job coaching
- on-the-job training
- help to move to the next level in your career
- software and mobility devices that can help you do your job
- interpreter or intervenor services
- transportation assistance
- assistive devices and training to use them
- tools and equipment you need for your job
- special clothing for your job
- specialized computer training
- other items you may need

You will work with a community service provider to figure out what kinds of supports you need to help you get and keep a job.

If your goal is to start up your own business, Employment Supports can help you. Here are some of the supports you may receive:

- help to develop and implement a business plan
- training in money management, record keeping and budgeting
- help with marketing your business
- mentoring
- financial help towards the costs of business tools, equipment and supplies, licenses and certification
- help getting work-related disability supports, such as assistive devices and technical equipment, interpreter, intervenor, reader and notetaker services.

Source: MCSS, 2015, para. 1–4.

Box 9.6: Job Development Strategies for Adults with ASD

Many individuals with ASD have characteristics that could make them attractive to potential employers, including punctuality, attention to detail, consistency, reliability, or good visual-spatial or mechanical skills. Whatever skills the person possesses, it is important to emphasize the strengths and the contributions (s)he could make to the business.

There are certain job development strategies that may be particularly useful and productive to prioritize when job searching with and for job seekers with ASD.

- **Person-centered planning** is vital in the job placement process and helps job developers identify both the strengths and support needs that a person with ASD brings to the job search. Several ICI publications on this topic can be downloaded for free from the web:
  - *Starting with Me: A Guide to Person-Centered Planning for Job Seekers*
    www.communityinclusion.org/article.php?article_id=54&type=topic&id=3
  - *More Than Just a Job: Person-Centered Career Planning*
    www.communityinclusion.org/article.php?article_id=16&type=topic&id=3
- **Career Exploration.** Many individuals with ASD may have to go through an extensive career exploration process, especially those with limited employment exposure and experience. Intensive counseling to identify options; spending time getting to know the neighborhood and community; participating in workplace tours and informational interviews; and trying out real job activities will help job seekers to hone in on employment interests and goals. Employment staff may also have to provide some individuals with alternative ways of expressing their preferences such as the use of AAC devices or by pointing to pictures or symbols.
- **Job Carving/Job Creation** can be an effective approach. It often makes sense to take advantage of a person's unique set of skills and interests by carving out or creating a job within an existing business. In doing so, job developers need to demonstrate to the employer that the job seeker can make their business more efficient or productive. For more information about how to go about this process, see the ICI publication:

> - *When Existing Jobs Don't Fit: A Guide to Job Creation*
>   www.communityinclusion.org/article.php?article_
>   id=126&type=topic&id=3
> - **Networking** has been proven to speed up the job search! Building on
>   the personal and professional business contacts of employment staff,
>   the job seeker, family members, neighbors, and friends is a far more
>   effective strategy for job development than making cold calls. This can
>   often enhance that vital opportunity by providing a foot in the door to
>   individuals with more significant barriers. For more information and
>   tips about the how-tos of networking, see ICI publications:
>   - *Networking: A Consumer Guide to an Effective Job Search*
>   www.communityinclusion.org/article.php?article_
>   id=62&type=topic&id=3
>   - *Making Networking Easier for Job Seekers: A Guide*
>   www.communityinclusion.org/article.php?article_id=138&type=
>   topic&id=3
>   - *Teaching Networking Skills: Paving a Way to Jobs and Careers*
>   *(manual)*
>   This manual provides a curriculum directly for use
>   with job seekers. It can be downloaded for free at www.
>   communityinclusion.org/article.php?article_id=251 or purchased
>   through the ICI Publications Office (see back page for ordering
>   information).
>
> *Source:* Jordan, 2008, para. 8.

RECREATION AND LEISURE

Recreation and leisure services vary significantly for many individuals. It is indicated, however, that this can often be a need, due to the inherent difficulty with social skills and making and keeping friends in the ASD population (Stoddart et al., 2013). In addition, the anxiety around attending various social groups can be overwhelming. Families have identified recreation supports for individuals as a necessity, as staying at home with family, watching TV, and being alone are isolating (Autism Ontario, 2008; Stoddart et al., 2013). A research study in central and southwestern Ontario demonstrated that there were some discrepancies relating to the quantity of services available. Professionals indicated more services were available than parents had stated, potentially demonstrating a disconnect between the advertising of the programs and the places where families sought programming information, or a lack of fit between the programs and the individuals with disabilities (White & Weiss, 2010). Nonetheless, the importance of quality of life is crucial. Garcia-Villamisar and Dattilo (2010) found that enrolling adults with ASD in a one-year recreation program significantly decreased stress and increased quality of life indicators (e.g., satisfaction, independence, competence, and social interaction) as compared to a control group, highlighting the importance of recreation and socialization.

Recreation programs for adults with ASD can have various forms and target various skills. Many programs focus on improving social skills due to the difficulties individuals face in such situations. There are numerous social programs. First, there are those that are informal and work on social skills naturally, through group activities in the community (e.g., dancing, bowling, going out for dinner, etc.). In addition, there are those that focus on teaching social skills, such as the PEERS Program, with a facilitator and participants. The PEERS Program, designed for high-functioning adolescents with ASD, is a parent-assisted program delivered over 14 weeks in 90-minute sessions (Laugeson, Frankel, Gantman, Dillon, & Mogil, 2012). It is being implemented in various places throughout the province through Autism Ontario and Woodview Mental Health and Autism Services.

Agencies for adults with developmental disabilities also offer regular programming in the day and evening that varies from cooking classes and art classes to daily living skill programs. These are usually on a first-come-first-served basis, and some have waiting lists. There are also recreation programs offered by local municipalities available to individuals with disabilities, either exclusively or in an integrated setting. In fact, many adults with ASD attend recreation activities available in their community, and bring a personal support worker for assistance when needed.

For those who may require additional support, day centres are available throughout the province that offer recreation and leisure programming for individuals during the day, while their primary caregivers are at work. Autism Ontario provides listings of local recreational groups and other community agencies that provide various recreation and leisure services to adults with ASD.

FINANCIAL SUPPORT

As indicated, Developmental Services Ontario (DSO) funding has recently been reformed to allow equal access to funding for adults with developmental disabilities (DSO, 2014). In order to receive funding, adults must have both a developmental disability and difficulty with adaptive functioning skills according to the DSO's assessment (DSO, 2014). After the assessments, and once approved for this funding, the DSO will provide a referral to agencies who can support the individual's needs, or put them on a waitlist until a spot is open. This support can include residential, respite, recreational, and other professional services. Alternatively, a direct funding option—called Passport—can be accessed to fund services for the adults with ASD to become actively involved in their community (MCSS, 2014). With this method, funds are reimbursed to the caregiver to help the individual with ASD become involved in community activities, to hire support workers, and to engage in person-centred planning (MCSS, 2014).

In addition to these major funding programs, there are a number of tax benefits available to Canadians with a disability or who are caring for a child with a disability. The Disability Tax Credit is available to help offset the extra costs of having a disability (Canada Revenue Agency [CRA], 2015). In fact, simplifying the application process is a current focus for the CRA (2015). For example, in 2015, $7,766 was available to be claimed for an individual with ASD, with an additional $4,530 for those under 18 and additional attendant care costs in other areas of tax claim (CRA, 2015). If the individual does not claim it, the caregiver may claim the amount. Other tax benefits include the Working Income Tax Benefit to assist those who are working but making low wages, which can be due in part to disability (CRA, 2015). Lastly, Registered Disability Saving Plans (RDSPs) are available for individuals with disabilities who have been approved for the Disability Tax Credit (RDSP, 2015). This allows families and the individual to save for the future with the government contributing, with the money growing while invested (RDSP, 2015). Canada is the first country in the world to have created RDSPs as an invested savings plan that can be taken out at any time for whatever the individual or family chooses, and does not affect disability payments (up to a certain amount) (RDSP, 2015). See Box 9.7 for more information on the RDSP.

Financial supports are also available for those attending post-secondary institutions. One of the most commonly utilized programs for Ontario students with disabilities is the Bursary for Students with Disabilities (BSWD) through the Ontario Student Assistance Program (OSAP) (MTCU, 2014). This bursary is available for those who apply for OSAP and are approved (Manett & Stoddart, 2012). Students are eligible for up to $2,000 per year to cover the additional costs of attending postsecondary school with a disability (MTCU, 2014). This could include the costs of additional computers or software that may be required, or the costs of psychological assessments (MTCU, 2014). The Repayment Assistance Plan for Borrowers with a Permanent Disability is another program that helps students with disabilities pay off their loans after finishing school (DisabilityAwards.ca, n.d.). Eligibility is based on income and

Box 9.7: All About the RDSP

The Registered Disability Savings Plan (RDSP) is a Canada-wide registered matched savings plan for people with disabilities. Here are some basics:

- For every $1 put in an RDSP account, the federal government will match it (if your family income is below $89,401) with up to $3! **This is the Canada Disability Savings Grant.**
- For people living on a low-income (less than $26,021), the federal government will invest $1000 each year for 20 years! **This is the Canada Disability Savings Bond.**
- People living on an income between $26,021 and $44,701 can still receive a partial bond.
- Anyone can contribute to an RDSP – family, friends, and even neighbours. This gives people who want to help a way to do so!
- RDSPs offer some of the best returns on investment available. Your money will grow. It might even triple in size!
- The RDSP is exempt from most provincial disability and income assistance benefits. The government will not claw this money back. (To find out how your province treats the RDSP, go to www.disabilitysavings. gc.ca.)
- There are no restrictions on how RDSP withdrawals are spent.

Source: RDSP, 2015, para. 1

disability-related costs (DisabilityAwards.ca, n.d.). Additional awards for post-secondary students with ASD may also be available through local agencies and within each individual post-secondary institution.

HOUSING

Housing is another area in high demand for adults with ASD in Ontario. Almost 60 percent of those partaking in Stoddart and colleague's (2013) Ontario survey lived with family. Only 13.6 percent were living on their own with no supports, and some lived on their own with help from family (5.9 percent), with professional support (2.3 percent), and in group homes (8.4 percent). The process of deinstitutionalization began in the 1950s with the movement away from institutions, where individuals with disabilities lived together and received specialized treatment (Davidson et al., 2001; Lamb & Bachrach, 2001). As institutions closed, individuals were moved into the community to receive individualized services (Davidson et al., 2001; Lamb & Bachrach, 2001). The provincial government began closing the institutions in Ontario in 1977, with the final closure in 2009 (Autism Ontario, 2008). This closing has also led to difficulties for those in the community, as the system has not been funded sufficiently, leading to fewer housing options for many, a lack of integration of services, and an abundance of individuals living with family (Autism Ontario, 2008; Lamb & Bachrach, 2001).

The various types of housing options are on a wide spectrum depending on the needs of the individual and their capacity to live independently. This can vary from living independently to living in group homes or nursing homes with constant care (see Table 9.2). The difficulty is that, although many individuals have typical cognitive functioning, they often lack skills in adaptive areas that are required for everyday living. Thus they often remain in family homes (Autism Ontario, n.d.; Stoddart et al., 2013). There are often options for those who are more severely affected by ASD, but supports for those who are almost independent are less common or inappropriate (Autism Ontario, n.d.). In addition, waiting lists are lengthy, and housing options are often found for those in crisis situations as a first priority (Autism Ontario, n.d.; Housing Study Group, 2013). In 2013, for example, the waiting list for housing for people with developmental disabilities was at 12,000 (Housing Study Group, 2013). Happily, this trend is changing, with $810 million dollars dedicated to assist in creating additional residential options for adults with disabilities over three years starting in 2015 (MCSS, 2014). The Developmental Services Housing Task Force is also investigating new and creative options for housing models (MCSS, 2014).

There are other creative, affordable, and sustainable options for individuals with disabilities (Housing Study Group, 2013). For example, Woodview Mental Health and Autism Services in Hamilton, Ontario provides a transitional housing support program in which individuals move from a residential teaching unit to supported independent living (SIL) (Woodview Mental Health and Autism Services, 2015). Individuals at a teaching unit learn independent living skills alongside other individuals with ASD. Once these skills have been attained, they move into one of the SIL townhouses where they share living space with three other friends and have access to the services that they require. For another example of a creative housing option, see Box 9.8.

Table 9.2: Housing Options for Adults with ASD

Option	Description
Independent options • Own • Lease • Rent • Co-op	There are many options for individuals with ASD to live on their own, as there are for other adults. However, this requires the individuals to have employment in order to support their house or to have families buy or rent it, which is difficult with the financial pressures of having a child with a disability.
Supported living	Supported living "offers services to individuals with disabilities who are able to live in a home or an apartment. The services, typically minimal in nature, are based on the individual's specific support needs and are provided by caregivers working under the direction of the individual" (Autism Speaks, 2011, p. 13).
Semi-independent living (SIL)	Twenty-four-hour supports are available for the individual, who lives either independently or with others. Support for independent living skills is provided by the staff at the residence.
Group homes	A group of unrelated people live in the home with staff support 24 hours a day, seven days a week. The home is owned by an agency, which hires staff. Staff provide instruction and activities in the home and community.
Group living/ ownership	Similar to a group home; however, the home is bought by a group of families who hire staff or contract an agency to hire staff.
Teaching family model (foster home living)	A professional family has one person or several people with a disability who live in the home.
Farmstead communities	A number of individuals live together, usually on a farm, with residential supports.
Assisted living	A care facility offers assistance with daily living skills and hygiene. It does not offer complex medical supports like a nursing home.
Nursing homes	Nursing homes provide complex care to individuals. The difficulty is that these are designed for the geriatric population, and unfortunately younger people are often placed here with no other options.
Developmental centre	Large centres for people with developmental disabilities living together.

Sources: Autism Ontario, 2008; Autism Speaks, 2011; Ombudsmen Ontario, 2014.

Read about it. Think about it. Write about it.

Research housing options for those with ASD in Ontario. Which models does each centre use?

Box 9.8: Celebrating Another Housing Option for Adults with Disabilities.

Years ago, when our family's now 18-year-old son, Robert, was dually diagnosed with PDD-NOS and Bipolar Disorder, we came across a website with housing options that looked interesting, but immediately discarded as impossible for us! For one thing, we were concerned that our son—who was then struggling in residential care at London's Child and Parent Resource Institute (CPRI) —would never be able to again live within our family unit; for another, I was apprehensive about the fit between this program and our city bylaws. Fast-forwarding to 2007, with the guidance of our realtor Karen Hobbs-Thomson of REMAX, my husband and I purchased a home with an "empty shell" in an outbuilding that was comprised of about 300 square feet, including a similarly tiny basement with full ceiling height. We purchased our home with the idea that this space could somehow be converted from its former use as the boiler room for commercial greenhouses, into a transitional living area that fit well with our prediction that our son would want some freedom by age 18—but not too much!

Immediately after purchasing our home, we began researching the options and checking out various possibilities that would align with our municipal regulations in the City of Brantford. After struggling for some time, we approached Brantford Housing, where Tom Hodgson enthusiastically reminded me of the Canadian Mortgage and Housing Corporation [CMHC] support for creative options in housing. Specifically, he kindly ordered and provided me with a copy of CMHC's "Residential Rehabilitation Assistance Program [RRAP]: Secondary/Garden Suite" application package. Within RRAP, the use of a Secondary/Garden Suite is described as follows: "Canada Mortgage and Housing Corporation (CMHC) offers financial assistance for the creation of a Secondary or Garden Suite for a low-income senior or adult with a disability—making it possible for them to live independently in their community, close to family and friends" (CMHC, 2010, para. 1).

What Is a Secondary Suite or a Garden Suite?
A secondary suite, sometimes called an in-law suite, is a self-contained separate unit within an existing home or an addition to a home. This means there are

full kitchen and bath facilities as well as a separate entrance. A garden suite is a separate living unit that is not attached to the principal residence, but built on the same property. Garden suites are sometimes referred to as "granny flats" because they were originally created to provide a home for an aging parent of a homeowner. Like a secondary suite, a garden suite is a self-contained unit. Regardless of which type of housing is chosen, secondary and garden suites must meet all applicable building code requirements as well as local municipal planning and zoning regulations.

Who Can Apply?

You may be eligible to receive assistance if: you are a homeowner or private entrepreneur owning residential property that would accommodate an affordable, self-contained rental unit for a low-income senior (65 years of age or more) or adult with a disability; your property meets with the applicable zoning and building requirements; you consent to enter into an Operating Agreement that establishes the rent that can be charged during the term of the Agreement; you also agree that the household income of the occupant(s) of the newly created self-contained unit will be below a CMHC set level. (Adapted from CHMC 2010, para. 1–6).

Our next step was to contact our city's planning department to see what proactive steps needed to be taken prior to the approval of a permit for this forgivable loan, described in detail above. During these lengthy and sometimes challenging processes, we were fortunate that our call for help came across the desk of Lucy Hives, a Senior Planner for the City of Brantford. Together, we researched various options; searched out paperwork, drawings, measurements, and plans; and reached various conclusions. First, we applied for a zoning change to allow the development of a fully self-contained unit on our property's outbuilding, currently zoned as a single-family dwelling space. Later, this option was discarded and we were requested to design and build a fully enclosed breezeway, which would join our main house together with our outbuilding. This joining together, along with full interior access to the unit for our son, would then allow us to obtain permit approval.

At this point, we were extremely privileged to have Rob Wilkie enter the scene, owner of Rob the Builder in Kitchener-Waterloo (robthebuilder@ primus.ca). Rob was able to take our vision and the city's regulations and craft them into a plan that worked for all involved. With this breezeway fully excavated, built, and finished with a series of shoe racks, coat hooks, and other storage devices to create delight in any mother—of a child with ASD or not—the second phase of constructing the living area could begin.

Years of planning went into several nail-biting weeks of preparing lengthy, detailed, and precise responses to a range of questions, inquires, and regulations put in place to support this CMHC program, as we prepared a package to be forwarded for approval. After several series of follow-up questions, answers, and more documentation, we received the "go ahead" letter! This was a day of celebration in our home!

Together with the unwavering support and ready assistance of Anne De Rosse, also of the Housing Department in the City of Brantford, we successfully navigated the step-by-step process of construction, approvals, and reimbursement. As of the time of this writing, we are awaiting only the last piece of the approval on the completion of our

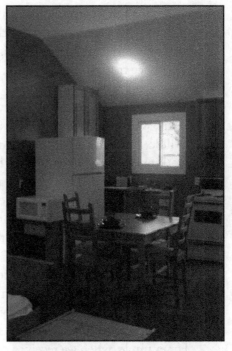

Figure 9.7: Robert's Apartment

extended living space from the Fire Marshall, the Electrical Safety Authority, CMHC, and the City of Brantford. We have been proud to be a part of Brantford's first use of this imaginative program.

This is what Tom Hodgson, RRAP Agent, very kindly had to say about the process:

> It was so exciting to receive the inquiry from Kimberly Maich with respect to CMHC's Secondary Suite program. I could tell after speaking with Kimberly for a short time that she was the perfect candidate for the program. The City of Brantford Housing Department had just recently taken over the administration of the program so we were thrilled about the possibility of seeing an application come to fruition. After visiting Kimberly and seeing the finished project it was obviously a resounding success. Kimberly's son Robert will be able to live independently but will also be close enough to family and friends to receive necessary support. Thanks Kimberly for your patience, determination and unwavering positive attitude throughout the process.

Consider CMHC's programs as an option for your son or daughter who is not quite ready to face the world with complete independence, but is ready to spread their wings slightly in the sight of his or her parents. Here are a few pieces of advice from one experience:

- Your work will be done on a very tight deadline—have your contractors ready, waiting and prepared for a quick turn-around. For example, Rob Wilkie, our dedicated builder, often slept in the living area itself while working (quietly) into the wee hours of the morning.
- Be prepared to deal with many details and to gather and share information from a variety of sources. Be patient and persistent!
- Photocopy everything you submit. Keep your information organized every step of the way. A clear proposal is a more readily accepted proposal.
- Don't be afraid to use the courier for speedy delivery!
- Ensure all your approvals are in place as soon as possible. Pay for your permit up front. Even though you may not be reimbursed for its cost, you will be prepared to start work as soon as your forgivable loan is approved. For example, when we received our approval letter, our work was to begin "immediately" and we were given a specific completion date.
- Be certain that your contractors know that they will be waiting for reimbursement for their work and that the program does not include up-front costs.
- Plan to have extra funds on hand for unexpected costs, as well as preparation costs. For example, prior to applying for this program, we paid close to $20,000 to waterproof the basement area and to build the breezeway required by municipal regulations.
- Keep in mind that you have a responsibility to maintain CMHC standards for a long period of time to fulfill the requirements for loan reimbursement.
- Finally, celebrate this program, an exceptional option for our grown sons and daughters with ASD or other disabilities.

Source: Maich, 2010.

A LOOK BACK

Chapter 9, "Supporting Ontario's Adults with Autism Spectrum Disorder," focused on:
- The current status of services for adults with ASD in Ontario, including a historical perspective and current Ministry investigations;
- A review of the most recent survey of adults with ASD in Ontario;
- An overview of post-secondary options for adults with ASD, including accommodations and advocating for one's education;
- A review of employment supports in Ontario and various support models that can be utilized;
- A brief overview of recreation, financial, and housing supports in Ontario.

A LOOK AHEAD

Chapter 10, "Supporting Ontario's Parents and Families," focuses on current and historical examinations of raising a child with ASD. It reviews topics such as:
- Negative historical views ascribed to parents of children with ASD;
- recent, positive models for understanding families which include children with ASD (e.g., levels of awareness);
- Examples of local, community-based, and provincial resources; and
- The importance of advocacy by and for families, and both well-established and emerging advocacy groups (e.g., Autism Ontario).

ADDITIONAL RESOURCES

- About the Services and Supports to Promote the Social Inclusion of Persons with Developmental Disabilities Act, 2008 (Ontario Ministry of Community and Social Services, 2012):
  www.mcss.gov.on.ca/en/mcss/publications/developmentalServices/services SupportsSocialInclusion.aspx
- Bursary for Students with Disabilities (Ontario Ministry of Training, Colleges, and Universities, 2014):
  www.osap.gov.on.ca/OSAPPortal/en/A-ZListofAid/PRDR008120.html
- Developmental Services in Ontario (Developmental Services Ontario, 2014):
  www.dsontario.ca
- Disability Offices for Ontario Colleges and Universities:
  www.cacuss.ca/disability_offices_ontario.htm

- *Diversity in Ontario's Youth and Adults with Autism Spectrum Disorder: Complex Needs in Unprepared Systems* (Stoddart, Burke, Muskat, Manett, Duhaime, Accardi, Burnham Riosa, & Bradley, 2013):
  www.redpathcentre.ca/sitebuildercontent/sitebuilderfiles/fullreport2013.pdf
- Ending the Wait: An Action Agenda to Address the Housing Crisis Confronting Adults with Developmental Disabilities (Housing Study Group, 2013):
  www.autismontario.com/Client/ASO/AO.nsf/object/Sep13ENews/$file/
  Ending+the+Wait+final+sep6.pdf
- *Forgotten: Ontario Adults with Autism and Adults with Asperger's* (Autism Ontario, 2008):
  www.autismsocietycanada.ca/images/dox/KeyReports/ForgottenReport
  AutismOntario.pdf
- Government Funding Ontario (DisabilityAwards.ca, n.d.):
  disabilityawards.ca/gov.php?ID=ON&lang=EN
- Housing and Residential Supports Tool Kit (Autism Speaks, 2011):
  www.autismspeaks.org/sites/default/files/housing_tool_kit_web2.pdf
- Ontario Disability Support Program: Employment Supports (Ontario Ministry of Training, Colleges, and Universities, 2013):
  www.mcss.gov.on.ca/en/mcss/programs/social/odsp/employment_support/
  index.aspx
- Registered Disability Saving Plan (RDSP, 2015):
  www.rdsp.com
- Spotlight on Transformation (Ontario Ministry of Community and Social Services):
  www.mcss.gov.on.ca/en/mcss/publications/spotlight.aspx
- Students with Disabilities (Ontario Ministry of Training, Colleges, and Universities, 2015):
  www.tcu.gov.on.ca/eng/postsecondary/careerplanning/disabilities.html#
  disabilities1
- The Youth KIT (CanChild, 2010):
  www.canchild.ca/en/canchildresources/youthkit_new_user.asp
- Transition Planning: A Resource Guide (Ontario Ministry of Education, 2002):
  www.edu.gov.on.ca/eng/general/elemsec/speced/transiti/transition.html
- What is Passport? (Ontario Ministry of Community and Social Services, 2014):
  www.mcss.gov.on.ca/en/mcss/programs/developmental/servicesupport/
  passport.aspx

REFERENCES

Accardi, C., & Duhaime, S. (2013). Finding and keeping employment. *Autism Matters, 61,* 1–3. Retrieved from autismontario.novosolutions.net/default.asp?id=153

Adreon, D. & Durocher, J. (2007). Evaluating the college transition needs of individuals with high-functioning autism spectrum disorder. *Intervention in School and Clinic, 42*(5), 271–279.

Alcorn MacKay, S. (2010). *Identifying trends and supports for students with autism spectrum disorder transitioning into postsecondary.* Toronto: Higher Education Quality Council of Ontario. Retrieved from http://www.heqco.ca/SiteCollectionDocuments/ASD.pdf

Allen, K. (2014, August 7). Adults with autism focus of new Ontario working group. *The Toronto Star.* Retrieved from www.thestar.com/news/world/2014/08/07/adults_with_autism_focus_of_new_ontario_working_group.html

American Psychiatric Association. (1994*). Diagnostic and statistical manual of psychiatric disorders* (4th ed.). Arlington, VA: American Psychiatric Publishing.

American Psychiatric Association. (2000). *Diagnostic and statistical manual: DSM IV-R* (4th ed.). Washington, DC: Author.

American Psychiatric Association. (2013). *Diagnostic and statistical manual: DSM-5* (5th ed.). Washington, DC: Author.

Autism Ontario. (n.d.). Ontario partnership for adults with Asperger's and autism comments to the minister of municipal affairs and housing Ontario's long term affordable housing strategy. Retrieved from www.autismontario.com/Client/ASO/AO.nsf/object/HousingSubmission/$file/Housing+Submission+Dec+31+2009.pdf

Autism Ontario. (2008). *Forgotten: Ontario adults with autism and adults with Aspergers.* Retrieved from www.autismsocietycanada.ca/images/dox/KeyReports/ForgottenReportAutismOntario.pdf

Autism Speaks. (2011). Housing and residential supports tool kit. Retrieved from www.autismspeaks.org/sites/default/files/housing_tool_kit_web2.pdf

Buck, T. R., Viskochil, J., Farley, M., Coon, H., McMahon, W. M., Morgan, J., & Bilder, D. A. (2014). Psychiatric comorbidity and medication use in adults with autism spectrum disorder. *Journal of Autism and Developmental Disorders, 44*(12), 3063–3071.

Burke, L. (2005). Psychological assessment of more able adults with autism spectrum disorder. In K. Stoddard (Ed.), *Children, youth, and adults with Asperger syndrome.* (pp. 211–225). London: Jessica Kingsley Publishers.

CanChild. (2010). The Youth KIT. Retrieved from www.canchild.ca/en/canchildresources/youthkit_new_user.asp

CBC News. (2013, May 1). The new definition of autism: Trying to make sense of a confusing world. CBC News Online. Retrieved from www.cbc.ca/news/health/the-new-definition-of-autism-1.1366823

Community Living Ontario. (2015). What is an intellectual disability? Retrieved from www.communitylivingontario.ca/about-us/what-intellectual-disability

Canada Revenue Agency. (2015). Tax credits and deductions for persons with disabilities. Retrieved from www.cra-arc.gc.ca/disability/

Davidson, L., Stayner, D. A., Nickou, C., Styron, T. H., Rowe, M., & Chinman, M. L. (2001). "Simply to be let in": Inclusion as a basis for recovery. *Psychiatric Rehabilitation Journal, 24*(4), 375–388.

Developmental Services Ontario. (2014). Developmental services in Ontario. Retrieved from www.dsontario.ca

DisabilityAwards.ca. (n.d.). Government funding Ontario. Retrieved from disabilityawards.ca/gov.php?ID=ON&lang=EN

García-Villamisar, D. A., & Dattilo, J. (2010). Effects of a leisure programme on quality of life and stress of individuals with ASD. *Journal of Intellectual Disability Research, 54*(7), 611–619.

Gordon, A. (2015, January 12). Agencies cite critical gaps in adult autism services. *The Toronto Star.* Retrieved from www.thestar.com/life/2015/01/12/agencies_cite_critical_gaps_in_adult_autism_services.html

Harper, A., Dyches, T. T., Harper, J., Roper, S. O., & South, M. (2013). Respite care, marital quality, and stress in parents of children with autism spectrum disorder. *Journal of Autism and Developmental Disorders, 43*(11), 2604–2616.

Housing Study Group. (2013). Ending the wait: An action agenda to address the housing crisis confronting adults with developmental disabilities. Retrieved from www.autismontario.com/Client/ASO/AO.nsf/object/Sep13ENews/$file/Ending+the+Wait+final+sep6.pdf

Jordan, M. (2008, December). Supporting individuals with autism spectrum disorder: Quality employment practices. *The Institute Brief, 25.* Retrieved from www.communityinclusion.org/article.php?article_id=266

Lamb, H. R., & Bachrach, L. L. (2001). Some perspectives on deinstitutionalization. *Psychiatric Services, 52*(8), 1039–1045.

Laugeson, E. A., Frankel, F., Gantman, A., Dillon, A. R., & Mogil, C. (2012). Evidence-based social skills training for adolescents with autism spectrum disorder: The UCLA PEERS program. *Journal of Autism and Developmental Disorders, 42*(6), 1025–1036.

Lombardo, M. V., & Baron-Cohen, S. (2011). The role of the self in mindblindness in autism. *Consciousness and cognition, 20*(1), 130–140.

Maich, K. (2010). Celebrating another housing option for adults with disabilities. *Autism Matters, 7*(4), 5–8.

Manett, J., & Stoddart, K. (2012). Facing the challenges of post-secondary education: Strategies for individuals with autism spectrum disorder (ASD). *Autism Matters, 46,* 1–3. Retrieved from www.autismontario.com/client/aso/ao.nsf/docs/149395542949b52a85257bc10060dbc6/$file/facing+the+challenges+of+post+secondary+education.pdf

Mansell, J., & Beadle-Brown, J. (2004). Person-centred planning or person-centred action? Policy and practice in intellectual disability services. *Journal of Applied Research in Intellectual Disabilities, 17*(1), 1–9.

Ombudsmen Ontario. (2012). Ontario ombudsman to investigate province's services for adults with developmental disabilities in crisis. Retrieved from www.ombudsman.on.ca/Newsroom/Press-Release/2012/Ontario-Ombudsman-to-investigate-provinces-servic.aspx?lang=en-CA

Ombudsmen Ontario. (2014). Adults with developmental disabilities in crisis: Ministry of Community and Social Services. Retrieved from ombudsman.on.ca/Investigations/SORT-Investigations/In-Progress/Adults-with-developmental-disabilities-in-crisis/Case-update---Annual-Report-2013-2014.aspx

Ombudsman Ontario. (2015). *Ombudsman Ontario: Ontario's watchdog; Annual report 2014–2015.* Toronto: Ombudsman Ontario. Retrieved from www.ombudsman.on.ca/Files/sitemedia/Documents/Resources/AR%202014-2015/AR14-15-EN_1.pdf

Ontario Statutes. (2008). *Services and Supports to Promote the Social Inclusion of Persons with Developmental Disabilities,* Chapter 14. Toronto: Queen's Printer. Retrieved from www.e-laws.gov.on.ca/html/statutes/english/elaws_statutes_08s14_e.htm

OntarioColleges.ca. (2015). Inclusive education programs at Ontario colleges. Retrieved from www.ontariocolleges.ca/SearchResults/EDUCATION-COMMUNITY-SOCIAL-SERVICES-INCLUSIVE-EDUCATION/_/N-lqjs

Ontario Ministry of Community and Social Services. (2012). About the services and supports to promote the social inclusion of persons with developmental disabilities act,

2008. Retrieved from www.mcss.gov.on.ca/en/mcss/publications/developmentalServices/servicesSupportsSocialInclusion.aspx

Ontario Ministry of Community and Social Services. (2014a). What is passport? Retrieved from www.mcss.gov.on.ca/en/mcss/programs/developmental/servicesupport/passport.aspx

Ontario Ministry of Community and Social Services. (2014b). Helping more people with ODSP employment supports. *Developmental Services: Spotlight on Transformation, 45,* 4. Retrieved from www.mcss.gov.on.ca/documents/en/mcss/publications/spotlight/DS-Spotlight_issue45_en.pdf

Ontario Ministry of Community and Social Services. (2015). Employment supports: What is available? Retrieved from http://www.mcss.gov.on.ca/en/mcss/programs/social/odsp/employment_support/available_supports.aspx

Ontario Ministry of Education. (2013). Policy/program memorandum 156: Supporting transitions for students with special education needs. Retrieved from https://www.edu.gov.on.ca/extra/eng/ppm/ppm156.pdf

Ontario Ministry of Training, Colleges, and Universities. (2013). Ontario disability support program: Employment supports. Retrieved from www.mcss.gov.on.ca/en/mcss/programs/social/odsp/employment_support/index.aspx

Ontario Ministry of Training, Colleges, and Universities (2014). Bursary for students with disabilities. Retrieved from osap.gov.on.ca/OSAPPortal/en/A-ZListofAid/PRDR008120.html

Ontario Ministry of Training, Colleges, and Universities. (2015). Students with disabilities. Retrieved from www.tcu.gov.on.ca/eng/postsecondary/careerplanning/disabilities.html#disabilities1

Poverty Free Ontario. (2015). Social assistance recipients. Retrieved from www.povertyfreeontario.ca/poverty-in-ontario/status-of-poverty-in-ontario/#_ftn1

RDSP. (2015). Registered disability saving plan. Retrieved from www.rdsp.com

Smith, L. E., Maenner, M. J., & Seltzer, M. M. (2012). Developmental trajectories in adolescents and adults with autism: The case of daily living skills. *Journal of the American Academy of Child & Adolescent Psychiatry, 51*(6), 622–631.

Stoddart, K. (2005). Introduction to Asperger syndrome: A developmental-lifespan perspective. In K. Stoddard (Ed.). *Children, youth, and adults with Asperger syndrome* (pp. 13–32). London: Jessica Kingsley Publishers.

Stoddart, K.P., Burke, L., Muskat, B., Manett, J., Duhaime, S., Accardi, C., Burnham Riosa, P. & Bradley, E. (2013). *Diversity in Ontario's Youth and Adults with Autism Spectrum Disorder: Complex Needs in Unprepared Systems.* Toronto, ON: The Redpath Centre. Retrieved from www.redpathcentre.ca/sitebuildercontent/sitebuilderfiles/fullreport2013.pdf

Woodview Mental Health and Autism Services. (2015). Hamilton. Retrieved from woodview.ca/autism/hamilton/

White, S. E., & Weiss, J. E. (2010). Brief report: Services for adults and adolescents with ASD in Ontario—parent and professional perspectives. *Journal on Developmental Disabilities, 16*(1), 34–39.

CHAPTER 10

SUPPORTING ONTARIO'S PARENTS AND FAMILIES

IN THIS CHAPTER:

- Historical Views of Parents, Families, and Disabilities
- Current Views of Parents, Families, and Disabilities
  - Levels of Awareness
- Resources
  - Information for Parents
  - Regionalized and Non-Exclusive Resources
- Advocacy

Chapter 10 focuses first on negative historical views ascribed to parents of children with ASD, moving to more recent frameworks, including the levels of awareness, which reflects more positive views of the parental journey. This chapter provides information about local, community-based, and provincial resources as well as multiple strong sources of parent and family advocacy and information within Ontario, such as Autism Ontario. Special features in chapter 10 include a parent story, the practices of the Huron-Perth Catholic District School Board, and the parent-created Special Needs Roadmap advocacy and information tool.

Like any other individual, every child, adolescent, and student with a disability comes along with a context. The child's parents and family or caregivers are part of such a context, what Hobbs (1978) referred to as an ecosystem or ecological system with the child in the centre, surrounded by clusters, such as family, community, neighbourhood, and school. It is clear that the family has an important place in the life of the child, that the child has a place of priority in the ecosystem of the family, that the child-parent relationship is an evolving, multi-directional relationship, and that if problems occur in the ecosystem of the child, the "efforts to help a child should address the system as a whole" (p. 757). However, current supportive, positive conceptions of children (at any age), family, and disability have not always existed—and have certainly not always been respected—in the fields of ASD, disability, and beyond.

Read about it. Think about it. Write about it.

Explain your experiences with the ecosystem of a child or adolescent with a disability, and how that affected outcomes, negative or positive.

HISTORICAL VIEWS OF PARENTS, FAMILIES, AND DISABILITIES

Phillip Ferguson (2002) states that how families react to children with disabilities is "inescapably embedded within a sociohistorical context" (p. 124), providing a patterned framework that shifts along with the cultural shifts that happen over time. According to Ferguson, the early 1800s to the early 1900s were characterized by blame: parents were to blame for the burden of childhood disability, due to their own (likely) disability, (poor) socioeconomic status, (female) gender, (lack of) morality, or (lack of) work ethic. From approximately 1920 to 1980, however, this blame on parental problems shifted to disability-led damage to the family context: an outcome that was intrinsic and inevitable and fit with the dominance of the medical model in the field, which still influences current attitudes and behaviours. Ferguson categorized these into four conceptions encompassing behavioural and attitudinal parental reactions as well as that seemingly inevitable damage (see Table 10.1).

These are but some of the many models that tended to blame parents or assign negativity, in some way, to parenting a child with a disability. Others are specific to families raising a child with ASD, such as Bettleheim's refrigerator mother (see Chapter 1); typically, they are aligned with a medical model of disability that focuses on ASD as a deficit-based issue that needs—along with the parents and families—to be fixed (Straus, 2013).

CURRENT VIEWS OF PARENTS, FAMILIES, AND DISABILITIES

The last two decades have, according to Ferguson (2002), brought with them "a dramatic evolution of our attitudes and supports for people with disabilities and their families" (p. 127), evidenced by changes in legislation and practices as well as movement to framing within a positive, social model of disability that frames

Table 10.1: Early Models of Parental Reactions to Disability

Model	Description
The neurotic parent	In this model, a pathological explanation is ascribed to any parental reaction no matter what, including passivity, guilt, and even anger: "justifiable anger toward an inadequate system of formal services is implicitly removed as an available parental response" (Ferguson, 2002, p. 126).
The dysfunctional parent	The presence of a child with a disability can cause significant damage to these parents, who are unable to successfully adjust to this life circumstance. This stress-based condition is named parentalplegia. Both of these initial models are found within a psychodynamic approach, and tend to focus on the child-mother relationship.
The suffering parent	This is found within the psychosocial approach, and is defined as the "interplay of parental emotions with the environmental circumstances in which the family found itself" (Ferguson, 2002, p. 126), such as grief, loneliness, and sorrow, or the emotional reactions from the child with a disability as an unexpected event in the typical life course of the family.
The powerless parent	The powerless parent is an interactionist approach, and also uncommon. In this outlook, parents are influenced by socially imposed outcomes such as stigma and disempowerment.

Source: Ferguson, 2002.

Read about it. Think about it. Write about it.

Do you see any of these models persisting in the way families of children with disabilities are perceived today? Explain.

disability as "socially constructed rather than biologically given" (Straus, 2013, p. 462). In Ontario schools, for example, this can be seen in broad legislative changes including more support for transition planning (e.g., *PPM 140*, *PPM 156*), a global focus on meeting diverse needs in inclusive classrooms (e.g., Universal Design for Learning, differentiated instruction) (Ontario Ministry of Education, 2005), and growth in advocacy groups and their initiatives (e.g., Autism Ontario).

Ferguson (2002) notes that more positive models have emerged throughout this time period, such as adapted, evolving, and supported families and the development of ready methods for measuring stress levels in order to determine appropriate family interventions (Weiss & Lunsky, 2011). Parents, likewise, have positive hopes for the future of their children with ASD. Watson, Hayes, Radford-Paz, and Coons (2013) reported that parents may be uncertain, concerned, anxious—even fearful—but also might have high expectations for improvement, and found that, in their Ontario parent sample, parents felt hope. They felt certain that, "despite life potentially being harder for them, their children could live fully independently, hold meaningful employment, and have their own families in the future" (p. 89). However, while this may hold true for some contexts (e.g., the general community), other contexts and situations may prove to be more challenging or stressful (Ferguson, 2002). Starr and Foy (2012), for example, found that their sample of Ontario parents were concerned about issues in school-based practice like behaviour management, professional education, communication, collaboration, and understanding (e.g. the attitudes of others, including other parents in the school community). Fletcher, Markoulakis and Bryden (2012) examined the financial, health, social, and lifestyle costs of raising a child with ASD from the perspective of married, female primary caregivers in Ontario, but found that:

> interestingly enough, regardless of the costs reported and the hardships endured by these families, all of the women expressed the positives that arose in their situations as well, a topic that has received limited exposure within the literature. This is certainly not meant to negate the costs reported by these mothers, but to show that these women were able to rise above the negatives and find the silver linings amidst the turmoil. As remarkable as these women are in the daily struggles they face with their children, it is evident that more resources and support are required to assist these women and their families. (p. 68)

Overall, then, even within positive models of the current context, "parents, especially mothers, are held individually responsible and accountable for 'problems' that occur within the family," even when their children, perhaps those with a developmental disability, are adults (Saaltink & Ouellette-Kuntz, 2014). Yet parents continue to persist with hopes and dreams for their children, even when others are not as forgiving. In fact, it has been demonstrated that "the hopes and goals for the parents of children with ASD are very similar to what all parents wish for their children regardless of disability" (Starr & Foy, 2012, p. 212).

Read about it. Think about it. Write about it.

Have you encountered a family who fits with any of these research outcomes? Explain some of the characteristics of this family, and the best-fit research that applies.

Box 10.1: Interview with Sadie

What does anyone starting in the field of ASD who is supporting parents and families need to understand and practice? This was easy for Sadie Smith, mother to 10-year-old Stella—now diagnosed with Asperger's—to answer succinctly, "Patience, compassion, and understanding." She continues, "If I could go back and tell myself, it would be to forget every single thing my mom ever did: to not yell, and to not expect a kid to know anything. The first thing Stella ever did that led me to believe something more was going on was her lack of ability to communicate that she wanted a peanut butter sandwich. But, I couldn't get it. There I was, forcing her to *tell* me, without knowing that she was autistic. She was three, and she would only point at the cupboard, even though she had the skills to communicate verbally, most times. Even if I opened it, she wouldn't tell me, but she would scream if I picked her up or put her down. At one point, I screamed back, 'WHAT DO YOU WANT?' and I was crying. I tried listing everything in the cupboard. She wouldn't even respond when I hit upon peanut butter: she just cried. But at one point she nodded while she was crying. She could speak, but she didn't ask. It didn't make sense to me: why could she do things one day, and not the other? I couldn't get it—I had no idea. I was so frustrated. She could speak, and she read "Hitachi" off the television when she was 18 months old. She could do all of these other things, so I thought she was being wilful or stubborn. So I made that peanut butter sandwich, put it on the coffee table with her juice, and went upstairs for 15 minutes and cried. And it clicked. There is something going on and she *couldn't* tell me. She couldn't communicate, and I felt like the worst person on the face of the earth."

Also resources: "Stella was three when it really started to show, though she had some characteristics when she was six and nine months old, like screaming, crying, not sleeping. There was always something. I think earlier diagnosis so that you can start this process sooner—even if it's in your own head. You don't necessarily need 1,001 resources and organizations. It more about what we know in our own heads. Sometimes you only need a paragraph of information, or information right from an adult with ASD." As Sadie emphasizes, it's not the quantity of information that is shared, but rather the quality.

And the fear—the fear of what will happen. "Just tell them it's not scary," Sadie recommends. "It can be frustrating, and hard, but it's not scary. The more accepting you are of the child and the diagnosis, the easier it is to deal with. The not-sleeping part and cleaning-the-poop-off-the-walls piece is frustrating, and it sucks, but if you can change it up in your head, and someone can tell you it will be all right," she says, "It will really help. If someone had told me this when she was as little as 18 months old, I would have really appreciated it. It's challenging, but not scary. Even stories can help." Though she does struggle, she admits, with some other parents of children with ASD who have self-pitying attitudes. "They think that they are suffering and their child is suffering," and she wonders, "Can you not even see one ounce of joy? And not just when they are sleeping." Just getting into a group is not enough.

"Be sure you know what ASD is," she stresses for those working with parents and families. "Not the ridiculous definitions you can find online. A group of autistic adults developed one, saying it's a neurological difference. The wiring is different. The perceptions are different. Then try to learn how to see things from that kind of perspective. As parents, we will never know exactly what it's like, but to know that it's different from what I do, and that it's everything—not just holding a pencil differently—it's the colour, light, texture, sound, everything." Looking back over her journey so far, she feels that her in-depth, empathetic understanding makes a significant difference: "If I had known that, I might not have reached my breaking point, but then I might not have reached an epiphany, either." Each moment, even tough moments, help along the pathway to understanding. And an educated, empathetic, understanding community can support that journey in a less painful, but equally enlightening manner.

Levels of Awareness

One unique model to support reconciliation of the differing interpretations of parents, families, and educators is "Levels of Awareness: A Closer Look at Communication between Parents and Professionals" (Ulrich & Bauer, 2003). These levels of awareness contrast with the accepted postulation of the grief cycle as the foundation experienced by emotionally bound parents in raising a child with exceptionalities (Anderegg, Vergason, & Smith, 1992). Anderegg and colleagues (1992) adapted the classic Kubler-Ross grief sequence to the immediate and extended families of children with disabilities, with the development of a three-stage model framed by confronting, adjusting, and adapting, and matched practical educator interventions to each component. Although the grief cycle model moves past the view of the parent as dysfunctional (Anderegg et al., 1992), it maintains an assumption of parental denial—an all too common vocalization by professionals working with parents which can be perceived as "condescending and patronizing" (p. 20). Alternatively, the levels-of-awareness approach suggests that parents move through four main levels of understanding, each with its own name and features (see Table 10.2).

Table 10.2: Levels of Awareness

Level	Phase name	Main feature
1	The ostrich phase	Lack of awareness, knowledge, or understanding
2	Special designation	Seeking services to meet special needs
3	Normalization	Minimizing differences; maximizing normality
4	Self-actualization	Reality, acceptance, and development of self-advocacy

Source: Ulrich & Bauer, 2003.

In this model, it is thought that parents will progress through these stages in a fairly linear fashion, moving to the next one when they have a transformational experience that elicits a change in thinking. For example, the authors share an example of a parent in the special designation phase who suddenly realized (an "Aha!" moment) that the constant, compensatory tutoring she was seeking and providing for her child (e.g., flash cards in the car) were negatively affecting her family's quality of life. This helped her to move on to the next phase, normalization, where seeking services was not such a focus. For professionals working with parents of children with special needs, understanding these levels can help foster empathy and communication. For example, if parent responses change over time, such change is reasonable, acceptable, and even beneficial within this model— rather than being a negative rationale for a critical response—as it underlies not an inconsistency but a movement through the levels of awareness towards self-actualization.

Read about it. Think about it. Write about it.

Share your reactions to the levels-of-awareness model. How might this change your perceptions of parental reactions?

Even with such a positive model of empathetic understanding in mind, however, conflict can happen. In response to concerns about effective resolution of such potential conflicts in the areas of special education—including students with ASD and their families—the Ontario Ministry of Education published *Shared Solutions: A Guide to Preventing and Resolving Conflicts Regarding Programs and Services for Students with Special Education Needs* (2007), noting its obligations as a service under the Ontario Human Rights Code.

The main components of this resource include Overview of Special Education, Understanding Conflict, Preventing Conflict, Resolving Conflict, and Collaborative Approaches to Resolving Conflict, all with the purpose of "work[ing] together to prevent conflicts, resolve them quickly, and allow students to develop their full potential and succeed in school" (2007, p. 5). According to this manual, conflict can be generated through planning processes, implementation processes, and issues with relationships, but many practical processes are available for resolving conflict: both proactively in a preventative manner, and after conflicts arise. *Shared Solutions* provides readers, who may be parents, teachers, school administrators, and others, with a specific framework for understanding themselves and others, and how to adjust responses to move towards optimal outcomes with concurrent positive change.

The Ontario Human Rights Code: The provincial Ontario Human Rights Code is described as a provision for "equal rights and opportunities without discrimination in specific social areas such as jobs, housing, services, facilities, and contracts or agreements. [Its] goal is to prevent discrimination and harassment because of race, sex, disability, and age" (Ontario Human Rights Commission, n.d., para. 1) across a total of 17 different areas. Other laws are then obligated to respect these areas. In the area of services—such as the education system—all people have the "right to equal treatment with respect to services, goods and facilities, without discrimination because of race, ancestry, place of origin, colour, ethnic origin, citizenship, creed, sex, sexual orientation, gender identity, gender expression, age, marital status, family status or disability" (Service Ontario e-laws, 2012, para. 3).

RESOURCES

Information for Parents

While access to the Internet has exponentially increased the ease of gathering information on almost any topic, serious information seekers—including parents

Box 10.2: The Huron Perth Catholic District School Board

In Charmaine Chadwick's fifth year in her role as the ABA Behaviour Resource Facilitator in Ontario's Huron Perth Catholic District School Board Support, she supports students who present with challenging behaviours, those who require skill-building, and those with ASD; she also provides staff training, consultation, resources, information (e.g., ASD, ABA), and behaviour planning and programming. "In our board," she emphasizes, "we have fully embraced the Connections process" (described in chapter 1). "Working collaboratively with parents, with IBI staff, and the whole team is a high priority for our board."

With only 18 schools, the HPCDSB is a small board, but a passionate one. They do not limit their support to what is happening within the walls of the board's schools, but will sometimes go to the homes of parents or caregivers—even community agencies—to model interventions and strategies, to collaborate on certain skills to prioritize, or to develop programming shared between school, agencies, and the home environment so that all settings are prepared. "Our board goes above and beyond," Charmaine reflected. "We don't put barriers up about whose role is whose. We don't need to have an extensive referral form; we just do what needs to be done to reach success!" Of course, she notes that she doesn't do it all on her own, but that everyone she works with understands ASD and understands behaviour, which is foundational to that success, which they support with individualized modelling and coaching. She also points out that the HPCDSB focuses on inclusive classes and tries to de-emphasize alternative programs beyond the government-mandated curriculum. "We have few students on alternative programs; the majority are on accommodated or modified programs. We have no self-contained programs. We embed developmental milestones into government curriculum as much as possible."

"We work on building capacity in all partners—including parents and families. If that means carefully crossing boundaries, then that's what we will do. For example, understanding the use of visual schedules and the difference between the Picture Exchange Communication System and a visual schedule. We know that behaviour is occurring for a reason and we need to teach skills to help support changing those behaviours using applied behaviour analysis. Parents are welcome to our training events. We have embraced this strategy and there is no second-guessing it: this is our common language." Charmaine also explains that a unique focus for supporting students and their families is through technology. "We use a lot of technology and equipment such as iPads," Charmaine emphasizes. "Our students also take them home so there isn't a need for parents to duplicate the costs of those resources. This initiative is across the board; these resources go back and forth."

Another bright light in their board-wide programming to support students with ASD—and their families—is the use of a peer-mediated program that began eight years ago, and has blossomed into seven schools and 180 students who use such an approach every day with evidence of long-term success. "We train peers about ASD and what inclusive practices are. We work together on identifying age-appropriate goals, then teach about prompting and reinforcement, and they do it! We've had long-term success. Using the locally developed PEER Pals (developed by Carmen and Charmaine) we train about 200 students each year."

Their next step is to develop even more consistency across the board: "We want to move pockets of excellence, celebrate, share, and learn from one another. We know what works; our interventions are effective. We just have to continue to fund and train and support. We are not totally there in every school but we are quite far; and we want to keep going: we don't ever want to be complacent."

of children with ASD—now have a new challenge: struggling with filtering through masses of dubious information to find suitable sources of correct information (e.g., evidence-based interventions). One appropriate source of online information in Ontario includes information packages and guiding practices provided through the provincial government. For example, the Special Needs: Autism section of the Ontario Ministry of Children and Youth Services website provides, among many other information, suggestions on how parents can best support the diagnostic process of ASD by preparing child-specific information (e.g., medications taken, behaviour change, play skills) or questions to ask (e.g., therapeutic support, medical care, etc.)

However, it is also possible to download a comprehensive kit from the same website, entitled *The Autism Parent Resource Kit* (Government of Ontario, n.d.). This kit is a fully online resource, covering topics ranging from kit-specific information (e.g., goals) to research outcomes. Beyond introductory information, the full range of focus areas are: ASD diagnosis and treatment, everyday living, common transitions, educational transition, family transitions, sensory development, physiological development, social development, emotional and mental health, encouraging your child, health care, family support, and ASD research, as well as a comprehensive glossary and complete references. Most chapters include helpful information, resources, practical visuals, and a "learn more" section with additional resources. Especially notable is the section on family support, which indicates that:

Box 10.3: How to Prepare for a Diagnostic Appointment

Before the appointment, it might be helpful to ...

- List all medications your child is taking (including vitamins, herbs or supplements, or any other over-the-counter medication).
- List any changes that you or anyone else has noticed in your child's behaviour. If your child has been evaluated by a pre-school or any other early childhood educator, bring their notes.
- Bring a video or photograph of behaviour, rituals, or routines displayed by your child. Many cell phones or digital cameras can be used to assist with this.
- If your child has siblings, try to make note of their siblings major developmental milestones to help spot differences and signs of development, which may indicate an ASD (such as the age they began talking).
- Make some notes about and be prepared to discuss how your child plays with other children, siblings, and parents.

Source: Ontario Ministry of Children and Youth Services, 2011, para. 3.

In addition to the challenges already discussed, parents of children with ASD must navigate other aspects of family life—such as caring for their other children, managing finances, building a career, and maintaining healthy relationships with their partners. It's important to find ways to look after your own needs as well as the needs of your children. (Government of Ontario, n.d., p. 92)

The family support section of the kit has explanations of many areas that affect family functioning once the initial emotional impact of the diagnostic processes concludes, such as family finances, employment issues, support for siblings, support groups—and much more. Page 93, for example, provides a helpful, concise overview of multiple programs of financial support, both provincial and federal (e.g., tax credits), including many practical elements, such as contact information.

Organization

A particularly practical recommendation is the creation of a child-specific binder or binders to easily compile and share printed documents, and to keep complex, important information readily available and organized. The kit suggests that contents should begin with a photo and a profile of the child with ASD, and include copies of government-issued identification (e.g., birth certificate), medical information (e.g., diagnosis, medications), education information (e.g., reports, IEP), contact information (e.g., therapy providers, physician), a related schedule of typical time commitments, and important financial and legal information (e.g., insurance policies). If parents are looking for a binder to use, rather than suggestions on its creation, McMaster University's CanChild Centre for Disability Research has created the The KIT: Keeping it Together. While The KIT (2015) is not ASD-specific, it is intended for parents of children with disabilities. This inexpensive answer to day-to-day organization is self-described as

> a way to organize information for your child, and to assist you when interacting with different service systems, for example health, education, and recreation. Included is a User's Guide that will help you through the initial process of how to use the KIT. It is useful for parents of children with a wide variety of special needs and all developmental ages from birth to 21 years. (para. 1)

A self-directed kit is also available for transition to adulthood, called the Youth KIT.

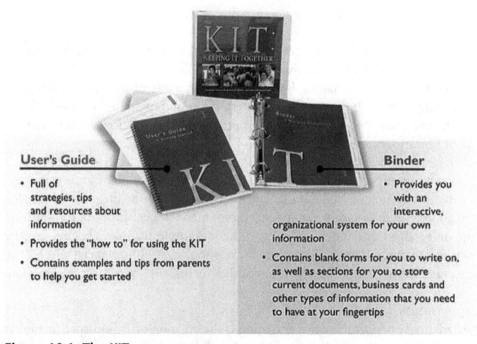

Figure 10.1: The KIT
Source: CanChild Centre for Disability Research, 2015.

Regionalized and Non-Exclusive Resources

Region- and community-specific information that includes provincial resources typically accessed by parents of children with ASD is also available, but not in a systematic or comprehensive manner. One example compiled for Ontario's Simcoe County through a collaboration between Autism Ontario's Simcoe County chapter, Simcoe County Preschool Speech and Language Program, and Children's Treatment Network of Simcoe York, is entitled *Next Steps ... A Resource Guide for Families of Children who have been Recently Diagnosed with an Autism Spectrum Disorder* (2012). With some similarities to Ontario's kit, *Next Steps* focuses on ASD, related financial help, available publicly and privately funded services, local support groups, educational and respite services, and a range of websites related to geographical supports.

Many other information resources are easily accessible online to support the needs of parents in turn supporting children with ASD, which are not specific to regional or provincial information, but are nonetheless helpful. One example is the *First 100 Days Kit: A Tool Kit to Assist Families in Getting the Critical Information They Need in the First 100 Days after an Autism Diagnosis* (Autism Speaks, 2008). The *First 100 Days Kit* is made up of 10 main sections, with a lengthy focus on treatments for children with ASD. The 10 components include About Autism; You, Your Family, and Autism; Getting Your Child Services; Treating Autism; and Making it Happen. In addition to this foundational information, it addresses other emotionally bound topics such as the question, "Is there a cure? Is recovery possible?" (Autism Speaks, 2008, p. 33). Parents will also find practical suggestions to managing this critical period, including a template for week-by-week planning, with embedded action plans appropriate to each phase. For example, in Week 1, initiating a phone log is suggested:

> Try to set aside some time each day to make the phone calls necessary to set up the evaluations and to start the process of getting services. There may be a waiting list for services and evaluations, so make the calls as soon as possible and follow up as needed—and don't hesitate to put your name on multiple lists so you can get the earliest appointment possible. Some of the professionals who provide services through Early Intervention or Special Education may take a specified number of days to complete evaluations or begin services. (Autism Speaks, 2008, p. 43)

Lastly, this resource provides more practical planning support, such as ideas for community awareness and safety concerns, emergency situations, (e.g., creating a personalized information page), informing neighbours, option of medical identification bracelet, a service provider planner, templates for contact information, assessment tracking, goal tracking, and a comprehensive glossary.

Read about it. Think about it. Write about it.
Which of these resources are new to you? Create a list.
Would any of these resources be helpful for families you support? Elaborate.

ADVOCACY

Information leads to knowledge; thus, accessing trustworthy information (such as the above examples) is essential in developing knowledgeable parents of children with ASD who can then make appropriate, informed choices (Matson & Williams, 2015). However, parents also work diligently on developing new skills to support their children with ASD and other disabilities, and one of these skills is advocacy. In the disability field in Ontario (and beyond) many advocacy groups exist, prompted by the political strength found in the parental groups of the 1960s (Bennett & Dworet, 2013).

In an Ontario-based study of parental experiences supporting adult children with intellectual and other disabilities, it is notable that even waiting takes effort; however, successful parental advocacy takes much more. Successful parents:

Advocacy: In the field of special education, an advocacy role may be taken on by the person with a disability (i.e., self-advocacy), by a parent (i.e., parental advocacy), or by a trained, experienced or untrained other who may or may not be advocating from a professional standpoint, also referred to as a "third party role" (Ontario Ministry of Education, 2007, p. 27). An advocate is a helper who may help to improve communication or decrease conflict. According to *Shared Solutions*, the advocacy role is maximized in the context of positive relationships, existing skills, and special education (e.g., programs, systems, services, policy, and legislations, etc.) (Ontario Ministry of Education, 2007).

Engaged intensively in the above described activities and benefitted from positive relationships with service providers who were able to advocate on their behalf, assist them in application processes, or provide them with flexible service options. These parents trusted that the services they had obtained or continued to seek would be able to meet their needs and their adult children's needs. (Saaltink & Ouellette-Kuntz, 2014)

Large, well-known groups support parents of children with disabilities (including ASD), but so do small groups that specialize in a particular area. One example of a smaller group that is available is The "Special Needs" Planning Group (SNPG). The purpose of this organization is to "give [parents] some of the basics necessary to the understanding and implementation of plans for the future of your family member with a disability" (Special Needs Planning Group, 2003, para. 1). One of the resources they provide is a yearly compilation of tax tips. Like many advocacy groups, SNPG was initiated and continues to be led by parents of individuals with special needs who have taken this life-changing pathway as a call to support others with similar needs. One very well-respected parental advocate in the province of Ontario was the late Lindsay Moir (1946–2012) of Comhnadh Consulting, well-known to struggling parents for not only his presentations and consultations, but for his tireless will to teach others how to best support children with exceptionalities, especially in Ontario's public school system. As a former insider to that system—a retired employee of the Ontario Ministry of Education—Lindsay Moir was called "an extraordinary advocate for students with special needs" (Ontario Association of Children's Rehabilitation Services, 2012, para. 1) and was hailed by Autism Ontario as an advocacy hero, described as follows:

> As with any effective advocate, not everyone agreed with all his views, but no one questioned Lindsay Moir's commitment to keeping the learning needs of the children in the forefront, or his passion for the sustained work of advocacy. He made the process of navigating the special education system in Ontario more understandable and he empowered parents to be their child's most effective advocate. He helped parents to not be afraid to insist on the best possible education for their child, and much of his work involved students with ASD. Autism Ontario is grateful to Lindsay Moir for his dedication to the field of autism, his listening ear, his practical and helpful ideas along with his commitment to families and their children. Lindsay made a positive difference in the lives of many people. (Spoelstra, 2012, p. 35)

One of Lindsay Moir's particularly well-loved initiatives was his readily accessed and responsive column: "Ask Lindsay." Though this column is no longer active, it remains hosted online by the Ontario Association of Children Rehabilitation Services: www.oacrs.com/en/asklindsay. "Ask Lindsay" responded to parent questions: oftentimes difficult, contentious ones. Some of the included, now-archived topics cover issues like school suspensions, school supports, and health care.

These responses not only answered parental questions, but taught important advocacy skills, and provided encouragement for the challenging job of parenting a child with special needs through the ages and stages of life. Larger groups with a strong overall advocacy component specific to ASD include the Asperger's Society, Autism Speaks Canada, and Autism Ontario (formerly Autism Society of Ontario).

The Asperger's Society of Ontario organized itself into a non-profit group in 2000, and has a 15-year record of service in the province. Like the SPNG, it was founded by parents; in this case, parents of children diagnosed with the former Asperger's, formally known as Asperger's disorder. One of its goals is to "improve public and professional awareness and understanding of the unique challenges, strengths and needs of individuals with Asperger Syndrome and their families" (n.d., para. 2). In keeping with such public advocacy goals—and more—the Asperger's Society provides phone-in resource support for questions specific to Asperger's. In addition, they have built, maintained, and shared a specialized resource library, a searchable resource database for region-specific services, such as workshops, employment supports, and treatment services, and an online list of frequently answered questions from a trusted source.

Autism Speaks Canada, like its high-profile US-based counterpart, raises awareness about ASD for the Canadian population, and takes advantage of regionally developed resources such as the aforementioned *First 100 Days Kit* (Autism Speaks, 2008) and other easily accessible online toolkits (e.g., Challenging Behaviours Tool Kit, Dental Tool Kit, etc.). Although these resources are not focused on Canadian legislation or Ontario needs, they have many areas of knowledge and skills that are not limited by geopolitical boundaries. Some are translated and available online in French. Autism Speaks Canada provides a helpful summary of all their Family Services Tool Kits, including those highlighted in Table 10.3.

One of the prominent and successful annual fundraising strategies utilized by Autism Speaks is its Walk Now for Autism Speaks Canada, described by this agency as "support[ing] Scientific Research, Services, Advocacy and Awareness. Yet, the Walks are more than a fundraiser, they provide an incredible opportunity for the ASD community to come together and make connections and feel the support" (para. 1). Its initiatives are recognized by its well-known bright blue puzzle piece, which has led to growing demonstrations of community support for ASD such as Light it Up Blue, encouraging outdoor illumination with this signature colour for World Autism Awareness Day on April 2nd, recognized in Canada since 2012 (Autism Speaks, 2015; Parliament of Canada, 2012). Another important resource for developing understanding about ASD is the unique online Video Glossary (2009). This one-of-a-kind tool allows open access to more than 100 video clips of both typically developing children and those with red flags for ASD, modeled by children diagnosed with ASD. Autism Speaks describes it as follows:

> Welcome to the ASD Video Glossary, an innovative web-based tool designed to help parents and professionals learn more about the early red

Table 10.3: Advocacy-Focused Tool Kits

Kit	Knowledge and Skills	Online link
Advocacy Tool Kit	• Advocacy skills (school, community) • Negotiation skills	www.autismspeaks.org/family-services/tool-kits/advocacy
A Parent's Guide to Autism	• ASD • Strategies, resources, support • Promoting positivity	www.autismspeaks.org/family-services/tool-kits/family-support-tool-kits#parents
A Sibling's Guide to Autism	• ASD • Feelings	www.autismspeaks.org/family-services/tool-kits/family-support-tool-kits#siblings
A Grandparent's Guide to Autism	• ASD • Supporting self and others • Developing relationships	www.autismspeaks.org/family-services/tool-kits/family-support-tool-kits#grandparents
A Friend's Guide to Autism	• ASD • Empathy, support, and relationships	www.autismspeaks.org/family-services/tool-kits/family-support-tool-kits#friends

Source: Autism Speaks Canada, 2015.

flags and diagnostic features of Autism Spectrum Disorder (ASD). This glossary contains over a hundred video clips and is available to you free of charge. Whether you are a parent, family member, friend, physician, clinician, childcare provider, or educator, it can help you see the subtle differences between typical and delayed development in young children and spot the early red flags for ASD. All of the children featured in the ASD Video Glossary as having red flags for ASD are, in fact, diagnosed with ASD.

Videos are categorized by inclusion in categories such as Overview, Social Communication/Social Interaction (e.g., nonverbal communication), Repetitive Behaviours and Restricted Interests (e.g., repetitive movements), and Associated Features (e.g., unusual motor skills). A recently added subdivision is Treatments. Accessing this option allows viewing of multiple examples of each of the 11 treatment options (e.g., positive behaviour support, pivotal response training, picture exchange communication system, the Lovaas model of ABA, discrete trial training, etc.), as well as helpful overviews of each option.

In Ontario, likely the most well-known parent advocacy group is the provincial multi-chaptered group: Autism Ontario. This group used to be known by its former name, the Autism Society of Ontario, which is still heard around the province. Autism Ontario's mission and vision are focused on individuals with ASD, but their areas of focus as an organization include public awareness and advocacy, and one of their strategic directions is educating educators and professionals. Autism Ontario is a well-governed organization with multiple chapters across Ontario, a board of directors, and a varied range of unique programs, described as "a primary source of information and referral on autism spectrum disorder (ASD) and one of the largest collective voices representing the autism community in the province" (McFee et al., 2012, p. 8). For example, public awareness is supported by many initiatives, including the public dissemination of *Autism Matters*, both in print and online, a flagship publication which includes focuses on features of local initiatives and programs, as well as resources reviews and creative contributions, in both English and French.

Unique programs that have been helpful for supporting parents in navigating supports and services for their children, youth, and adults with ASD include Spirale, Abacus, and Calypso. All three programs help parents to connect to appropriate services of care, education, and support for those with ASD by service type, geographical region, and more.

The Potential Programme (formerly Realize Community Potential) is yet

Table 10.4: Specialized Program Access through Autism Ontario

Program	Focus	Online link
Spirale	• Professional services	www.autismontario.com/client/aso/spirale.nsf/web/Home?OpenDocument
Abacus	• ABA providers	www.abacuslist.ca/
Calypso	• Camp programs	www.autismontario.com/client/aso/calypso.nsf/web/Home?OpenDocument

Source: Autism Ontario, 2015.

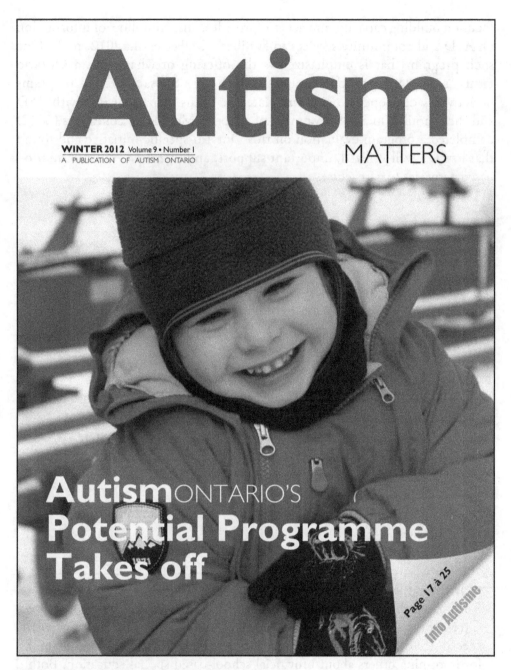

Figure 10.2: *Autism Matters,* **Winter 2012**
Source: Autism Ontario, 2012.

another successful, ongoing initiative through Autism Ontario (2015) that provides direct, skilled clinical interventions to families (e.g., workshops) with a focus on building capacity, and acts to "provide a 'one stop shop' of information on ASD and community services to families" (McFee et al., 2012, p. 9). One such program that is emphasized is the offering of what Autism Ontario terms "social learning opportunities," which are necessary, desired programs or activities developed to accommodate the needs of participants with ASD and their families in an environment of support. McFee and colleagues (2012) completed a program evaluation on this Ontario-specific initiative and found that it was a well-utilized, important support, and increased Autism Ontario–based activities (e.g., events).

Read about it. Think about it. Write about it.

Explain your experiences with one or more of these individuals and groups that support parental advocacy in Ontario.

Box 10.4: The Ontario Special Needs Roadmap for School

> Recent Social Media Statistics on The Ontario Special Needs Roadmap for School:
> Tweets: 20.8 K
> Following: 9,183
> Followers: 10.6 K
> Likes: 7,491
> Lists: 27

If getting information out there is the goal, The Ontario Special Needs Roadmap is already a success. Kim Peterson and Heather Rose, two innovative Ottawa-based advocates for parents and families supporting students with special needs, have been busily supporting the growth of their unique tool for informing others about provincial school-based special education. Both bilingual federal government employees, Kim (an IT project manager) and Heather (a programmer) worked together over a dozen years ago, and as time progressed, had children, took leaves, and eventually worked together once again. As friendly colleagues, their conversations naturally veered to their families, and Kim, one day, shared that her son, Ryder, had ASD. In turn, Heather shared concerns about daughter Molly, who was also eventually diagnosed with ASD. Kim, then, shared information that she had learned about the complex systems of service provision and school-based services, more than overwhelming areas to navigate. As time passed, they thought about taking their experiences and pulling together a tool that might help others in this journey without being at the mercy of a service provider, committed to making a roadmap for service navigation, and inevitably, also smoothing the pathway toward self-advocacy.

"We didn't really know how things worked—we had no idea! We heard horror stories, one after another, of things lacking. We went to everything, saw everyone, and talked to everyone we could talk to, but mostly other parents." What these self-described "just two moms" found was anxiety, uncertainty, and waiting lists, so they researched, printed, read, talked, and studied even more. It was, and continues to be, "lots of work and research," but they are motivated by the significant needs of other parents.

"So we just started sketching where you go, what you do, these are the services, without any money, but with an awful lot of social media followers: about 4,000 right now! We made a lot of rough drafts, and we made a roadmap!" So far, Heather and Kim have devoted 18 months of time, meeting three or four times a week, and their recently shared roadmap, "has been downloaded thousands of times, has started to go in local doctors' offices, has been introduced at meetings; we have taken it to workshops, and we go to workshops and presentations to learn more to make it even better." They excitedly reported: "70 percent of our followers are in the education field: THEY are now coming to US with questions! Most recently, we received an email from a family moving from Korea to Ontario." When asked what was next, Kim and Heather overflowed with plans about French translations and supporting newcomers to Canada. "Our end game," they shared, "is to go across Canada and do this in every province and territory." It is quite evident that these "two moms" are going to make it all happen.

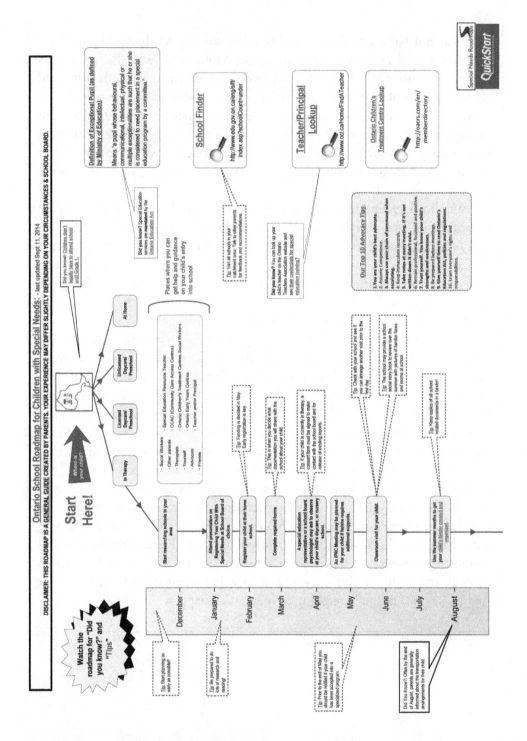

Figure 10.3: One Component of The Ontario Special Needs Roadmap
Source: Special Needs Roadmaps, 2014, p. 1.

> **Read about it. Think about it. Write about it.**
>
> Would you recommend this roadmap to a parent who is trying to navigate the system for a student with ASD? Why or why not?

A LOOK BACK

Chapter 10, "Supporting Ontario's Parents and Families," focused on historical and current examinations of raising a child with ASD. It reviewed topics such as:

- Negative historical views ascribed to parents of children with ASD;
- Recent, positive models for understanding families that include children with ASD (e.g., the levels of awareness);
- Examples of local, community-based, and provincial resources; and
- The importance of advocacy by and for families, and both well-established and emerging advocacy groups (e.g,. Autism Ontario).

ADDITIONAL RESOURCES

- "Ask Lindsay" (Ontario Association of Children's Rehabilitation Services, 2012):
  www.oacrs.com/en/asklindsay
- Asperger's Society of Ontario:
  www.aspergers.ca/
- Autism Ontario:
  www.autismontario.com/
- Autism Speaks Canada:
  www.autismspeaks.ca/
- Autism Speaks Family Services Tool Kits:
  www.autismspeaks.ca/_autismspeaksca/assets/File/Tool%20Kit%20
  Documents/2014%20Family%20Services%20Tool%20Kits%20List%20
  FINAL%20SECURED.pdf
- The Autism Parent Resource Kit (Government of Ontario, n.d.):
  www.children.gov.on.ca/htdocs/English/documents/topics/specialneeds/
  autism/aprk/Autism_Parent_Resource_Kit.pdf
- Autism Speaks Video Glossary (Autism Speaks, 2009):
  http://resources.autismnavigator.com/

- The KIT: Keeping it Together (CanChild Centre for Childhood Disability Research):
  www.canchild.ca/en/canchildresources/parents_kit.asp
- First 100 Days Kit: A Tool Kit to Assist Families in Getting the Critical Information They Need in the First 100 Days after an Autism Diagnosis (Autism Speaks, 2008):
  www.autismspeaks.org/docs/family_services_docs/100_day_kit.pdf
- Next Steps ... A Resource Guide for Families of Children who have been Recently Diagnosed with an Autism Spectrum Disorder (Autism Ontario Simcoe County Chapter, Simcoe County Preschool Speech and Language Program, and Children's Treatment Network of Simcoe York, 2012):
  www.autismontario.com/client/aso/ao.nsf/docs/d3485d3bb8e27c3f85257a4 600574199/$file/next+steps+march+2012.pdf
- Ontario Human Rights Code (Service Ontario e-laws, 2012):
  www.e-laws.gov.on.ca/html/statutes/english/elaws_statutes_90h19_e.htm
- Ontario Special Needs Roadmap for School:
  static1.squarespace.com/static/54038db5e4b0a7034afb87b6/t/5411cacae4b 08f31227afd08/1410452170231/School+Roadmap_landscape_Sept+10.pdf
- *Shared Solutions* (Ontario Ministry of Education, 2007):
  www.edu.gov.on.ca/eng/general/elemsec/speced/shared.pdf
- The "Special Needs" Planning Group:
  www.specialneedsplanning.ca/

REFERENCES

Asperger's Society of Ontario. (n.d.) Retrieved from www.aspergers.ca/

Anderegg, M. L., Vergason, G. A., & Smith, M. C. (1992). A visual representation of the grief cycle for use by teachers with families of children with disabilities. *Remedial & Special Education*, *13*(2), 17–23.

Autism Ontario. (2012). *Autism matters*: Winter 2012. Retrieved from www.autismontario.com/ Client/ASO/AO.nsf/object/AMWinter2012/$file/AM+Winter+2012.pdf

Autism Ontario. (2015). About Us. Retrieved from http://www.autismontario.com/client/aso/ ao.nsf/web/About+Us

Autism Ontario's Simcoe County Chapter, Simcoe County Preschool Speech and Language Program, & Children's Treatment Network of Simcoe York. (2012). Next steps ... a resource guide for families of children who have been recently diagnosed with an autism spectrum disorder. Retrieved from www.autismontario.com/client/aso/ao.nsf/docs/d3485d3bb8e27c3 f85257a4600574199/$file/next+steps+march+2012.pdf

Autism Speaks. (2008). First 100 days kit: A tool kit to assist families in getting the critical information they need in the first 100 days after an autism diagnosis. Retrieved from www. autismspeaks.org/docs/family_services_docs/100_day_kit.pdf

Autism Speaks Canada. (2009). Autism speaks video glossary. Retrieved from http://resources. autismnavigator.com/

Autism Speaks Canada. (2015). Retrieved from http://www.autismspeaks.ca/

Bennett, S. & Dworet, D. (2013). *Special education in Ontario schools* (7th ed.). Niagara-on-the-Lake, ON: Highland Press.

CanChild Centre for Childhood Disability Research. (2015). The KIT: Keeping it Together. Retrieved from www.canchild.ca/en/canchildresources/parents_kit.asp

Ferguson, P. M. (2002). A place in the family: an historical interpretation of research on parental reactions to having a child with a disability. *Journal of Special Education, 36*(3), 124–130.

Fletcher, P. C., Markoulakis, R., & Bryden, P. J. (2012). The costs of caring for a child with an autism spectrum disorder. *Issues in comprehensive pediatric nursing, 35*(1), 45–69.

Government of Ontario. (n.d.). The autism parent resource kit. Retrieved from www.children.gov.on.ca/htdocs/English/documents/topics/specialneeds/autism/aprk/Autism_Parent_Resource_Kit.pdf

Hobbs, N. (1978). Families, schools, and communities: An ecosystem for children. *Teachers College Record, 79*(4), 756–766.

Matson, J. L., & Williams, J. L. (2015). The curious selection process of treatments for autism spectrum disorder. *Research in Autism Spectrum Disorder, 9*(2015), 21–25.

McFee, K. H., Schroeder, J. H., Bebko, J. M., Thompson, M., Spoelstra, M., Verbeek, L., & ... Casola, S. (2012). Building capacity: Autism Ontario's realize community potential program. *Journal on Developmental Disabilities, 18*(3), 8–20.

Ontario Association of Children's Rehabilitation Service. (2012). Ask Lindsay. Retrieved from www.oacrs.com/en/asklindsay

Ontario Human Rights Commission. (n.d.). Human rights in Ontario. Retrieved from www.ohrc.on.ca/en

Ontario Ministry of Children and Youth Services. (2011). ASD diagnosis and treatment. Retrieved from www.children.gov.on.ca/htdocs/English/topics/specialneeds/autism/aprk/asd-diagnosis-and-treatment/diagnosis.aspx

Ontario Ministry of Education. (2005). *Education for all: The report of the expert panel on literacy and numeracy instruction for students with special education needs, Kindergarten to grade 6.* Toronto, ON: Queen's Printer. Retrieved from www.edu.gov.on.ca/eng/document/reports/speced/panel/speced.pdf

Ontario Ministry of Education. (2007). *Shared solutions: A guide to preventing and resolving conflicts regarding programs and services for students with special education needs.* Toronto, ON: Queen's Printer for Ontario. Retrieved from www.edu.gov.on.ca/eng/general/elemsec/speced/shared.pdf

Parliament of Canada. (2012). Senate public bill S-206: An act respecting world autism day. Retrieved from www.parl.gc.ca/LegisInfo/BillDetails.aspx?Language=E&Mode=1&Bill=S206&Parl=41&Ses=1

Service Ontario e-laws. (2012). Human rights code. Retrieved from www.e-laws.gov.on.ca/html/statutes/english/elaws_statutes_90h19_e.htm

Saaltink, R., & Ouellette-Kuntz, H. (2014). "You did everything": Effort, motherhood, and disability in parents' narratives of their attempts to obtain services. *Journal on Developmental Disabilities, 20*(2), 44–54.

Special Needs Planning Group. (2003). The "special needs" planning group. Retrieved from http://www.specialneedsplanning.ca

Special Needs Roadmaps. (2014). Ontario school roadmap for children with special needs. Retrieved from www.specialneedsroadmaps.ca/

Spoelstra, M. (2012). Ontario loses a hero: Lindsay Moir (1946–2012). *Autism Matters, 19*(1), 1–40. Retrieved from www.autismontario.com/Client/ASO/AO.nsf/object/AMWinter2012/$file/AM+Winter+2012.pdf

Starr, E. M., & Foy, J. B. (2012). In parents' voices: The education of children with autism spectrum disorder. *Remedial & Special Education, 33*(4), 207–216. doi:10.1177/0741932510383161

Straus, J. N. (2013). Autism as culture. In L. J. Davis (Ed.), *The disability studies reader* (460–475). New York, NY: Routledge.

Ulrich, M. E., & Bauer, A. E. (2003). Levels of awareness: A closer look at communication between parents and professionals. *TEACHING Exceptional Children, 35*(6), 20–23.

Watson, S., Hayes, S., Radford-Paz, E., & Coons, K. (2013). "I'm hoping, I'm hoping ....": Thoughts about the future from families of children with autism or fetal alcohol spectrum disorder in Ontario. *Journal on Developmental Disabilities, 19*(3), 76–93.

Weiss J, & Lunsky Y. (2011). The brief family distress scale: A measure of crisis in caregivers of individuals with autism spectrum disorder. *Journal of Child & Family Studies, 20*(4), 521–528. doi:10.1007/s10826-010-9419-y

COPYRIGHT ACKNOWLEDGEMENTS

CHAPTER 1

Table 1.1: Blacher, J., & Christensen, L. (2011). Sowing the seeds of the autism field: Leo Kanner (1943). *Intellectual & Developmental Disabilities, 49*(3), 172–191. doi:10.1352/1934-9556-49.3.172. Used by permission of the authors.

CHAPTER 2

Figure 2.1: Thompson, T. (2013). Autism research and services for young children: History, progress and challenges. *Journal of Applied Research in Intellectual Disabilities, 26*, 81–107. Used by permission of John Wiley & Sons.

Figures 2.2 and 2.3: Thames Valley Children's Centre. (2008). *Paving the Way for Success: A Supplementary Guide for Educators of Students with Autism Spectrum Disorder*. London, ON: Author. Used by permission of the Thames Valley Children's Centre.

Figure 2.4: Grzadzinski, R., Huerta, M., & Lord, C. (2013). DSM-5 and autism spectrum disorders (ASDs): An opportunity for identifying ASD subtypes. *Molecular Autism, 4*(1), 1-6. doi:10.1186/2040-2392-4-12. Published by BioMed Central. Used by permission of the authors.

CHAPTER 3

Figure 3.3: Thames Valley Children's Center & Greater Essex County District School Board. (2008). *Structured Learning Environment Work Tasks: A Guide for the Elementary Educator* (2nd ed.). London, ON: Author. Retrieved from http://www.ncdsb.net/education/student_services/work_task/ch1-2%20intro.pdf. Used by permission of the Thames Valley Children's Center.

Figure 3.4: Image by David Shane Smith for Gillespie-Lynch, K. (2013, May 1). Response to and initiation of joint attention: Overlapping but distinct roots of development in autism? *OA Autism, 1*(2), 13. Retrieved from www.oapublishinglondon.com/article/596. Used by permission of David Shane Smith.

Figure 3.5: Byom, L.J., and Mutlu, B. (2013). Theory of mind: Mechanisms, methods, and new directions. *Frontiers in Human Neuroscience, 7*, 413. doi: 10.3389/fnhum.2013.00413. Used by permission of the authors.

Figure 3.6: Innovative Learning Concepts. (2013). How it works: Math for all senses. TouchMath Memory Cue Poster. Retrieved from https://www.oncoursesystems.com/school/webpage/12712431/1242281. Used by permission of Innovative Learning Concepts.

Table 3.4: Wong, C., Odom, S.L., Hume, K. Cox, A.W., Fettig, A., Kucharczyk, S., ... Schultz, T.R. (2014). *Evidence-Based Practices for Children, Youth, and Young Adults with Autism Spectrum Disorder*. Chapel Hill: The University of North Carolina, Frank Porter Graham Child Development Institute, Autism Evidence-Based Practice Review Group. Used by permission of the authors.

CHAPTER 4

Figure 4.6: AssistiveWare. (2014). Proloquo2Go. Retrieved from www.assistiveware.com/product/proloquo2go. Used by permission of AssistiveWare.

Table 4.5: Koegel, R. L., Camarata, S., Koegel, L.K., Ben-Tall, A., & Smith, A.E. (1998). Increasing speech intelligibility in children with autism. *Journal of Autism and Developmental Disorders*, 28(3), 241–251. Used by permission of Springer Science and Business Media.

CHAPTER 5

Figure 5.1: Spence, S. H. (1995). *Social Skills Training: Enhancing Social Competence with Children and Adolescents*. London: NFER-Nelson. Retrieved from http://www.scaswebsite.com/1_54_.html. Used by permission of the author.

Figure 5.7: Wolfberg, P., Bottema-Beutel, K., & DeWitt, M. (2012). Including children with autism in social and imaginary play with typical peers: Integrated play groups model. As published in Volume 5, Issue 1, of The Strong's *American Journal of Play*. © The Strong. Used by permission of the authors and publisher.

Table 5.2: Aimes, M., & Weiss, J. (2013). Cognitive behavioural therapy for a child with autism spectrum disorder and verbal impairment: A case study. *Journal of Developmental Disabilities*, 19(1), 61–69. Used by permission of the Ontario Association on Developmental Disabilities.

Table 5.6: Thiemann, K. (2006, April). Comprehensive social communication interventions for elementary students with ASD. Paper presented at ASD-School Support Program 2nd Annual Conference, Niagara Falls, ON. Used by permission of the author.

Table 5.7: Gulick, R.F., & Kitchen, T.P. (2007). *Effective Instruction for Children with Autism: An Applied Behavior Analytic Approach*. Erie, PA: The Dr. Gertrude A. Barber National Institute. Used by permission of the Barber National Institute.

Table 5.10: Wolfberg, P., Bottema-Beutel, K., & DeWitt, M. (2012). Including children with autism in social and imaginary play with typical peers: Integrated play groups model. As published in Volume 5, Issue 1, of The Strong's *American Journal of Play*. © The Strong. Used by permission of the authors and publisher.

CHAPTER 6

Figure 6.1: Mancil, G.R., & Pearl, C.E. (2008). Restricted interests as motivators: Improving academic engagement and outcomes of children on the autism spectrum. *TEACHING Exceptional Children Plus*, 4(6). Retrieved from escholarship.bc.edu/education/tecplus/vol4/iss6/art7. Used by permission of the authors.

Figure 6.2: Busick, M., & Neitzel, J. (2009). *Self-Management: Steps for Implementation*. Chapel Hill, NC: National Professional Development Center on Autism Spectrum Disorder, Frank Porter Graham Child Development Institute, The University of North Carolina. Retrieved from http://csesa.fpg.unc.edu/sites/csesa.fpg.unc.edu/files/ebpbriefs/SelfManagement_Steps. pdf. Used by permission of the publisher.

Table 6.1: Lanou, A., Hough, L., & Powell, E. (2012). Case studies on using strengths and interests to address the needs of students with autism spectrum disorder. *Intervention in School and Clinic, 47*(3), 175–182. Used by permission of the authors.

Table 6.4: Neitzel, J. (2009b). *Steps for Implementation: Response Interruption/Redirection*. Chapel Hill, NC: The National Professional Development Center on Autism Spectrum Disorder, Frank Porter Graham Child Development Institute, The University of North Carolina. Retrieved from http://csesa.fpg.unc.edu/sites/csesa.fpg.unc.edu/files/ebpbriefs/ResponseInterruption_Steps. pdf. Used by permission of the publisher.

CHAPTER 9

Figures 9.1–9.6: Stoddart, K.P., Burke, L., Muskat, B., Manett, J., Duhaime, S., Accardi, C., Burnham Riosa, P. & Bradley, E. (2013). *Diversity in Ontario's Youth and Adults with Autism Spectrum Disorder: Complex Needs in Unprepared Systems*. Toronto, ON: The Redpath Centre. Retrieved from www.redpathcentre.ca/sitebuildercontent/sitebuilderfiles/fullreport2013.pdf. Used by permission of The Redpath Centre.

Table 9.1: Alcorn MacKay, S. (2010). *Identifying Trends and Supports for Students with Autism Spectrum Disorder Transitioning into Postsecondary*. Toronto: Higher Education Quality Council of Ontario. Retrieved from http://www.heqco.ca/SiteCollectionDocuments/ASD.pdf. Used by permission of the Higher Education Quality Council of Ontario.

CHAPTER 10

Figure 10.2: Autism Ontario. (2012). *Autism Matters: Winter 2012*. Retrieved from www.autismontario.com/Client/ASO/AO.nsf/object/AMWinter2012/$file/AM+Winter+2012.pdf. Used by permission of Autism Ontario.

INDEX